ANATOMY, PHYSIOLOGY, AND PATHOPHYSIOLOGY

for Allied Health

SECOND EDITION

ANATOMY, PHYSIOLOGY, AND PATHOPHYSIOLOGY

for Allied Health

Kathryn A. Booth, RN-BSN, MS, RMA, RPT
Total Care Programming, Inc.
Palm Coast, Florida

Terri D. Wyman, CMRS
UMASS Memorial Medical Center
Worcester, Massachusetts

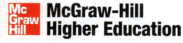

**McGraw-Hill
Higher Education**

Boston   Burr Ridge, IL   Dubuque, IA   New York   San Francisco   St. Louis
Bangkok   Bogotá   Caracas   Kuala Lumpur   Lisbon   London   Madrid   Mexico City
Milan   Montreal   New Delhi   Santiago   Seoul   Singapore   Sydney   Taipei   Toronto

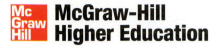

ANATOMY, PHYSIOLOGY, AND PATHOPHYSIOLOGY FOR ALLIED HEALTH
Published by McGraw-Hill, a business unit of The McGraw-Hill Companies, Inc., 1221 Avenue of the Americas, New York, NY, 10020.
Copyright © 2009 by The McGraw-Hill Companies, Inc. All rights reserved. Previous edition © 2008. No part of this publication may be reproduced or distributed in any form or by any means, or stored in a database or retrieval system, without the prior written consent of The McGraw-Hill Companies, Inc., including, but not limited to, in any network or other electronic storage or transmission, or broadcast for distance learning.

Some ancillaries, including electronic and print components, may not be available to customers outside the United States.

This book is printed on acid-free paper.

1 2 3 4 5 6 7 8 9 0 WCK/WCK 0 9 8

ISBN 978-0-07-337395-9
MHID 0-07-337395-8

Vice President/Editor in Chief: *Elizabeth Haefele*
Vice President/Director of Marketing: *John E. Biernat*
Senior sponsoring editor: *Debbie Fitzgerald*
Managing developmental editor: *Patricia Hesse*
Developmental editor: *Connie Kuhl*
Executive marketing manager: *Roxan Kinsey*
Lead media producer: *Damian Moshak*
Media producer: *Marc Mattson*
Director, Editing/Design/Production: *Jess Ann Kosic*
Lead project manager: *Susan Trentacosti*
Senior production supervisor: *Janean A. Utley*
Designer: *Srdjan Savanovic*
Senior photo research coordinator: *Carrie K. Burger*
Photo researcher: *Pam Carley*

Media project manager: *Mark A. S. Dierker*
Cover design: *Jenny El-Shamy*
Typeface: *10/12 Slimbach*
Compositor: *ICC Macmillan Inc.*
Printer: *Quebecor World Versailles Inc.*
Cover credits: *Heart: ©Getty Images; skull x-ray: ©Getty Images/ Steve Allen; man's back: The McGraw-Hill Companies, Inc./Eric Wise, photographer; photomicrograph of muscular artery: ©The McGraw-Hill Companies, Inc./Al Telser, photographer; hips and legs: ©The McGraw-Hill Companies, Inc./Photo by JW Ramsey; background: David Gould, ©Gettyimages*
Credits: The credits section for this book begins on page 277 and is considered an extension of the copyright page.

Library of Congress Cataloging-in-Publication Data
Booth, Kathryn A., 1957-
    Anatomy, physiology, and pathophysiology for allied health / by Kathryn A. Booth
and Terri D. Wyman. — 2nd ed.
        p. ; cm.
    Includes index.
    ISBN-13: 978-0-07-337395-9 (alk. paper)
    ISBN-10: 0-07-337395-8 (alk. paper)
    1. Human anatomy. 2. Human physiology. 3. Physiology, Pathological. 4. Allied health personnel. I. Wyman, Terri D. II. Title.
    [DNLM: 1. Anatomy. 2. Allied Health Personnel. 3. Pathology. 4. Physiology.
QS 4 B7245a 2009]
QM23.2.B66 2009
612—dc22

2007049736

www.mhhe.com

Brief Contents

APPENDIXES

Contents

APPENDIXES

Preface

Anatomy, Physiology, and Pathophysiology for Allied Health, Second Edition, is an introductory book to the body systems for medical assisting and other allied health students. It aquaints students with basic information about all the body systems. The book speaks directly to the student, with chapter introductions, case studies, and chapter summaries written to engage the student's attention.

When referring to patients in the third person, we have alternated between passages that describe a male patient and passages that describe a female patient. Thus, the patient will be referred to as "he" half the time and as "she" half the time. The same convention is used to refer to the physician. The medical assistant or allied health professional is consistently addressed as "you."

Patient Education

Throughout the book we provide the reader with information needed to educate patients so the patients can participate fully in their health care.

There is a particular focus on patient education. It is always desirable for patients to be as knowledgeable as possible about their health. Patients who do not understand what is expected of them may become confused, frightened, angry, and uncooperative; educated patients are better able to understand why compliance is important.

We have also made a consistent effort to discuss patients with special needs. These groups include the following:

- **Elderly patients.** Special care is often required with elderly patients. The body undergoes many changes with age, and patients may have difficulty adjusting to their changing physical needs. Several chapters deal with the changes that occur to the body throughout the aging process, including changes in the skin, musculoskeletal system, and the eyes and ears. Additionally, Chapter 13 includes an Educating the Patient feature on preventing falls in the elderly.

- **Children.** Throughout these A&P chapters we discuss the changes that occur to the body during childhood and adolescence. The Pathophysiology sections also highlight many of the diseases and conditions that arise during childhood, combined with the signs and symptoms of each, to make you aware of the hallmarks of some of these common childhood conditions. Included are special sections on bone, muscle

development, and nervous system development, as well as sections in Chapter 13 describing the normal developmental changes to look for in infants and children regarding the senses of sight and hearing.

- **Patients with disabilities.** Many different diseases and disabilities require extra effort or consideration on the part of the medical assistant or other allied health care worker. Patients in wheelchairs and patients with diabetes, hemophilia, or visual or hearing impairments all require specific accommodations. Throughout these A&P chapters, particularly in the Pathophysiology and Educating the Patient areas, we discuss accommodating our patients who are differently abled.

- **Patients from other cultures.** Communicating with patients from other cultures, especially when language barriers are involved, poses a special challenge. In addition, people from different cultures and areas of the world are prone to different types of diseases and conditions. In the Pathophysiology sections, we point out the cultures and peoples who are at higher risk for diseases such as hypertension, stroke, cardiovascular disease, and certain types of cancer.

Organization of the Text

Anatomy, Physiology, and Pathophysiology for Allied Health, Second Edition, provides the student with information on anatomy, physiology, and pathophysiology, beginning with a chapter on the organization of the body; each chapter that follows addresses a particular body system. These chapters also include information on the most common diseases and disorders of each body system.

Each chapter opens with a list of key terms, the chapter outline, and the learning outcomes the student can expect to achieve after completing the chapter. The main text of each chapter begins with an overview of chapter content and includes a case study for students to consider as they read the chapter. Chapters are organized by body system and discuss first the structure (anatomy) of the body system, how the individual parts work together when healthy (physiology), and then discuss the diseases that most often occur within that body system (pathophysiology). Throughout the chapter we have strived to make the information "student friendly" with terminology and anatomy hints to help the student understand the presented information instead of memorizing it. Expanded color photographs, anatomic and technical drawings, tables, charts, and mnemonic features help educate the student about various aspects of the human body in health and in disease. The text features, set off in boxes within the text, include the following:

- **Case Studies** are provided at the beginning of all chapters. They represent situations similar to those that the medical assistant may encounter in daily practice. Students are encouraged to consider the case study as they read each chapter. Case Study Questions in the end-of-chapter review check students' understanding and application of chapter content.
- **Educating the Patient** boxes focus on ways to instruct patients about caring for themselves outside the medical office.
- **Career Opportunities** boxes provide the student with information on various specialized medical professions or duties related to the medical assistant's role within the health-care team.
- **Pathophysiology** boxes provide students with a list of the most common diseases and disorders of each body system and include information on the causes, common signs and symptoms, treatment, and, where possible, the prevention of each disease.

Each chapter closes with a summary of the chapter material, focusing on why it is important for the medical assistant or other allied health professional to have a clear understanding of the body system not only when it is functioning correctly, but also when a condition or disease process is suspected or known. Preventive measures for patient education are also stressed, as is the idea of the allied health professional as a role model for good health. The summary is followed by an end-of-chapter review that consists of the following elements:

- Case Study Questions
- Discussion Questions
- Critical Thinking Questions
- Application Activities
- Virtual Fieldtrip

These questions and activities allow students to practice specific skills.

A list of further readings, including related books and journal articles, will be provided for each chapter within the Instructor's Manual and on McGraw-Hill's medical assisting Online Learning Center. The end-of-chapter questions and activities, as well as the additional online resources, provide supplementary information about the subjects presented in the chapter and allow students to practice specific skills.

The book also includes a glossary and several appendixes for use as reference tools. The glossary lists all the words presented as key terms in each chapter along with a pronunciation guide and the definition of each term. The

appendixes include the American Association of Medical Assistants (AAMA) and the Commission on Accreditation of Allied Health Education Programs (CAAHEP) competencies for the medical assistant, the American Medical Technologists (AMT) Registered Medical Assistant (RMA) certified exam topics, the National Healthcareer Association (NHA) medical assisting duty/task list, commonly used prefixes and suffixes, Latin and Greek terms, abbreviations and symbols used in medical terminology, and a comprehensive list of professional organizations and agencies.

Ancillary Material

Instructor Productivity CD-ROM. The Instructor Productivity CD-ROM provides easy-to-use resources for class preparation. The Instructor Productivity CD-ROM includes the following:

- EZTest test generator with answer rationales and correlations to CMA and RMA competencies
- PowerPoint® Presentations
- Course syllabi
- An Instructor's Manual that consists of
  - A complete lesson plan for each chapter, including an introduction to the lesson, teaching strategies, pathophysiology review, alternate teaching strategies, case studies, chapter close, resources, and an answer key to the student textbook.

Together the student edition, the online learning center, and the instructor's CD-ROM form a complete teaching and learning package.

Online Learning Center. The Online Learning Center (OLC) is a text-specific website that offers an extensive array of learning and teaching tools. This site includes a special link for students on the main menu called A&P where numerous drag and drop activities are available for each chapter using the same figures as found in the textbook. These activities provide plenty of review as well as chapter quizzes with immediate feedback, links to relevant websites, and many more study resources. Log on at www.mhhe.com/medicalassisting3.

Reviewer Acknowledgments

Roxane M. Abbott, MBA
    Sarasota County Technical Institute
    Sarasota, FL
Dr. Linda G. Alford, Ed.D.
    Reid State Technical College
    Evergreen, AL
Suzzanne S. Allen
    Sanford Brown Institute
    Garden City, NY

Ann L. Aron, Ed.D.
Aims Community College
Greeley, CO

Emil Asdurian, MD
Bramson ORT College
Forest Hills, NY

Rhonda Asher, MT, ASCP, CMA
Pitt Community College
Greenville, NC

Adelina H. Azfar, DPM
Total Technical Institute
Brooklyn, OH

Joseph H. Balatbat, MD, RMA, RPT, CPT
Sanford Brown Institute
New York, NY

Mary Barko, CMA, MAED
Ohio Institute of Health Careers
Elyria, OH

Katie Barton, LPN, BA
Savannah River College
Augusta, GA

Kelli C. Batten, NCMA, LMT
Medical Assisting Department Chair
Career Technical College
Monroe, LA

Nina Beaman, MS, RNC, CMA
Bryant and Stratton College
Richmond, VA

Kay E. Biggs, BS, CMA
Columbus State Community College
Columbus, OH

Norma Bird, M.Ed., BS, CMA
Medical Assisting Program Director/Master Instructor
Pocatello, ID

Kathleen Bode, RN, MS
Flint Hills Technical College
Emporia, KS

Natasha Bratton, BSN
Beta Tech
North Charleston, SC

Karen Brown, RN, BC, Ed.D
Kirtland Community College
Roscommon, MI

Kimberly D. Brown, BSHS, CHES, CMA
Swainsboro Technical College
Swainsboro, GA

Nancy A. Browne, MS, BS
Washington High School
Kansas City, KS

Teresa A. Bruno, BA
EduTek College
Stow, OH

Marion I. Bucci, BA
Delaware Technical and Community College
Wilmington, DE

Michelle Buchman, BSN, RNC
Springfield College
Springfield, MO

Michelle L. Carfagna, RMA, ST, BMO, RHE
Brevard Community College
Cocoa, FL

Carmen Carpenter, RN, MS, CMA
South University
West Palm Beach, FL

Pamela C. Chapman, RN, MSN
Caldwell Community College and Technical Institute
Hickory, NC

Patricia A. Chappell, MA, BS
Director, Clinical Laboratory Science
Camden County College
Blackwood, NJ

Phyllis Cox, MA Ed, BS, MT(ASCP)
Arkansas Tech University
Russellville, AR

Stephanie Cox, BS, LPN
York Technical Institute
Lancaster, PA

Christine Cusano, CMA, CPhT
Clark University–CCI
Framingham, MA

Glynna Day, M.Ed
Dean of Education
Academy of Professional Careers
Boise, ID

Anita Denson, BS
National College of Business and Technology
Danville, KY

Leon Deutsch, RMA, BA, MA Ed
Keiser College
Orlando, FL

Walter R. English, MA, MT(AAB)
Akron Institute
Cuyahoga Falls, OH

Dennis J. Ernst MT(ASCP)
Center for Phlebotomy Education
Ramsey, IN

C.S. Farabee, MBA, MSISE
High-Tech Institute Inc.
Phoenix, AZ

Deborah Fazio, CMAS, RMA
Sanford Brown Institute–Cleveland
Middleburg Heights, OH

William C. Fiala, BS, MA
University of Akron
Akron, OH

Cathy Flores, BHS
Central Piedmont Community College
Charlotte, NC

Brenda K. Frerichs, MS, MA, BS
   Colorado Technical University
   Sioux Falls, SD

Michael Gallucci, PT, MS
   Assistant Professor of Practice,
   Program in Physical Therapy,
   School of Public Health,
   New York Medical College
   Valhalla, NY

Susan C. Gessner, RN, BSN, M Ed
   Laurel Business Institute
   Uniontown, PA

Bonnie J. Ginman, CMA
   Branford Hall Career Institute
   Springfield, MA

Robyn Gohsman, RMA, CMAS
   Medical Career Institute
   Newport News, VA

Cheri Goretti, MA, MT(ASCP), CMA
   Quinebaug Valley Community College
   Danielson, CT

Jodee Gratiot, CCA
   Rocky Mountain Business Academy
   Caldwell, ID

Marilyn Graham, LPN
   Moore Norman Technology Center
   Norman, OK

Donna E. Guisado, AA
   North-West College
   West Covina, CA

Debra K. Hadfield, BSN, MSN
   Baker College of Jackson
   Jackson, MI

Carrie A. Hammond, CMA, LPRT
   Utah Career College
   West Jordan, UT

Kris A. Hardy, CMA, RHE, CDF
   Brevard Community College
   Cocoa, FL

Toni R. Hartley, BS
   Laurel Business Institute
   Uniontown, PA

Brenda K. Hartson, MS, MA, BS
   Colorado Technical University
   Sioux Falls, SD

Marsha Perkins Hemby, BA, RN, CMA
   Pitt Community College
   Greenville, NC

Linda Henningsen, RN, MS, BSN
   Brown Mackie College
   Salina, KS

Carol Hinricher, MA
   University of Montana College of Technology
   Missoula, MT

Elizabeth A. Hoffman, MA Ed., CMA
   Baker College of Clinton Township
   Clinton Township, MI

Gwen C. Hornsey, BS
   Medical Assistant Instructor
   Tulsa Technology Center, Lemley Campus
   Tulsa, OK

Helen J. Houser, MSHA, RN, RMA
   Phoenix College
   Phoenix, AZ

Melody S. Irvine, CCS-P, CPC, CMBS
   Institute of Business and Medical Careers
   Ft. Collins, CO

Kathie Ivester, MPA, CMA(AAMA), CLS(NCA)
   North Georgia Technical College
   Clarkesville, GA

Josephine Jackyra, CMA
   The Technical Institute of Camden County
   Sicklerville, NJ

Deborah Jones, BS, MA
   High-Tech Institute
   Phoenix, AZ

Karl A. Kahley, CHE, BS
   Instructor, Medical Assisting
   Ogeechee Technical College
   Statesboro, GA

Barbara Kalfin Kalish
   City College, Palm Beach Community College
   Ft Lauderdale, FL

Cheri D. Keenan, MA Instructor, EMT-B
   Remington College
   Garland, TX

Barbara E. Kennedy, RN, CPhT
   Blair College
   Colorado Springs, CO

Tammy C. Killough, RN, BSN
   Texas Careers Vocational Nursing Program Director
   San Antonio, TX

Jimmy Kinney, AAS
   Virginia College at Huntsville
   Huntsville, AL

Karen A. Kittle, CMA, CPT, CHUC
   Oakland Community College
   Waterford, MI

Diane M. Klieger, RN, MBA, CMA
   Pinellas Technical Education Centers
   St. Petersburg, FL

Mary E. Larsen, CMT, RMA
   Academy of Professional Careers
   Nampa, ID

Nancy L. Last, RN
   Eagle Gate College
   Murray, UT

Holly Roth Levine, NCICS, NCRMA, BA, BSN, RN
   Keiser College
   West Palm Beach, FL

Christine Malone, BS
   Everett Community College
   Everett, WA

Janice Manning
   Baker College
   Jackson, MI

Loretta Mattio-Hamilton, AS, CMA, RPT, CCA, NCICS
   Herzing College
   Kenner, LA

Gayle Mazzocco, BSN, RN, CMA
   Oakland Community College
   Waterford, MI

Patti McCormick, RN, PHD
   President, Institute of Holistic Leadership
   Dayton, OH

Heidi M. McLean, CMA, RMA, BS, RPT, CAHI
   Anne Arundel Community College
   Arnold, MD

Stephanie R. McGahee, AATH
   Augusta Technical College
   Thomson, GA

Tanya Mercer, BS, RN, RMA
   KAPLAN Higher Education Corporation
   Roswell, GA

Sandra J. Metzger, RN, BSN, MS. Ed
   Red Rocks Community College
   Lakewood, CO

Joyce A. Minton, BS, CMA, RMA
   Wilkes Community College
   Wilkesboro, NC

Grace Moodt, RN, BSN
   Wallace Community College
   Dothan, AL

Sherry L. Mulhollen, BS, CMA
   Elmira Business Institute
   Elmira, NY

Deborah M. Mullen, CPC, NCMA
   Sanford Brown Institute
   Atlanta, GA

Michael Murphy, CMA
   Berdan Institute @ The Summit Medical Group
   Union, NJ

Lisa S. Nagle, CMA, BS.Ed,
   Augusta Technical College
   Augusta, GA

Peggy Newton, BSN, RN
   Galen Health Institute
   Louisville, KY

Brigitte Niedzwiecki, RN, MSN
   Chippewa Valley Technical College
   Eau Claire, WI

Thomas E. O'Brien, MBA, BBA, AS, CCT
   Central Florida Institute
   Palm Harbor, FL

Linda Oliver, MA
   Vista Adult School
   Vista, CA

Linda L. Oprean, BSN
   ACT College
   Manassas, VA

Holly J. Paul, MSN, FNP
   Baker College of Jackson
   Jackson, MI

Shirley Perkins, MD, BSE
   Everest College
   Dallas, TX

Kristina Perry, BPA
   Heritage College
   Las Vegas, NV

James H. Phillips, BS, CMA, RMA
   Central Florida College
   Winter Park, FL

Carol Putkamer, RHIA, MS
   Alpena Community College
   Alpena, MI

Mary Rahr, MS, RN, CMA-C
   Northeast Wisconsin Technical College
   Green Bay, WI

David Rice, AA, BA, MA
   Career College of Northern Nevada
   Reno, NV

Dana M. Roessler, RN, BSN
   Southeastern Technical College
   Glennville, GA

Cindy Rosburg, MA
   Wisconsin Indian Technical College
   New Richmond, WI

Deborah D. Rossi, MA, CMA
   Community College of Philadelphia
   Philadelphia, PA

Donna Rust, BA
   American Commercial College
   Wichita Falls, TX

Ona Schulz, CMA
   Lake Washington Technical College
   Kirkland, WA

Amy E. Semenchuk, RN, BSN
   Rockford Business College
   Rockford, IL

David Lee Sessoms, Jr. M.Ed., CMA
   Miller-Motte Technical College
   Cary, NC

Susan Shorey, BA, MA
   Valley Career College
   El Cajon, CA

Lynn G. Slack, BS
    ICM School of Business and Medical Careers
    Pittsburgh, PA

Patricia L. Slusher, MT(ASCP), CMA
    Ivy Tech State College
    Kokomo, IN

Deborah H. Smith, RN, CNOR
    Southeastern Technical College
    Vidalia, GA

Kristi Sopp, AA
    MTI College
    Sacramento, CA

Nona K. Stinemetz, Practical Nurse
    Vatterott College
    Des Moines, IA

Patricia Ann Stoddard, MS, RT(R), MT, CMA
    Western Business College
    Vancouver, WA

Sylvia Taylor, BS, CMA, CPC-A
    Cleveland State Community College
    Cleveland, TN

Cynthia H. Thompson, RN, MA
    Davenport University
    Bay City, MI

Geiselle Thompson, M. Div.
    The Learning Curve Plus
    Cary, NC

Barbara Tietsort, M. Ed.
    University of Cincinnati, Raymond Walters
    Cincinnati, OH

Karen A. Trompke, RN
    Virginia College at Pensacola
    Pensacola, FL

Marilyn M. Turner, RN, CMA
    Ogeechee Technical College
    Statesboro, GA

L. Joleen VanBibber, AS
    Davis Applied Technology College
    Kaysville, UT

Lynette M. Veach, AAS
    Columbus State Community College
    Columbus, OH 43215

Antonio C. Wallace, BS
    Sanford Brown Institute
    Atlanta, GA

Jim Wallace, MHSA
    Maric College
    Los Angeles, CA

Denise Wallen, CPC
    Academy of Professional Careers
    Boise, ID

Mary Jo Whitacre, MSN, RN
    Lord Fairfax Community College
    Middletown, VA

Donna R. Williams, LPN, RMA
    Tennessee Technology Center
    Knoxville, TN

Marsha Lynn Wilson, BS, MS (ABT)
    Clarian Health Sciences Education Center
    Indianapolis, IN

Linda V. Wirt, CMA
    Cecil Community College
    North East, MD

Dr. MaryAnn Woods, PhD, RN
    Prof. Emeritus,
    Fresno City College
    Fresno, CA 93741

Bettie Wright, MBA, CMA
    Umpqua Community College
    Roseburg, OR

Mark D. Young, DMD, BS
    West Kentucky Community and Technical College
    Paducah, KY

Cynthia M. Zumbrun, MEd, RHIT, CCS-P
    Allegany College of Maryland
    Cumberland, MD

Previous Edition Reviewers

Kaye Acton, CMA
    Alamance Community College
    Graham, NC

Jannie R. Adams, Ph.D, RN, MS-HAS, BSN
    Clayton College and State University,
    School of Technology
    Morrow, GA

Cathy Kelley Arney, CMA, MLT (ASCP), AS
    National College of Business and Technology
    Bluefield, VA

Joseph Balabat, MD
    Drake Schools
    Astoria, NY

Marsha Benedict, CMA-A, MS, CPC
    Baker College of Flint
    Flint, MI

Michelle Buchman
    Springfield College
    Springfield, MO

Patricia Celani, CMA
    ICM School of Business and Medical Careers
    Pittsburgh, PA

Theresa Cyr, RN, BN, MS
    Heald Business College
    Honolulu, HI

Barbara Desch
    San Joaquin Valley College
    Visalia, CA

Herbert J. Feitelberg, BA, DPM
King's College
Charlotte, NC

Geri L. Finn
Remington College, Dallas Campus
Garland, TX

Kimberly L. Gibson, RN, DOE
Sanford Brown Institute
Middleburg Heights, OH

Barbara G. Gillespie, MS
San Diego & Grossmont Community College Districts
El Cajon, CA

Cindy Gordon, MBA, CMA
Baker College
Muskegon, MI

Mary Harmon
MedTech College
Indianapolis, IN

Glenda H. Hatcher, BSN
Southwest Georgia Technical College
Thomasville, GA

Helen J. Hauser, RN, MSHA, RMA
Phoenix College
Phoenix, AZ

Christine E. Hetrick
Cittone Institute
Mt. Laurel, NJ

Beulah A. Hoffmann, RN, MSN, CMA
Ivy Tech State College
Terre Haute, IN

Karen Jackson
Education America
Garland, TX

Latashia Y. D. Jones, LPN
CAPPS College, Montgomery Campus
Montgomery, AL

Donna D. Kyle-Brown, PhD, RMA
CAPPS College, Mobile Campus
Mobile, AL

Sharon McCaughrin
Ross Learning
Southfield, MI

Tanya Mercer, BS, RMA
Kaplan Higher Education Corporation
Roswell, GA

T. Michelle Moore-Roberts
CAPPS College, Montgomery Campus
Montgomery, AL

Linda Oprean
Applied Career Training
Manassas, VA

Julie Orloff, RMA, CMA, CPT, CPC
Ultrasound Diagnostic School
Miami, FL

Delores W. Orum, RMA
CAPPS College
Montgomery, AL

Katrina L. Poston, MA, RHE
Applied Career Training
Arlington, VA

Manuel Ramirez, MD
Texas School of Business
Friendswood, TX

Beatrice Salada, BAS, CMA
Davenport University
Lansing, MI

Melanie G. Sheffield, LPN
Capps Medical Institute
Pensacola, FL

Kristi Sopps, RMA
MTI College
Sacramento, CA

Carmen Stevens
Remington College, Fort Worth Campus
Fort Worth, TX

Deborah Sulkowski, BS, CMA
Pittsburgh Technical Institute
Oakdale, PA

Fred Valdes, MD
City College
Ft. Lauderdale, FL

Janice Vermiglio—Smith, RN, MS, PhD
Central Arizona College
Apache Junction, AZ

Erich M. Weldon, MICP, NREMT-P
Apollo College
Portland, Oregon

Guided Tour

Case studies present situations similar to those that a medical assistant may encounter in daily practice.

CHAPTER 5

The Cardiovascular System

KEY TERMS

agglutination
agranulocyte
albumins
anemia
aneurysm
aortic semilunar valve
arrhythmia
atherosclerosis
atria
atrioventricular node
atrioventricular septum
baroreceptors
basophil
bicuspid valve
bilirubin
biliverdin
bundle of His
capillary
carboxyhemoglobin
carditis
cerebrovascular accident
chordae tendineae
chylomicron
coagulation
coronary sinus
deoxyhemoglobin
diapedesis
diastolic pressure
embolus
endocardium
eosinophil
epicardium
erythroblastosis fetalis
erythrocyte
erythropoietin

CHAPTER OUTLINE

- The Heart
- Blood Vessels
- Blood Pressure
- Circulation
- Blood

LEARNING OUTCOMES

After completing Chapter 5, you will be able to:

5.1 Describe the structure of the heart and the function of each part.
5.2 Trace the flow of blood through the heart.
5.3 List the most common heart sounds and what events produce them.
5.4 Explain how heart rate is controlled by the electrical conduction system of the heart.
5.5 List the different types of blood vessels and describe the functions of each.
5.6 Define blood pressure and tell how it is controlled.
5.7 Trace the flow of blood through the pulmonary and systemic circulation.
5.8 List the major arteries and veins of the body and describe their locations.

KEY TERMS (Concluded)

fibrinogen	lymphocyte	Rh antigen
globulins	megakaryocytes	RhoGAM
granulocyte	mitral valve	serum
hematocrit	monocyte	sinoatrial node
hemocytoblast	murmur	systemic circuit
hemolytic anemia	myocardial infarction	systolic pressure
hemostasis	myocardium	thalassemia
hepatic portal system	neutrophil	thrombocytes
hypertension	oxyhemoglobin	thrombophlebitis
interatrial septum	parietal pericardium	thrombus
interventricular septum	pericardium	tricuspid valve
leukemia	platelets	varicose veins
leukocyte	pulmonary circuit	vasoconstriction
leukocytosis	pulmonary semilunar valve	vasodilation
leukopenia	pulmonary trunk	ventricle
lipoprotein	Purkinje fibers	visceral pericardium

66

Chapter Openers

Every chapter opens with a Chapter Outline, Learning Outcomes, Key Terms, and an Introduction that prepares students for the learning experience.

Tables

Tables provide students with important information in an easy-to-read format.

Introduction

Bones and joints do not themselves produce movement. By alternating between contraction and relaxation, muscles cause bones and supported structures to move. The human body has more than 600 individual muscles. Although each muscle is a distinct structure, muscles act in groups to perform particular movements. This chapter focuses on the differences among three muscle tissue types, the structure of skeletal muscles, muscle actions, and the names of skeletal muscles.

CASE STUDY

Five days ago, a 40-year-old woman came to the doctor's office where you work as a medical assistant. She complained about pain in her back and right leg. Because this patient had a history of disc damage in her spine, she was sent home with pain medication and an order for bed rest for a 24-hour period. Two days later, she returned to the office with nausea, a severe headache, muscle twitching in her legs and arms, severe back pain, and tightness in her chest. The doctor once more asked the patient to elaborate on her activities the day before she fell ill. He was told that she had sprayed her furniture and carpets with an organophosphate insecticide to get rid of fleas in her house. She had also dipped her cats and dogs with the same insecticide. The doctor explained that organophosphates block acetylcholinesterase and immediately transferred her to the hospital for respiratory therapy and medicine to combat the insecticide poisoning.

As you read this chapter, consider the following questions:

1. What is the function of acetylcholinesterase?
2. Why does this patient exhibit muscle twitching and back pain?
3. What type of respiratory therapy will this patient require?
4. What precautions should a person take when using insecticides that contain organophosphates?
5. Why is it important for patients to give their doctor a complete account of their activities prior to an illness?

Functions of Muscle

Muscle tissue is unique because it has the ability to contract. It is this contraction that allows muscles to perform various functions. In addition to allowing the human body to move, muscles provide stability, the control of body openings and passages, and warming of the body.

Movement

Skeletal muscles are attached to bones by tendons. Because skeletal muscles cross joints, when these muscles contract, the bones they attach to move. This allows for various body motions, such as walking or waving your hand. Facial muscles are attached to the skin of the face, so when they contract, different facial expressions are produced, such as smiling or frowning. Smooth muscle is found in the walls of various organs, such as the stomach, intestines, and in these organs such as the m tine or the bir uterus. Cardia

ventricular contractions that pump blood into the blood vessels.

Stability

You rarely think about it, but muscles are holding your bones tightly together so that your joints remain stable. There are also very small muscles holding your vertebrae together to make your spinal column stable.

Control of Body Openings and Passages

Muscles also form valve-like structures called **sphincters** around various body openings and passages. These sphincters control the movement of substances into and out of these passages. For example, a urethral sphincter prevents urination until you relax it to permit urination.

52

TABLE 10-1	Cancer Staging
Stage	**Description**
Stage 0	Very early cancer. Cancer cells are localized in a few cell layers.
Stage I	Cancer cells have spread to deeper cell layers, or some may have spread to surrounding tissues.
Stage II	Cancer cells have spread to surrounding tissues but are considered contained in the primary cancer site.
Stage III	Cancer cells have spread beyond the primary cancer site to nearby areas.
Stage IV	Cancer cells have spread to other organs of the body.
Recurrent	Cancer cells have reappeared after treatment.

diagnostic tests include blood counts, an analysis of blood chemistry, and x-rays.

Signs and Symptoms. The symptoms of different types of cancer vary but the following are usually observed in most types: fever, chills, unintended weight loss, fatigue, and a general sense of not feeling well.

Treatment. The treatment of cancer differs depending on the type and stage of cancer. The stage of cancer refers to how large a tumor is and how far cancer cells have spread throughout the body. Table 10-1 provides a summary of cancer staging.

If tumors are localized and have not spread, the cancer can often be successfully treated by surgically removing the tumor. Other treatment options are chemotherapy and radiation therapy. Even if a cancer cannot be cured, its progression can sometimes be slowed, allowing patients to live additional years.

Allergies

An allergic reaction is an immune response to a substance, such as pollen, that is not normally harmful to the body. An allergy can also be an excessive immune response. Substances that trigger allergic responses are called **allergens.** Allergic reactions involve IgE antibodies and mast cells. When IgE antibodies bind to allergens, they cause mast cells to release histamine and heparin. These chemicals trigger allergic reactions. A patient receiving allergy shots is being injected with tiny amounts of the allergen. This causes the body to produce IgG antibodies that will prevent IgE antibodies from binding to the allergen. IgG antibodies do not trigger immune responses because they do not activate mast cells.

Most allergies do not cause life-threatening conditions, but some do. One life-threatening condition that can result is **anaphylaxis.** In this condition, blood vessels dilate so quickly that blood pressure drops too quickly for organs to adjust. Without treatment, patients may go into anaphylactic shock and die.

Signs and Symptoms. The signs and symptoms of allergies vary depending on what part of the body is exposed to allergens. Allergens that are inhaled often cause a runny nose, sneezing, coughing, or wheezing. An allergen that is ingested causes nausea, diarrhea, or vomiting. Skin allergens cause rashes. Allergens in the blood, such as penicillin for people who are allergic to it, are often the most life-threatening because they can affect many organ systems.

Treatment. Many allergies are effectively treated with over-the-counter medications called **antihistamines.** Prescription-strength antihistamines are also available. Various types of nasal sprays and decongestants can also reduce the symptoms of allergies. When a person experiences anaphylaxis, an injection of **epinephrine** is usually an effective treatment. Epinephrine causes vasoconstriction, which increases blood pressure.

Pathophysiology

Common Diseases and Disorders of the Immune System

As science and medicine develop a better understanding of the immune system and its relationship to causing disease, multiple diseases and disorders involving many body systems are now thought to have an *autoimmune* component. An **autoimmune disease** is one where the body begins to attack its own antigens. Examples of autoimmune diseases include scleroderma (Chapter 24), rheumatoid arthritis (Chapter 25), multiple sclerosis

continued —

158   CHAPTER 10

Educating the Patient boxes
Educating the Patient boxes give the medical assistant important information to share with the patients for self-care outside the medical office.

**New—added Caution acronym to emphasize information important to the subject.

Pathophysiology boxes
Pathophysiology section at the end of each chapter lists common diseases and disorders associated with that body system.

Review
Each chapter ends with a review section with case studies, discussion questions, critical thinking questions, application activities, and an Internet activity to reinforce the information that was just learned.

Educating the Patient

Snoring

Snoring occurs when the muscles of the palate, tongue, and throat relax. Airflow then causes these soft tissues to vibrate. These vibrating tissues produce the harsh sounds characteristic of snoring.

Snoring causes daytime sleepiness and is sometimes associated with a condition known as obstructive sleep apnea (OSA). In OSA, the relaxed throat tissues cause airways to collapse, which prevent a person from breathing. Snoring affects approximately 50% of men and 25% of women older than the age of 40 years. The common causes of snoring include:

- Enlargement of the tonsils or adenoids
- Being overweight
- Alcohol consumption
- Nasal congestion
- A deviated (crooked) nasal septum

The severity of snoring varies among people. The Mayo Clinic's Sleep Disorders Center uses the following scale to determine the severity of snoring:

- Grade 1: Snoring can be heard from close proximity to the face of the snoring person.
- Grade 2: Snoring can be heard from anywhere in the bedroom.
- Grade 3: Snoring can be heard just outside the bedroom with the door open.
- Grade 4: Snoring can be heard outside the bedroom with the door closed.

You can educate patients about making lifestyle modifications and using aids to help reduce their snoring:

- Lose weight
- Change the sleeping position from the back to the side
- Avoid the use of alcohol and medications that cause sleepiness
- Use nasal strips to widen the nasal passageways
- Use dental devices to keep airways open

In addition, patients may benefit from a CPAP (continuous positive airway pressure) machine, which uses a mask attached to a pump that forces air into their passageways while they sleep. If these therapies are not effective, patients may need surgery to trim excess tissues in the throat, such as an **uvulotomy**, or laser surgery to remove a portion of the soft palate.

Pathophysiology

Common Diseases and Disorders of the Respiratory System

Allergic rhinitis is a hypersensitivity reaction to various airborne allergens.

- **Causes.** There are many causes, which may be seasonal such as with hay fever or continual as those caused by dust, molds, colognes, cigarette smoke, animal dander, and mites.
- **Signs and symptoms.** There are numerous signs and symptoms, which may include sneezing; itchy, watery eyes; red, swollen eyelids; congested nasal mucus mem...

the assistance of an allergist for desensitization injections may be an option for long-term management.

Asthma is a condition in which the tubes of the bronchial tree become obstructed as a result of inflammation.

- **Causes.** The causes can include allergens (pollen, pets, dust mites, etc.), cigarette smoke, pollutants, perfumes, cleaning agents, cold temperatures, and exercise (in susceptible individuals).
- **Signs and symptoms.** Symptoms include difficulty

Pathophysiology

Common Diseases and Disorders of the Skeletal System

Arthritis is a general term meaning joint inflammation. Although there are more than 100 types of arthritis, we will discuss the two most common types.

Osteoarthritis, which is also known as degenerative joint disease (DJD), primarily affects the weight-bearing joints of the hips and knees. The cartilage between the bones and the bones themselves begin to break down.

- **Causes.** Research points to inflammatory processes or metabolic disorders as the etiology of DJD.
- **Signs and symptoms.** These include joint stiffness, and aching and pain, especially with weather changes. There is often fluid around the joint and grating noises with joint movement.
- **Treatment.** Anti-inflammatory drugs, including aspirin and NSAIDS (nonsteroidal anti-inflammatory drugs) such as naproxen and Feldene, may be used. Intra-articular steroid injections may be tried for severe cases. In some cases, a series of injections of medications containing hyaluronic acid are used when other treatments do not work. These injections serve as joint fluid replacement. Some success has been found with transplanting harvested cartilage cells from the patient's healthy knee cartilage, which are then grown in the lab and reinjected into the patient's diseased joint. Surgical scraping of the joint may also be done to remove deteriorated bone fragments. As a last resort, joint replacement may be recommended.

Rheumatoid arthritis (RA) is a chronic systemic inflammatory disease that attacks the smaller joints, typically of the hands and feet, as well as the surrounding tissues of those joints. There may be flares or attacks of pain and inflammation followed by periods of remission. RA is much more common in women than in men.

- **Causes.** RA is believed to be autoimmune in nature, triggering the joint inflammation.
- **Signs and symptoms.** In this disease, the synovial membrane is attacked, causing edema and congestion. Tissue becomes granular and thick, eventually destroying the joint capsule and bone. Scar tissue forms, bones atrophy, and visible deformities become apparent due to the bone malalignment and immobility. Patients also have moderate to severe pain in the affected joints.
- **Treatment.** Treatment includes anti-inflammatory drugs, exercise, heat or cold treatments, and cortisone injections. Researchers are working with genetic techniques to block the immune system reaction. Low-impact aerobic exercise may be helpful and some patients find warm water exercises beneficial as well.

Bursitis is inflammation of a bursa, which is a fluid-filled sac that cushions tendons. It occurs most commonly in the elbow, knee, shoulder, and hip.

- **Causes.** Overuse of, and trauma to, joints are the most common causes of this condition. Bacterial infections can also cause bursitis.
- **Signs and symptoms.** Signs and symptoms include joint pain and swelling as well as tenderness in the structures surrounding the joint.
- **Treatment.** The most common treatments are bed rest, pain medications, steroid injections, aspiration of excess fluid from the bursa, and antibiotics.

Carpal tunnel syndrome occurs when the median nerve in the wrist is excessively compressed. Typists, assembly-line workers, painters, and people who play sports such as racquetball are most likely to develop carpal tunnel syndrome.

- **Causes.** Overuse of the wrist is a common cause of this syndrome.
- **Signs and symptoms.** Weakness and numbness in the hand, and pain in the wrist, hand, or elbow are common symptoms.
- **Treatment.** This condition can be treated with wrist splints, pain medications, and steroid injections and by having the patient change work habits to better position and support the wrists. If these treatments do not improve the patient's condition, surgery to reduce the pressure on the nerves may be needed.

Ewing's family of tumors (EFT) is a group of tumors that affect different tissue types. However, the tumors primarily affect bone.

- **Causes.** Causes of EFT are not clear, but it most often affects Caucasians, the long bones of the body, and people between the ages of 10 and 20.
- **Signs and symptoms.** Fever, pain in the tumor location, fractures, and bruises in the tumor location are the primary symptoms.
- **Treatment.** Treatment options include surgery, chemotherapy, radiation therapy, a bone marrow transplant, or a stem cell transplant.

Gout, also known as gouty arthritis, is a type of arthritis that usually occurs more frequently with age.

- **Causes.** Gout is caused by deposits of uric acid crystals in the joints. People with gout cannot break down uric acid properly and remove it from their bloodstream.
- **Signs and symptoms.** Symptoms include sudden or chronic joint pain, commonly in the great toe, joint swelling and stiffness, and fever.

continued →

REVIEW
CHAPTER 6

CASE STUDY QUESTIONS

Now that you have completed this chapter, review the case study at the beginning of the chapter and answer the following questions:

1. Why is the patient wheezing?
2. Is asthma a life-threatening condition?
3. What is the advantage of using a nebulizer to deliver the bronchodilator?
4. Why did the doctor refer the patient for allergy testing?

Discussion Questions

1. Explain the importance of mucus, cilia, and stomach acid in protecting the respiratory system.
2. List the various respiratory volumes that are commonly measured in the clinical setting. What does each volume represent?
3. Explain the importance of surfactant in respiration. Why is it that premature infants and low-birth weight infants are at higher risk of RDS?

Critical Thinking Questions

1. Smoking destroys cilia in the respiratory tract. Describe how smoking damages the lungs. What causes the "barrel chest" that is characteristic of many patients with emphysema?
2. What effect would breathing in a paper bag have on oxygen concentrations in the blood? Would this be helpful for a person who is hyperventilating? Why or why not?

Application Activities

1. Give the name of the structure for each of the descriptions noted below.
   a. Contains the esophagus, trachea, and larynx
   b. Moves air in and out of trachea; produces sound
   c. The small branches within the lungs
   d. The protective, double-walled sac around the lungs
   e. The pulmonary parenchyma
   f. Keeps us from aspirating while eating or drinking

2. Explain how the cardiovascular system is interrelated with the respiratory system.
3. How many lobes does the left lung have? The right lung? Why are they different in size?

Virtual Fieldtrip

Visit the McGraw-Hill Higher Education Medical Assisting website at www.mhhe.com/medicalassisting3 to complete the following activity:

Cigarette smoking affects all of us, children most of all, and often the tobacco industries target young people to develop new consumers. The site for this exercise has been developed so that parents and others can keep young people safe from the dangers of cigarettes. Once you enter the site's home page, find the icon on the left side labeled "The Tobacco Toll." Choose your state from the list and get the current statistics for your state regarding the following:

- Number of high school students who smoke
- Number of male high school students who use smokeless or spit tobacco
- Number of children (younger than age 18) who become new daily smokers each year
- Number of children (younger than age 18) exposed to secondhand smoke at home
- Number of cigarette packs bought or smoked by children (younger than age 18) each year
- Number of adults in your state who smoke
1. What are the death statistics in your state from smoking?
2. What are the monetary costs to your state related to smoking?

Open the CD and complete this chapter's practice activities, play the games, listen to the key terms, and test yourself with the interactive review. E-mail, print, and/or save your results to document your proficiency.

ANATOMY, PHYSIOLOGY, AND PATHOPHYSIOLOGY

for Allied Health

CHAPTER 1

Organization of the Body

KEY TERMS

acids
active transport
allele
anabolism
anaphase
anatomical position
anatomy
anterior
atoms
autosome
bases
biochemistry
catabolism
caudal
cell membrane
cells
centrioles
chemistry
chromosome
cilia
complex inheritance
compound
connective tissue
cranial
cytokinesis
cytoplasm
deep
diaphragm
diffusion
distal
DNA
dorsal
electrolytes
endocrine gland
endoplasmic reticulum

CHAPTER OUTLINE

- The Study of the Body
- Organization of the Body
- Body Organs and Systems
- Anatomical Terminology
- Body Cavities and Abdominal Regions
- Chemistry of Life
- Cell Characteristics
- Movement Through Cell Membranes
- Cell Division
- Genetic Techniques
- Heredity
- Major Tissue Types

LEARNING OUTCOMES

After completing Chapter 1, you will be able to:

1.1 Describe body organization from simple to more complex levels.
1.2 List the body organ systems, their general functions, and the major organs contained in each.

KEY TERMS *(Concluded)*

epithelial tissue
exocrine gland
femoral
filtration
flagellum
frontal
gene
Golgi apparatus
homologous chromosome
inferior
inorganic
interphase
ions
lateral
lysosomes
matrix
matter
medial

meiosis
metabolism
metaphase
midsagittal
mitochondria
mitosis
molecule
muscle tissue
mutation
nervous tissue
neuroglial cells
neurons
nucleus
organ
organelle
organic
organism
organ systems

osmosis
ovum
phenylketonuria (PKU)
physiology
posterior
prophase
proximal
ribosomes
RNA
sagittal
sex chromosome
sex-linked trait
superficial
superior
telophase
tissue
transverse
ventral

1.3 Define the anatomical position and explain its importance.

1.4 Use anatomical terminology correctly.

1.5 Name the body cavities and the organs contained in each.

1.6 Explain the abdominal regions and quadrants.

1.7 Explain why a basic understanding of chemistry is important in studying the body.

1.8 Describe important molecules and compounds of the human body.

1.9 Label the parts of a cell and list their functions.

1.10 List and describe the ways substances move across a cell membrane.

1.11 Describe the stages of cell division.

1.12 Explain how mutations occur and what effects they may produce.

1.13 Describe the uses of the genetic techniques, DNA fingerprinting, and the polymerase chain reaction.

1.14 Describe the different patterns of inheritance.

1.15 Describe the locations and characteristics of the four main tissue types.

1.16 Describe the signs and symptoms of various genetic conditions.

Introduction

The human body is complex in its structure and function. This chapter provides an overview of the human body. It introduces you to the way the body is organized from the chemical level all the way up to the organ system level. You will also learn important terminology used in the clinical setting to describe body positions and parts. This chapter also focuses on how diseases develop at the genetic and organism levels.

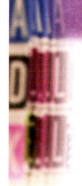

CASE STUDY

The parents of a 2-year-old boy have come to the hematologist's office because their son constantly seems to be covered in bruises, even at the slightest touch. Additionally, he has had frequent bleeds and joint pain for no apparent reason. The child's mother tells you that she feels guilty "for causing my son's problems."

After consulting with the physician and review of their son's medical record and lab work, a diagnosis is made.

As you read this chapter, consider the following questions:

1. Did the child's parents harm their child?
2. What is the child's probable diagnosis?
3. If the child was born with this condition, why would his mother be feeling guilty?
4. How will this little boy be treated?
5. Will the physician be able to cure their son?

The Study of the Body

Anatomy is the scientific term for the study of body structure. For example, the heart may be described as a hollow, cone-shaped organ that is an average of 14 centimeters long and 9 centimeters wide. Understanding anatomy also allows us to understand the normal position of body structures and how to describe these positions precisely and correctly. **Physiology** is the term used for the study of the function of the body's organs. For example, the physiology of the heart can be described by saying that the heart pumps blood into blood vessels to transport nutrients throughout the body.

Anatomy and physiology are commonly studied together because they are always related. For example, the anatomy of the heart (a hollow, muscular organ) allows it to do its function (pump blood into tubular blood vessels). If the heart was not hollow, it could not allow blood to flow into it. If the heart was not muscular, it not could pump blood.

Knowledge of anatomy and physiology will help you grasp the meaning of diagnostic and procedural codes. It can also help you understand the clinical procedures you will perform as a medical assistant. It can make it easier to see how and why certain diseases develop. Diseases develop in the body when homeostasis is not maintained.

Homeostasis is defined as the relative consistency of the body's internal environment. Body conditions that must remain within a stable range include body temperature, blood pressure, and the concentration of various chemicals within the blood. Individual cells must also maintain homeostasis. For example, if chemicals within a cell change the deoxyribonucleic acid (DNA) or genetic makeup of the cell, that cell can become cancerous.

Organization of the Body

The body's structure can be divided into different levels of organization. The chemical level is the simplest level. It refers to the billions of atoms and molecules in the body. **Atoms** are the simplest units of all matter and many are essential to life. **Matter** is anything that takes up space and has weight. The four most common atoms in the human body are carbon, hydrogen, oxygen, and nitrogen. **Molecules** are made up of atoms that bond together. Proteins and carbohydrates are examples of molecules that consist of hundreds of atoms.

Molecules join together to form **organelles,** which can be thought of as cell parts. Organelles combine to form cells such as leukocytes (white blood cells), erythrocytes (red blood cells), neurons (nerve cells), and adipocytes (fat cells). **Cells** are considered to be the smallest living units in the body. When the same types of cells organize together, they form **tissues.** The four major types of body tissue are epithelia, connective, nervous, and muscle. Two or more tissue types combine to form **organs,** and organs arrange to form **organ systems.** Finally, organ systems combine to form an **organism.** Figure 1-1 illustrates the organization of the body's organ systems.

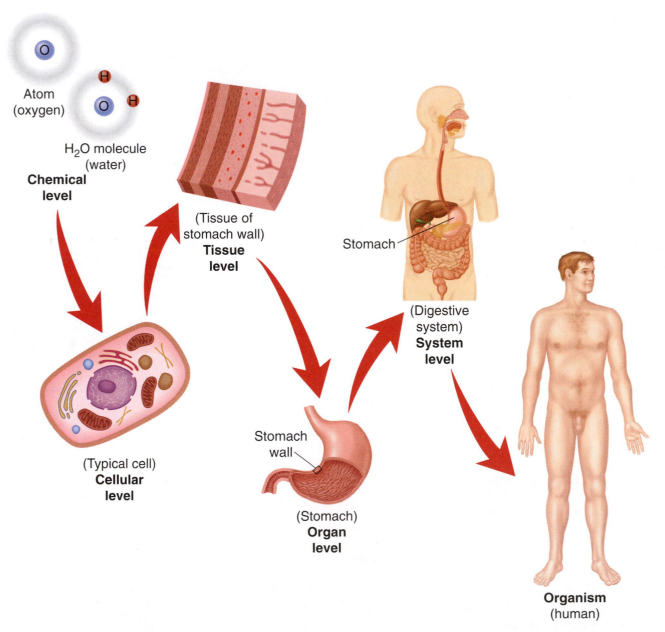

Atom
(oxygen)

H₂O molecule
(water)
**Chemical
level**

(Tissue of
stomach wall)
**Tissue
level**

Stomach

(Digestive
system)
**System
level**

(Typical cell)
**Cellular
level**

Stomach
wall

(Stomach)
**Organ
level**

Organism
(human)

Figure 1-1. The human body is organized in levels, beginning with the chemical level and progressing to the cellular, tissue, organ, system, and organism (whole body) levels.

Body Organs and Systems

Organs are structures formed by the organization of two or more different tissue types that work together to carry out specific functions. For example, the heart is made of cardiac muscle tissue, connective tissue, and epithelial tissue. These tissues work together to carry out the function of the heart, which is to effectively pump blood into blood vessels. Organ systems are formed when organs join together to carry out vital functions. For example, the heart and blood vessels unite to form the cardiovascular system. The organs of the cardiovascular system function to circulate blood throughout the body to ensure that all body cells receive enough nutrients. See Figure 1-2 for a

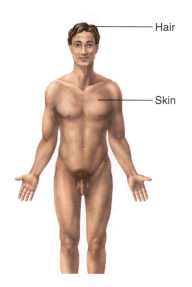

Integumentary System

Serves as a sense organ for the body, provides protection, regulates temperature, prevents water loss, and produces vitamin D precursors. Consists of skin, hair, nails, and sweat glands.

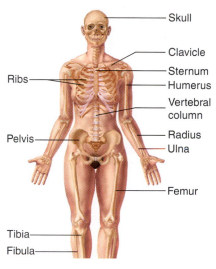

Skeletal System

Provides protection and support, allows body movements, produces blood cells, and stores minerals and fat. Consists of bones, associated cartilages, ligaments, and joints.

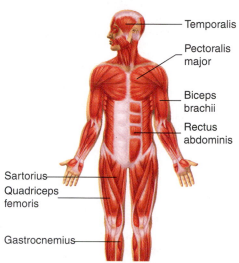

Muscular System

Produces body movements, maintains posture, and produces body heat. Consists of muscles attached to the skeleton by tendons.

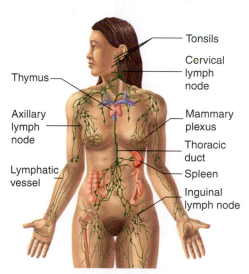

Lymphatic System

Removes foreign substances from the blood and lymph, combats disease, maintains tissue fluid balance, and absorbs fats from the digestive tract. Consists of the lymphatic vessels, lymph nodes, and other lymphatic organs.

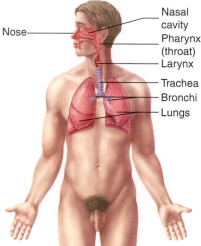

Respiratory System

Exchanges oxygen and carbon dioxide between the blood and air and regulates blood pH. Consists of the lungs and respiratory passages.

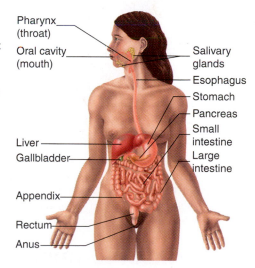

Digestive System

Performs the mechanical and chemical processes of digestion, absorption of nutrients, and elimination of wastes. Consists of the mouth, esophagus, stomach, intestines, and accessory organs.

Figure 1-2. Organ systems of the body.

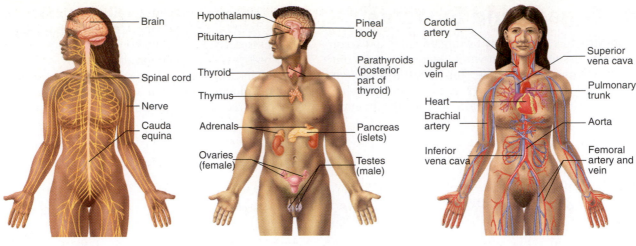

Nervous System

A major regulatory system that detects sensations and controls movements, physiologic processes, and intellectual functions. Consists of the brain, spinal cord, nerves, and sensory receptors.

Endocrine System

A major regulatory system that influences metabolism, growth, reproduction, and many other functions. Consists of glands, such as the pituitary, that secrete hormones.

Cardiovascular System

Transports nutrients, waste products, gases, and hormones throughout the body; plays a role in the immune response and the regulation of body temperature. Consists of the heart, blood vessels, and blood.

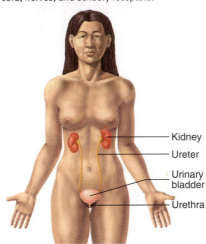

Urinary System

Removes waste products from the blood and regulates blood pH, ion balance, and water balance. Consists of the kidneys, urinary bladder, and ducts that carry urine.

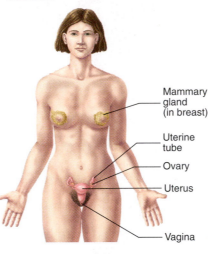

Female Reproductive System

Produces oocytes and is the site of fertilization and fetal development; produces milk for the newborn; produces hormones that influence sexual function and behaviors. Consists of the ovaries, vagina, uterus, mammary glands, and associated structures.

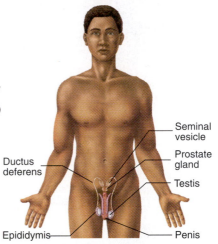

Male Reproductive System

Produces and transfers sperm cells to the female and produces hormones that influence sexual functions and behaviors. Consists of the testes, accessory structures, ducts, and penis.

Figure 1-2. (*concluded*)

summary of the organ systems of the human body, their general functions, and the organs within each.

Anatomical Terminology

Anatomical terms are used to describe the location of body parts and various body regions. In order to correctly use these terms, it is assumed that the body is in the anatomical position. In the **anatomical position,** a body is standing upright and facing forward with the arms at the sides and the palms of the hands facing forward. Even if patients are lying down, for consistency and correct communication when you use anatomical terms, always refer to patients as if they are in the anatomical position. (Figure 1-5 demonstrates the anatomical position.)

Directional Anatomical Terms

The directional anatomical terms are **cranial, caudal, ventral, dorsal, medial, lateral, proximal, distal, superficial,** and **deep.** They are used to identify the position of body structures compared to other body structures. For example, the eyes are medial to the ears but lateral to the nose. See Table 1-1 and Figure 1-3 for an explanation and illustration of these important directional terms.

TABLE 1-1 Directional Anatomical Terms

Term	Definition	Example
Superior (cranial)	Above or close to the head	The thoracic cavity is superior to the abdominal cavity.
Inferior (caudal)	Below or close to the feet	The neck is inferior to the head.
Anterior (ventral)	Toward the front of the body	The nose is anterior to the ears.
Posterior (dorsal)	Toward the back of the body	The brain is posterior to the eyes.
Medial	Close to the midline of the body	The nose is medial to the ear.
Lateral	Farther away from the midline of the body	The ears are lateral to the nose.
Proximal	Close to a point of attachment or to the trunk of the body	The knee is proximal to the toes.
Distal	Farther away from a point of attachment or from the trunk of the body	The fingers are distal to the elbow.
Superficial	Close to the surface of the body	Skin is superficial to muscles.
Deep	More internal	Bones are deep to skin.

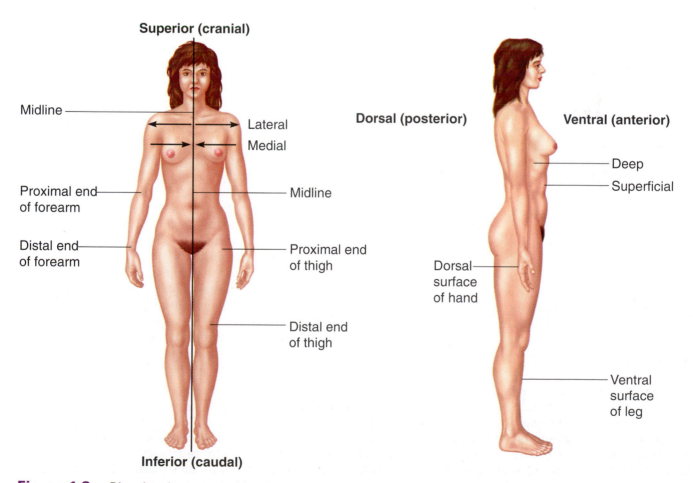

Figure 1-3. Directional terms provide mapping instructions for locating organs and body parts.

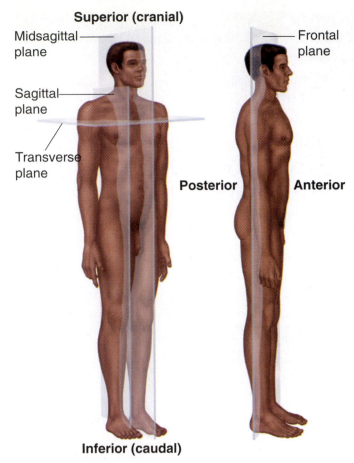

Superior (cranial)

Midsagittal plane

Sagittal plane

Transverse plane

Frontal plane

Posterior   Anterior

Inferior (caudal)

Figure 1-4. Spatial terms are based on imaginary cuts or planes through the body.

Anatomical Terms Used to Describe Body Sections

Sometimes in order to study internal body parts, it helps to imagine the body as being divided into sections. Medical professionals often use the following terms to describe how the body is divided into sections: sagittal, transverse, and frontal (coronal).

A **sagittal** plane divides the body into left and right portions. A **midsagittal** plane runs lengthwise down the midline of the body and divides it into equal left and right halves. A **transverse** plane divides the body into **superior** (upper) and **inferior** (lower) portions. A **frontal,** or coronal, plane divides the body into **anterior** (frontal) and **posterior** (rear) portions. Figure 1-4 illustrates these planes.

Anatomical Terms Used to Describe Body Parts

Many other anatomical terms are used to describe different regions or parts of the body. For example, the term *brachium* refers to the arm and the term **femoral** refers to the thigh. Figure 1-5 illustrates many of the common anatomical terms used to describe body parts.

Body Cavities and Abdominal Regions

The largest body cavities are the dorsal cavity and the ventral cavity. The dorsal cavity is divided into the cranial cavity and the spinal cavity. The cranial cavity houses the brain and the spinal cavity contains the spinal cord. The ventral cavity is divided into the thoracic cavity and the abdominopelvic cavity. The muscle called the **diaphragm** separates the thoracic and abdominopelvic cavities. The lungs, heart, esophagus, and trachea are contained in the thoracic cavity. The abdominopelvic cavity is divided into a superior abdominal cavity and an inferior pelvic cavity. The stomach, small and large intestines, gallbladder, liver, spleen, kidneys, and pancreas are located in the abdominal cavity. The bladder and internal reproductive organs are located in the pelvic cavity. Figure 1-6 depicts these cavities. The abdominal area is further divided into nine regions or four quadrants, which are illustrated in Figure 1-7.

Chemistry of Life

The chemical level is the lowest level of organization. It includes all the chemical elements that make up matter. Liquids, solids, and gases are all matter. **Chemistry** is the study of what matter is made of and how it changes. It is important to have a basic understanding of chemistry when studying anatomy and physiology because body structures and functions result from chemical processes that occur within body cells or fluids.

When two or more atoms are chemically combined, a molecule is formed. Molecules are the basic units of compounds. A **compound** is formed when two or more atoms of more than one element are combined. An example of a molecule is water, which is composed of two hydrogen atoms and one oxygen atom. Water is also an example of a compound because its molecules are made up of atoms of two different elements—hydrogen and oxygen. Water is critical to both chemical and physical processes in human physiology, and it accounts for approximately two-thirds of a person's body weight.

Metabolism is the overall chemical functioning of the body. The two processes of metabolism are **anabolism** and **catabolism.** In anabolism, small molecules combine to form larger ones (for example, when amino acids combine to form proteins). In catabolism, larger molecules are broken down into smaller ones (for example, when stored glycogen is converted to glucose molecules for energy).

Electrolytes

When put into water, some substances release **ions,** which are either positively or negatively charged particles; these substances are called **electrolytes.** For example, NaCl (sodium chloride) is an electrolyte. When you put NaCl in

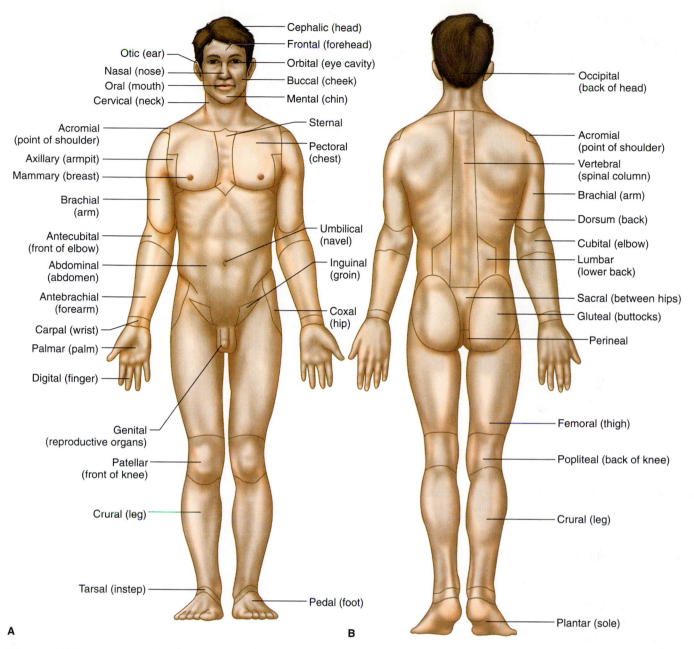

Figure 1-5. Numerous anatomical terms are used to describe regions of the body: (A) anterior view and (B) posterior view.

water, it releases the sodium ion (Na) and the chloride ion (Cl). Electrolytes are critical because the movements of ions into and out of body structures regulate or trigger many physiologic states and activities in the body. For example, electrolytes are essential to fluid balance, muscle contraction, and nerve impulse conduction.

Acids and Bases. **Acids** are a type of electrolyte. These electrolytes release hydrogen ions (H) in water. Many acids, such as lemon juice and vinegar, have a sour taste. **Bases** are also a type of electrolyte. They release hydroxyl ions (OH) in water. A basic substance may also be referred to as an alkali. Many basic substances are slippery

and bitter to the taste. Detergents are examples of basic substances.

Testing Acids and Bases. In the clinical setting, litmus paper or a pH meter is often used to determine if a substance is acidic or basic. An acidic substance will turn blue litmus paper red, and a basic substance will turn red litmus paper blue. The pH scale runs from 0 to 14. If a solution has a pH of 7, the solution is neutral, which means that it is neither acidic nor basic. If a solution has a pH less than 7, the solution is acidic. If a solution has a pH greater than 7, it is basic, or alkaline. The more acidic a solution is, the higher the concentration of hydrogen

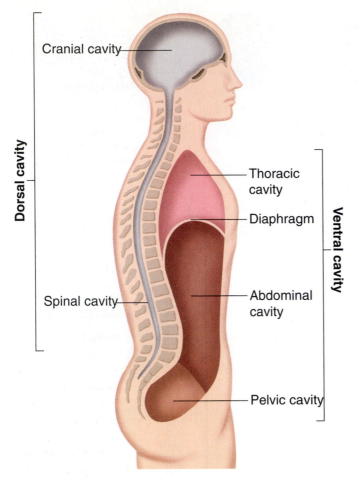

Figure 1-6. The two main body cavities are dorsal and ventral.

Cranial cavity

Dorsal cavity

Spinal cavity

Thoracic cavity

Diaphragm

Abdominal cavity

Pelvic cavity

Ventral cavity

ions it contains. The pH values of some common substances are shown in Figure 1-8.

Biochemistry

Biochemistry is the study of matter and chemical reactions in the body. Matter can be divided into two large categories—organic and inorganic matter. **Organic** matter contains carbon and hydrogen, and tends to be large. **Inorganic** matter generally does not contain carbon and hydrogen; these molecules tend to be small. Examples of inorganic substances are water, oxygen, carbon dioxide, and salts such as sodium chloride. Water is the most abundant inorganic compound in the body. The four major classes of organic matter in the body are carbohydrates, lipids, proteins, and nucleic acids.

Carbohydrates. Body cells depend on carbohydrate molecules to make energy. The most common carbohydrate used by body cells is glucose. Starches are a type of carbohydrate commonly found in potatoes, pastas, and breads, which is broken down into glucose when needed.

Lipids. Lipids are fats. There are three types of lipids found in the body: triglycerides, phospholipids, and steroids. Triglycerides are used to store energy for cells, and phospholipids are primarily used to make cell membranes. Butter and oils are composed of triglycerides, and the body stores these molecules in adipose tissue (fat). Steroids are very large lipid molecules used to make cell membranes and some hormones. Cholesterol is an example of an essential steroid for body cells.

Proteins. Proteins have many functions in the body. Many proteins act as structural materials for the building

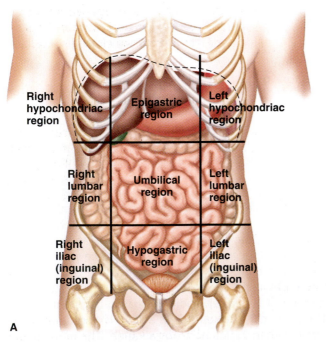

Right hypochondriac region

Epigastric region

Left hypochondriac region

Right lumbar region

Umbilical region

Left lumbar region

Right iliac (inguinal) region

Hypogastric region

Left iliac (inguinal) region

A

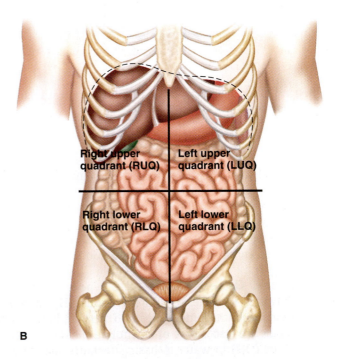

Right upper quadrant (RUQ)

Left upper quadrant (LUQ)

Right lower quadrant (RLQ)

Left lower quadrant (LLQ)

B

Figure 1-7. (A) The abdominal area divided into nine regions and (B) the abdominal area divided into four quadrants.

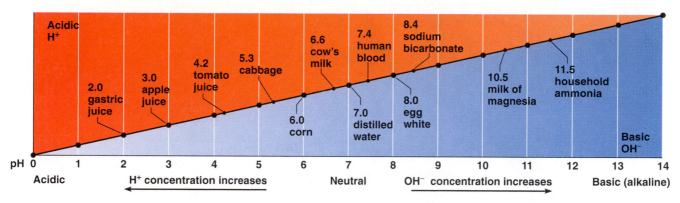

Figure 1-8. pH scale. As the concentration of hydrogen ions (H) increases, a solution becomes more acidic and the pH decreases. As the concentration of hydroxyl ions (OH) increases, a solution becomes more basic and the pH increases.

of solid body parts. Other proteins act as hormones, enzymes, receptors, and antibodies.

Nucleic Acids. DNA (deoxyribonucleic acid) and RNA (ribonucleic acid) are two examples of nucleic acids. DNA contains the genetic information of cells, and RNA is used to make proteins.

Cell Characteristics

Chemicals react to form the complex substances that make up cells, the basic unit of life. The human body is composed of millions of cells. There are many kinds of cells, and each type has a specific function. Most cells have three main parts: cell membrane, cytoplasm (containing each cell's organelles), and the nucleus. Figure 1-9 shows the structure of a composite cell.

Cell Membrane

The **cell membrane** is the outer limit of a cell. It is very thin and is selectively permeable, which means that it allows some substances to pass through it while preventing other substances from passing through. The cell membrane is composed of two layers of phospholipids, different types of proteins, cholesterol, and a few carbohydrates.

Cytoplasm and Its Organelles

The **cytoplasm** of a cell is the "inside" of the cell. It is mostly made up of water, proteins, ions, and nutrients. The cytoplasm houses organelles that perform many functions for the cell and therefore for system and body functions. These organelles include cilia, the flagellum, ribosomes, the endoplasmic reticulum, mitochondria, the Golgi apparatus, lysosomes, and centrioles.

- Many cells contain hair-like projections on the outside of the cell membrane called **cilia.** Cilia assist with propelling matter throughout the body tracts, such as within the respiratory system. Cells with cilia are often found in the mucus membranes.

- A **flagellum** is a tail-like structure found on the human sperm cell and provides its "swimming" type of locomotion.
- **Ribosomes** are responsible for protein synthesis.
- The **endoplasmic reticulum** comes in two forms—smooth and rough. The rough endoplasmic reticulum is named for the presence of ribosomes on its surface, which give it a bumpy or rough appearance. Both types of endoplasmic reticulum form networks or passageways to transport substances throughout the cytoplasm.
- **Mitochondria** provide energy for the cell and are the centers for cell respiration. There may be only one mitochondrion in a cell or many, depending on how much energy is required for each cell type.
- The cell's **Golgi apparatus** is known to synthesize or produce carbohydrates. It's also thought to prepare and store secretions for discharge from the cell.
- The organelles known as **lysosomes** perform the digestive function for the cell.
- The **centrioles** are two cylindrical organelles near the nucleus. They are essential to cell division because they equally distribute chromosomes to the resultant "daughter" cells.

Nucleus

The **nucleus** of a cell is typically round in structure and is placed near the center of a cell. It is enclosed by a nuclear membrane that contains nuclear pores so that larger substances can move into and out of the nucleus. It contains **chromosomes,** which are thread-like structures made up of DNA.

Movement Through Cell Membranes

The selectively permeable cell membrane controls what moves into and out of cells. Some substances move across the cell membrane without the use of energy. These

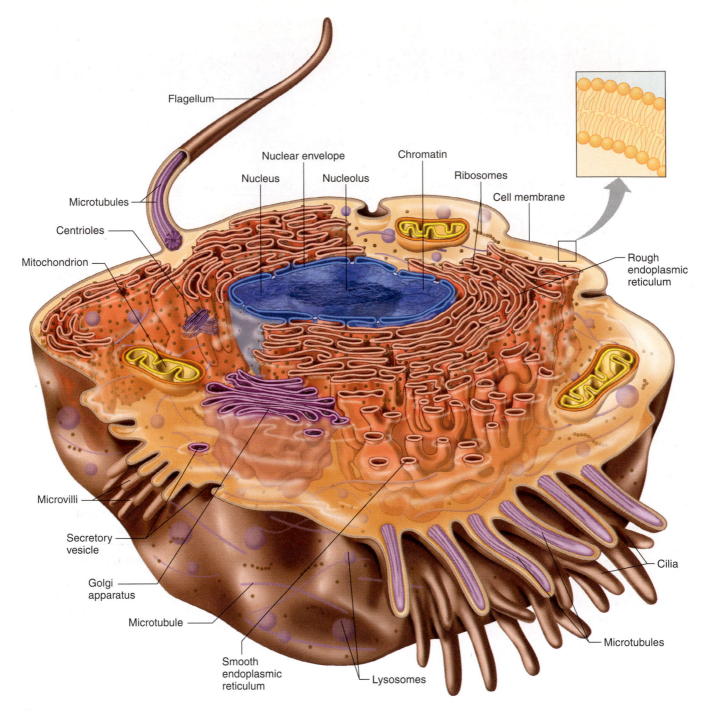

Figure 1-9. Composite cell.

Diffusion

Diffusion is the movement of a substance from an area of high concentration to an area of low concentration—it can be described as the spreading out of a substance. Substances that easily diffuse across the cell membrane include gases such as oxygen and carbon dioxide.

Osmosis

Osmosis is the diffusion or movement of water across a semi-permeable membrane, such as a cell membrane. You should remember that water will always try to diffuse or move toward the higher concentration of solutes (solids in solution).

movements are called passive mechanisms. Sometimes the cell has to use energy to move a substance across its membrane, in movements known as active mechanisms.

Filtration

In **filtration,** some type of pressure, such as gravity or blood pressure, forces substances across a membrane that acts like a filter. Filtration separates substances in solutions. For example, you could separate sand from water by pouring the sand/water mixture through a filter. In the body, capillaries in the kidneys act as filters to separate components of blood.

Active Transport

In **active transport,** substances move across the cell membrane with the help of carrier molecules. The substances move from an area of low concentration to an area of high concentration. In other words, substances are gathered together, which is the opposite of diffusion. Some substances that are moved across the cell membrane through active transport include sugars, amino acids, potassium, calcium, and hydrogen ions.

Cell Division

Cells can become damaged, diseased, or worn out, and replacements must be made. Also, new cells are needed for normal growth. Cells reproduce by cell division, a process that involves splitting the nucleus, through **mitosis** or **meiosis,** and splitting the cytoplasm, called **cytokinesis.**

A cell that carries out its normal daily functions and is not dividing is said to be in **interphase.** For example, if a liver cell is in interphase, it is making liver enzymes, detoxifying blood, and processing nutrients. During interphase, a cell prepares for cell division by duplicating its DNA and cytoplasmic organelles. For most body cells, each daughter cell will have the exact same copy of DNA and organelles as the original mother cell. Sometimes when the DNA is duplicated, errors called **mutations** occur. These mutations will be passed on to the descendants (daughter cells) of that cell and may or may not affect the cells in harmful ways.

Mitosis

Following interphase, a cell may enter mitosis, a part of cell division in which the nucleus divides. During this process, the cell membrane constricts to divide the cytoplasm of the cell. The result is that the organelles of the original cell get distributed almost evenly into the two new cells. The stages of mitosis are listed here and pictured in Figure 1-10.

- **Prophase** occurs when the centrioles that have replicated just prior to the onset of mitosis move to opposite ends of the cell. As they separate, they create spindle fibers between them.
- During **metaphase,** the chromosomes line up in the middle of the cell between the centrioles on these spindle fibers.

- During **anaphase,** the centromeres divide, pulling the chromatids, now chromosomes, toward the centrioles at opposite sides of the cell.
- The final stage is called **telophase.** As the chromosomes reach the centrioles, each with its complete set, cytokinesis or division of the cytoplasm takes place and mitosis is complete.

Remember that during mitosis, the nucleus makes a complete copy of all 23 of its chromosome pairs (46 chromosomes altogether). As the cell divides, each new cell receives a complete set of chromosome pairs. The resulting cells are identical to each other.

Meiosis

Meiosis is reproductive cell division. It takes place only in the reproductive organs when the male and female sex cells are formed. During meiosis, the nucleus copies all 23 chromosome pairs, but two divisions take place. The four cells that are formed each contains only one of each chromosome pair, for a total of 23 chromosomes. This type of cell division must occur so that when the sex cells combine during fertilization, the resulting cell contains the usual number of chromosomes (46).

Genetic Techniques

DNA is the primary component of genes and is found in the nucleus of most cells within the body. A **gene** is a segment of DNA that determines a body trait. Genetic techniques involve using or manipulating genes.

The chemical structure of every person's DNA is the same. The only difference among people is the order of the nitrogen bases. The unique sequence of the nucleotides determines the characteristics of an individual. One DNA molecule will contain hundreds or thousands of genes. Each gene occupies a particular location on the DNA molecule, making it possible to compare the same gene in a number of different samples. Two widely used genetic techniques in the clinical setting are the polymerase chain reaction (PCR) and DNA fingerprinting.

Polymerase Chain Reaction

The polymerase chain reaction (PCR) is a quick, easy method for making millions of copies of any fragment of DNA. This technique has been revolutionary in the study of genetics and has very quickly become a necessary tool for improving human health.

PCR can produce millions of gene copies from tiny amounts of DNA, even from just one cell. This method is especially useful for detecting disease-causing organisms that are impossible to culture, such as many kinds of bacteria, fungi, and viruses. It can, for example, detect the AIDS virus sooner—during the first few weeks after infection—than other tests. PCR is also more accurate than

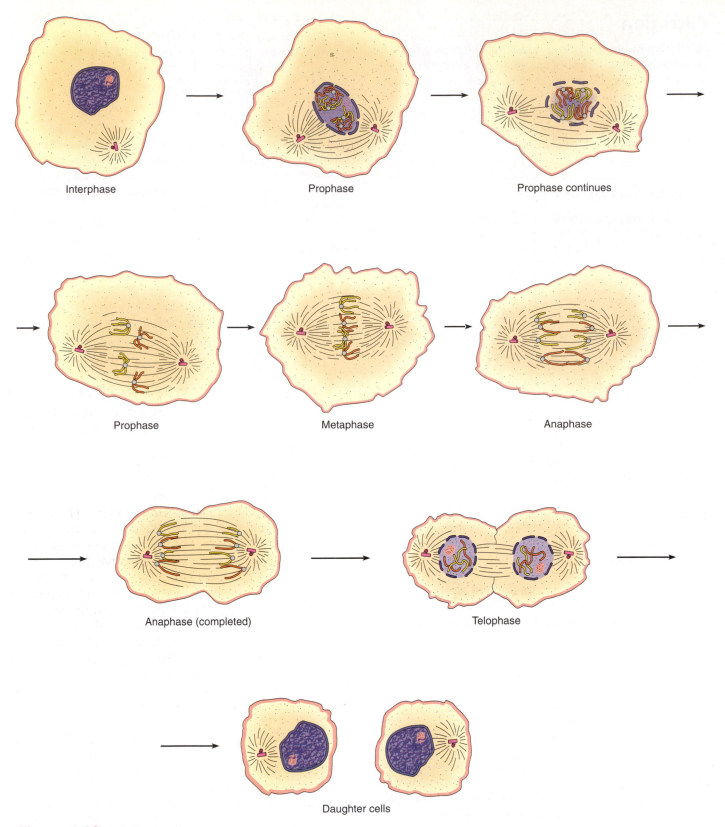

Figure 1-10. Cell mitosis.

standard tests. The technique can detect bacterial DNA in children's middle ear fluid, which indicates an infection, even when culture methods fail to detect bacteria. Other diseases diagnosed through PCR include Lyme disease, stomach ulcers, viral meningitis, hepatitis, tuberculosis, and many sexually transmitted diseases (STDs), including herpes and chlamydia.

PCR is also leading to new kinds of genetic testing because it can easily distinguish among the tiny variations in DNA that all people possess. This testing can diagnose people who have inherited disorders or who carry mutations that could be passed to their children. PCR is also used in tests that determine who may develop common disorders such as heart disease and various types of cancer. This knowledge helps individuals take steps to prevent those diseases.

DNA Fingerprinting

A DNA "fingerprint" refers to the unique sequences of nucleotides in a person's DNA and is the same for every cell, tissue, and organ of that person. Consequently, DNA fingerprinting is a reliable method for identifying and distinguishing among human beings to establish paternity and identify suspects in criminal cases. It is also used to diagnose genetic disorders such as cystic fibrosis, hemophilia, Huntington's disease, familial Alzheimer's, sickle cell anemia, thalassemia, and many others. Detecting genetic diseases early, or in utero, allows patients and medical staff to prepare for proper treatment. Researchers also use this information to identify DNA patterns associated with genetic diseases.

Heredity

Heredity is the transfer of genetic traits from parent to child. When a sperm cell and an **ovum** (egg) unite, a cell called a zygote forms. The zygote has 46 chromosomes, or 23 chromosomal pairs. One half of each pair came from the sperm, and the other half from the ovum. The first 22 pairs, which are the same size and shape, are called **homologous chromosomes,** also known as **autosomes.** The 23rd pair are called **sex chromosomes.** If the sex chromosomes are an X chromosome and a Y chromosome, the child is a male. If the sex chromosomes are both X chromosomes, the child is a female. Although the sex chromosomes determine the gender of the child, they also determine other body traits. However, the autosomes determine most body traits.

Each chromosome possesses many genes. Homologous chromosomes carry the same genes that code for a particular trait, but the genes may be of different forms, which are called **alleles.** Many times only one allele is actually expressed as a trait even if another allele is present. The allele that is always expressed over the other is called a dominant allele. The one that is not expressed is called recessive. The only way a recessive allele can be expressed is if there is no dominant allele present.

Detached earlobes are an example of a trait that is determined by a dominant allele. If a child inherits a dominant allele for this trait from one parent but inherits the recessive allele from the other parent, the child will have detached earlobes. If the child inherits recessive alleles from both parents, then he or she will have attached earlobes.

Most traits in the body are determined by multiple alleles. For example, hair color, height, skin tone, eye color, and body build are each determined by many different genes. **Complex inheritance** is the term used to describe inherited traits that are determined by multiple genes. It explains why different children within the same family can each have different characteristics.

Sex-linked traits are carried on the sex chromosomes, X and Y. The Y chromosome is much smaller than the X chromosome and does not carry many genes. Therefore, if the X chromosome carries a recessive allele, it is likely to be expressed because there is usually no corresponding allele on the Y chromosome. For example, red-green color blindness is determined by the presence of a recessive allele that is always found on the X chromosome. This disorder (like most sex-linked disorders) primarily affects males because the corresponding Y chromosome does not have any allele to prevent the expression of the recessive allele.

Genetic influences are known to contribute to many thousands of different health conditions. We will discuss some of the more common genetic diseases and disorders later in the Pathophysiology section found at the end of this chapter.

Major Tissue Types

As you learned earlier in the chapter, tissues are groups of cells that have similar structures and functions. The four major tissue types in the body are epithelial, connective, muscle, and nervous.

Epithelial Tissue

When you think of **epithelial tissue,** you should think of a covering, lining, or gland. Epithelial tissue covers the body and most organs. Epithelial tissue also lines tubes of the body, such as blood vessels and the esophagus, as well as hollow organs of the body, such as the stomach and heart. This type of tissue also lines body cavities, such as the thoracic cavity and the abdominopelvic cavity. Glandular tissue is also classified as a type of epithelial tissue.

Glandular epithelium is composed of cells that make and secrete (give off) substances. If a gland secretes its product into a duct, such as with a sweat or oil (sebaceous) gland, it is called an **exocrine gland.** If a gland secretes its product directly into tissue fluids or blood, it is called an **endocrine gland.** Endocrine glands do not have ducts, so they have to secrete their products into surrounding tissue fluids or blood. The pancreas and thyroid are considered endocrine glands because they release their hormones directly into the bloodstream.

Epithelial tissues are avascular, which means that they lack blood vessels. However, these tissues have a nerve supply and are very mitotic—they divide constantly. In addition, the cells within epithelial tissues are packed together tightly. Epithelial tissues have many different functions, depending on their location in the body. For example, those covering the body protect against invading pathogens and toxins. Those that line the digestive tract secrete a variety of enzymes needed for digestion. They

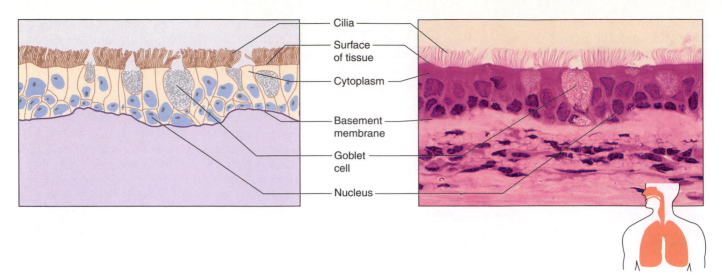

Figure 1-11. Epithelial tissue lining the respiratory tract.

often possess microvilli, which allow the body to absorb nutrients. Epithelial tissues lining the respiratory tract have cilia and goblet cells. The goblet cells produce mucus that traps small particles that enter the respiratory tract. The cilia constantly push the mucus and trapped particles away from the lungs (Figure 1-11). Epithelial cells within the kidneys act as filters that help to remove waste products from blood.

Connective Tissue

Connective tissues are the most abundant tissues in the body. The cells of connective tissues are not packed together tightly. Instead, a **matrix** separates the cells. Think of the matrix simply as the matter that is between the cells of connective tissue. It contains fibers, water, proteins, inorganic salts, and other substances. The components of the matrix vary, depending on the type of connective tissue. Connective tissues generally have a rich blood supply, except for cartilage and some dense connective tissues that contain a very poor blood supply.

Many different cell types are located in connective tissues. The most common cell types are fibroblasts, mast cells, and macrophages. Fibroblasts make fibers, and mast cells secrete substances such as heparin and histamine that promote inflammation when tissue is damaged. Macrophages are cells that destroy unwanted material, such as bacteria or toxins.

Blood. This tissue is composed of red blood cells, white blood cells, platelets, and plasma. Plasma is the matrix of blood. Unlike other connective tissues, this matrix does not contain fibers. Blood functions to transport substances throughout the body. Blood and its cell functions will be discussed in depth in Chapters 5 and 10.

Osseous (Bone) Tissue. The matrix of osseous tissue contains mineral salts that make it a very hard tissue.

Contrary to popular belief, bone tissue is a living tissue and is therefore metabolically active.

Cartilage. The matrix of cartilage is rigid, although it is not as hard as osseous tissue. Cartilage gives shape to structures such as the ears and nose. It also protects the ends of long bones and forms the discs between the vertebrae of the neck and spine.

Dense Connective Tissue. The matrix of dense connective tissue is packed with tough fibers that make it a soft but very strong tissue. Ligaments, tendons, and joint capsules have large amounts of this tissue type. Ligaments connect bones to bones, tendons connect muscles to bones, and joint capsules surround moveable joints in the body. Dense connective tissues also make up a large part of the dermis of skin. When skin is damaged, this tissue "fills" in the space of damage and forms a scar.

Adipose (Fat) Tissue. Within adipose tissue, unique cells—adipocytes—store fats. This tissue type stores energy for body cells, cushions body parts and organs, and insulates the body against excessive heat or cold (Figure 1-12).

Muscle Tissue

Muscle tissue is a specialized type of tissue that contracts and relaxes. The three types of muscle tissue are skeletal, visceral (smooth), and cardiac. Skeletal muscle tissue, as its name suggests, is attached to the skeleton. This type of muscle tissue is voluntary because we can consciously control its movement. For example, we can consciously decide to contract the skeletal muscles attached to our arm bones and make them move. It is also referred to as being striated because the cells of this muscle tissue type have striations or stripes in their cytoplasm (Figure 1-13).

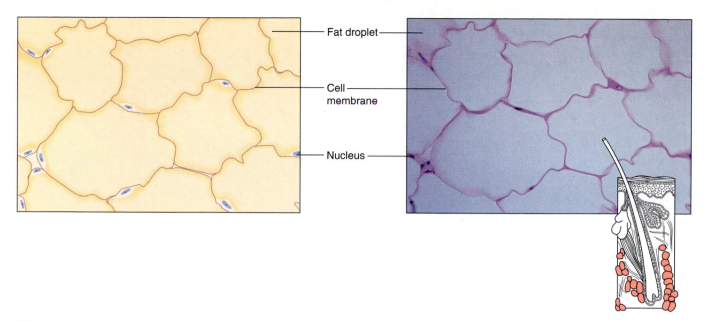

Figure 1-12. Adipose tissue.

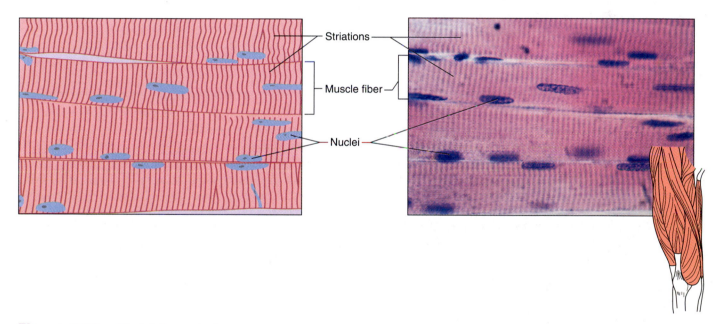

Figure 1-13. Skeletal muscle tissue.

Visceral (smooth) muscle tissue is located in the walls of hollow organs (except the heart), the walls of blood vessels, and the dermis of skin. It is involuntary because we cannot consciously control its movement. For example, you do not consciously decide when the visceral muscle of your stomach contracts. This tissue is also called smooth because its cells do not possess striations in their cytoplasm.

Cardiac muscle tissue is the specialized muscle tissue located in the wall of the heart. Like skeletal muscle tissue, cardiac muscle is striated. Like smooth muscle tissue, it is not under voluntary control and so is also referred to as being involuntary.

Nervous Tissue

Nervous tissue is located in the brain, spinal cord, and peripheral nerves. This tissue specializes in sending impulses or electrical messages to the neurons, muscles, and glands in the body. Nervous tissue contains two types of cells: **neurons** and **neuroglial cells.** Neurons are the largest cells and are the cells that transmit impulses. Although neuroglial cells are smaller, they are more abundant and act as support cells for the neurons. They do not transmit impulses (Figure 1-14).

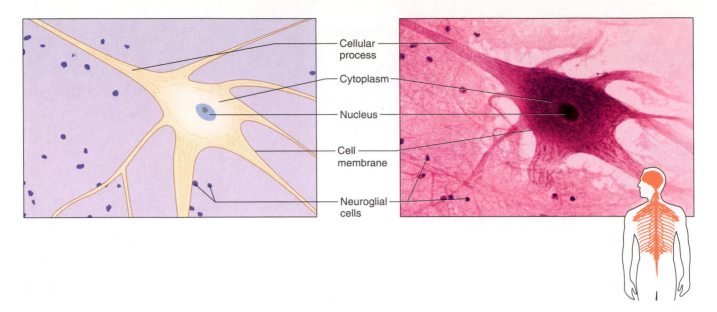

Figure 1-14. Nervous tissue.

Pathophysiology

Common Genetic Disorders

Albinism is a condition in which a person is born with little or no pigmentation in the skin, eyes, or hair. Albinism affects all races, and in most cases there is no family history.

- **Causes.** At least six different genes are involved with pigment production. This condition develops when a person inherits one or more faulty genes that do not produce the usual amounts of a pigment.
- **Signs and symptoms.** People with the condition experience visual problems and sun-sensitive skin.
- **Treatment.** Although there is no cure, treatments are available to help the symptoms. Prenatal testing for the condition is available.

Cystic fibrosis is a life-threatening disease that mainly affects the lungs and pancreas. This disease is one of the most common inherited life-threatening disorders among white people in the United States.

- **Causes.** Inheritance is autosomal recessive, so if both parents are carriers, there is a 25% chance that each child born to them will develop cystic fibrosis.
- **Signs and symptoms.** Patients with this disorder have increasing problems with breathing. Thick secretions eventually block passageways in the air, and these secretions may become infected.
- **Treatment.** There is no cure, but treatments are available to help patients live with the complications associated with this disorder. Newborn babies are commonly screened for the disease because the sooner treatment begins, the healthier the child can be. Parents are also

commonly screened for the gene to determine the likelihood of having a child with cystic fibrosis.

Down syndrome, also called Trisomy 21, is a disorder that causes mental retardation and physical abnormalities.

- **Causes.** This disorder occurs when a person has three copies of chromosome 21 instead of two. This condition can be diagnosed through prenatal tests such as amniocentesis. The risk of having a child with Down syndrome increases with the age of the mother.
- **Signs and symptoms.** The signs of Down syndrome include a flat facial profile, protruding tongue, oblique slanting eyes, abundant neck skin, short broad hands, and poor muscle tone. Heart, digestive, hearing, and visual problems are also common in people with this condition. Learning difficulties are common in Down syndrome and can range from moderate to severe.
- **Treatment.** There is no cure, but support programs and the treatment of health problems allow many patients with Down syndrome to live a relatively normal life.

Fragile X syndrome is the most common inherited cause of learning disability. All races and ethnic groups seem to be affected equally by this syndrome.

- **Causes.** In this disorder, one of the genes on the X chromosome is defective and makes the chromosome susceptible to breakage. This sex-linked disorder affects boys more severely than girls. It is estimated that approximately 1 in 300 females is a carrier for this disorder.

continued ⟶

Common Genetic Disorders *(concluded)*

- **Signs and symptoms.** Mental impairment, learning disabilities, attention deficit disorder, a long face, large ears, and flat feet are some of the signs and symptoms. Fragile X syndrome can be easily diagnosed using prenatal tests such as amniocentesis.
- **Treatment.** There is no cure, but some treatments and support groups are available to patients with this disorder.

Hemophilia is a group of inheritable blood disorders. Each condition may be severe to mild.

- **Causes.** In each type, an essential clotting factor is low or missing. Most types of hemophilia are X-linked recessive disorders; therefore, this disorder primarily affects males. Carriers of the gene can be identified with a blood test, and prenatal tests can diagnose the condition in the fetus.
- **Signs and symptoms.** Symptoms include easy bruising, spontaneous bleeding, and prolonged bleeding. Repeated bleeding in the joints leads to arthritis and permanent joint damage.
- **Treatment.** Treatment includes injections of the missing clotting factors, often Factor VIII.

Klinefelter's syndrome is a chromosomal abnormality that affects males.

- **Causes.** Males with this disorder have an extra X chromosome.
- **Signs and symptoms.** Tall stature, pear-shaped fat distribution, small testes, sparse body hair, and infertility are the most common signs and symptoms. Thyroid problems, diabetes, and osteoporosis are also common in patients with this syndrome.
- **Treatment.** There is no cure, but treatments such as testosterone replacement therapy can decrease the risk of osteoporosis and produce more male characteristics.

Muscular dystrophy is a group of genetic disorders that primarily affect the muscular and nervous systems. It most often affects males.

- **Causes.** Most types involve mutations in the genes responsible for producing muscle proteins. Some types of muscular dystrophy are inherited as an X-linked disorder, but some are caused by gene mutations.
- **Signs and symptoms.** In this disorder, muscle cells gradually break down, causing progressive muscle weakness.
- **Treatment.** There is no cure, and few treatments are available to slow down the loss of muscle cells. Prenatal genetic tests are available for some types of muscular dystrophies.

Phenylketonuria (PKU) develops if a person cannot synthesize the enzyme that converts phenylalanine to tyrosine. Phenylalanine is an essential amino acid, but too much of it can be harmful, so the body regularly converts it to tyrosine.

- **Causes.** This condition is inherited as an autosomal recessive disorder.
- **Signs and symptoms.** If phenylalanine builds up in the blood, it can lead to irreversible organ damage, including the brain.
- **Treatment.** Phenylalanine is found in many proteins, so meats and other protein-rich foods must be avoided. Early detection of PKU is important in order to prevent developmental delays. There is no cure for PKU, but special diets allow a person to lead a normal life. Most newborns are tested for PKU, and prenatal diagnosis is also available.

Turner's syndrome is a disorder that almost exclusively affects females.

- **Causes.** This disease results when an X chromosome is completely or partially missing.
- **Signs and symptoms.** The signs and symptoms may include web neck, broad chest, widely spaced nipples, low hairline, short stature, and infertility. Prenatal tests can diagnose the condition, but most girls are diagnosed in late childhood when they fail to start menstruating.
- **Treatment.** There is no cure for Turner's syndrome, but treatments with growth hormone replacements can increase the height of the patient.

Summary

The human body is divided into several levels of organization, from the simplest to the most complex. These levels are chemical, cellular, tissue, organ, organ system, and organism. Anatomy is the study of the structure of the human body and physiology is the study of its functions. Cells multiply through mitosis and meiosis. Understanding these processes assists with the concept that one mutant cell can lead to multiple illnesses and birth defects. Directional terms are used to describe the location of body parts and regions, allowing for specificity when describing locations. These terms always relate to the anatomic position. It is important to understand the relationship between the body levels as well as the basics of the organization of the human body and the relationships found within each organization, before studying the individual systems.

REVIEW

CASE STUDY QUESTIONS

Now that you have completed this chapter, review the case study at the beginning of the chapter and answer the following questions:

1. Did the child's parents harm their child?
2. What is the child's probable diagnosis?
3. If the child was born with this condition, why would his mother be feeling guilty?
4. How will this little boy be treated?
5. Will the physician be able to cure their son?

Discussion Questions

1. Explain the function of the four types of tissues in one of the body systems.
2. Describe the four abdominal quadrants and the nine abdominal regions. What is the importance of knowing these areas in the clinical setting?
3. What are acids and bases? Describe the pH scale.

Critical Thinking Questions

1. Diseases develop when homeostasis is not maintained. What treatments can bring the following conditions back to normal: high body temperature, dehydration, and high blood pressure?
2. Body systems have distinct functions, but at least several are closely interrelated. When considering a patient experiencing an MI (myocardial infarction), what are some of the symptoms the patient may have? What body systems create each of the symptoms?
3. Genetic testing has become more common for both expectant parents and persons with strong family histories of genetic disorders. How does genetic testing assist these people? What questions may remain if the results of such tests are positive for diseases like CF, Down syndrome, Alzheimer's disease, or even some cancers?

Application Activities

1. Referring back to the discussion of genetics within this chapter, explain how it is possible for blue-eyed parents with straight, blond hair to produce the following children: one with blonde hair and green eyes; one with brown hair and blue eyes; and one with dark, curly hair and brown eyes.
2. Using your knowledge of body terminology, answer the following questions:
   a. What upper-arm joint is proximal to the elbow joint?
   b. What joint(s) are distal to the ankle?
   c. What does the term *mediolateral* mean?
   d. What organs are found in the abdominal cavity?

Virtual Fieldtrips

Visit the McGraw-Hill Higher Education Medical Assisting website at www.mhhe.com/medicalassisting3 to complete the following activity:

Use the CDC website and answer the following questions:

- Click the "About the CDC" tab. What is the purpose of the CDC?
- Return to the home page, enter the topic "birth defects," and then use the quick link to genetics. Now choose the pediatric genetic FAQ, "My child was screened as a newborn for genetic conditions—why was this done?" What tests are commonly done in this screening?
- How many infants are tested yearly? How many severe disorders are found?
- What does this early screening accomplish?

Now use the A-Z index and look up Down syndrome. What is its other name? What is the only well-established risk factor for this disease? What combination of factors increases the risk of Down syndrome with younger moms?

Open the CD and complete this chapter's practice activities, play the games, listen to the key terms, and test yourself with the interactive review. E-mail, print, and/or save your results to document your proficiency.

The Integumentary System

CHAPTER OUTLINE

- Functions of the Integumentary System
- Skin Structure
- Skin Color
- Skin Lesions
- Accessory Organs
- Skin Healing
- Skin and Aging

LEARNING OUTCOMES

After completing Chapter 2, you will be able to:

- **2.1** List the functions of skin.
- **2.2** Explain the role of skin in regulating body temperature.
- **2.3** Describe the layers of skin and the characteristics of each layer.
- **2.4** Explain the factors that affect skin color.
- **2.5** Identify and describe common skin lesions.
- **2.6** List the accessory organs of skin and describe their structures and functions.
- **2.7** Explain the process of skin healing, including scar production.
- **2.8** Describe the effects of aging on skin.
- **2.9** List the different types of burns and describe their appearances and treatments.
- **2.10** Describe the causes, signs and symptoms, and treatments of various types of skin cancer.
- **2.11** Describe the causes, signs and symptoms, and treatments of common skin disorders.
- **2.12** Explain the ABCD rule and its use in evaluating melanoma.
- **2.13** Using the acronym *CAUTION,* list the seven warning signs of cancer.

KEY TERMS

alopecia
apocrine gland
arrector pili
cellulitis
cyanosis
dermatitis
dermatome
dermis
eccrine gland
eczema
epidermis
follicle
folliculitis
hemoglobin
herpes simplex
herpes zoster
hypodermis
impetigo
keratin
keratinocyte
lunula
melanin
melanocyte
nail bed
oxygenated
pediculosis
psoriasis
rosacea
scabies
sebaceous
sebum
stratum basale
stratum corneum
stratum germinativum
subcutaneous
sudoriferous

Introduction

The integumentary system consists of skin and its accessory organs. The accessory organs of skin are hair follicles, nails, and skin glands. Skin is the body's outer covering and is its largest multifunctioning organ.

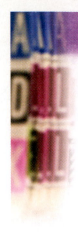
Last Independence Day, a 19-year-old man came to the urgent care facility where you work as a medical assistant. He had been in an accident involving fireworks and was diagnosed with partial-thickness (second-degree) burns to his anterior torso as well as full-thickness (third-degree) burns to his right hand.

As you read this chapter, consider the following questions:

1. Using the rule of nines, estimate the total percentage of the patient's body surface that was affected by this burn.
2. What percentage of his body was affected by partial-thickness (second-degree) burns? What percentage was affected by full-thickness (third-degree) burns?
3. What layers of skin have been affected by each of the burn types?
4. What functions of the skin are lost by each of these injuries?
5. What types of treatments does each burn require?

Functions of the Integumentary System

People are often interested in the appearance of their skin but rarely consider its functions. The integumentary system serves many purposes, including these important functions:

- Protection. As long as skin is intact and not inflamed, it is our first line of defense against the entry of bacteria and viruses. It also protects underlying structures from ultraviolet (UV) radiation and dehydration.
- Body temperature regulation. Skin plays a major role in regulating body temperature. When a person is hot, dermal blood vessels dilate, which is why a person's skin becomes pinkish. Because the dermal blood vessels are dilated, more blood than normal passes through the skin. This is beneficial because blood carries a lot of the heat in the body. When the blood gets close to the surface of the body (to skin), the heat can escape. Conversely, if a person is cold, the dermal blood vessels constrict, preventing the heat in blood from escaping.
- Vitamin D production. When exposed to sunlight, the skin produces a molecule that is turned into vitamin D. The body needs vitamin D for calcium absorption.
- Sensation. The skin is packed with sensory receptors that can detect touch, heat, cold, and pain.
- Excretion. Small amounts of waste products, such as water and salts, are lost through skin when a person perspires. This is why hydration is so important when exercising or during exposure to high temperatures, when the amount of perspiration increases and higher amounts of water and salts are lost.

Skin Structure

The skin is a complex organ that consists of two layers: the **epidermis** (top layer) and the **dermis** (middle layer). These skin layers sit on a third layer called the **subcutaneous** layer or **hypodermis** (Figure 2-1).

Epidermis

The epidermis is the most superficial layer of skin. It is made up of many layers of tightly packed cells. The epidermis can be divided into two layers: the stratum corneum and the stratum basale.

The **stratum corneum** is the most superficial layer of the epidermis. Most of the cells in this layer are dead and very flat. Because they have accumulated keratin, the cells in this layer stick together and form an impermeable layer for skin. Most bacteria, viruses, and water cannot penetrate the stratum corneum.

The **stratum basale,** also known as the **stratum germinativum,** is the deepest layer of the epidermis. The cells in this layer are constantly dividing (or germinating), and constantly push older cells up toward the stratum corneum.

The most common cell type in the epidermis is the **keratinocyte.** This cell makes and accumulates the protein keratin. **Keratin** is a durable protein that makes the epidermis waterproof and resistant to bacteria and viruses. Another cell type of the epidermis is the **melanocyte,** which makes the pigment **melanin.** Melanin is deposited throughout the layers of the epidermis. This pigment traps UV radiation from sunlight and prevents the radiation from harming structures in the underlying layers of skin.

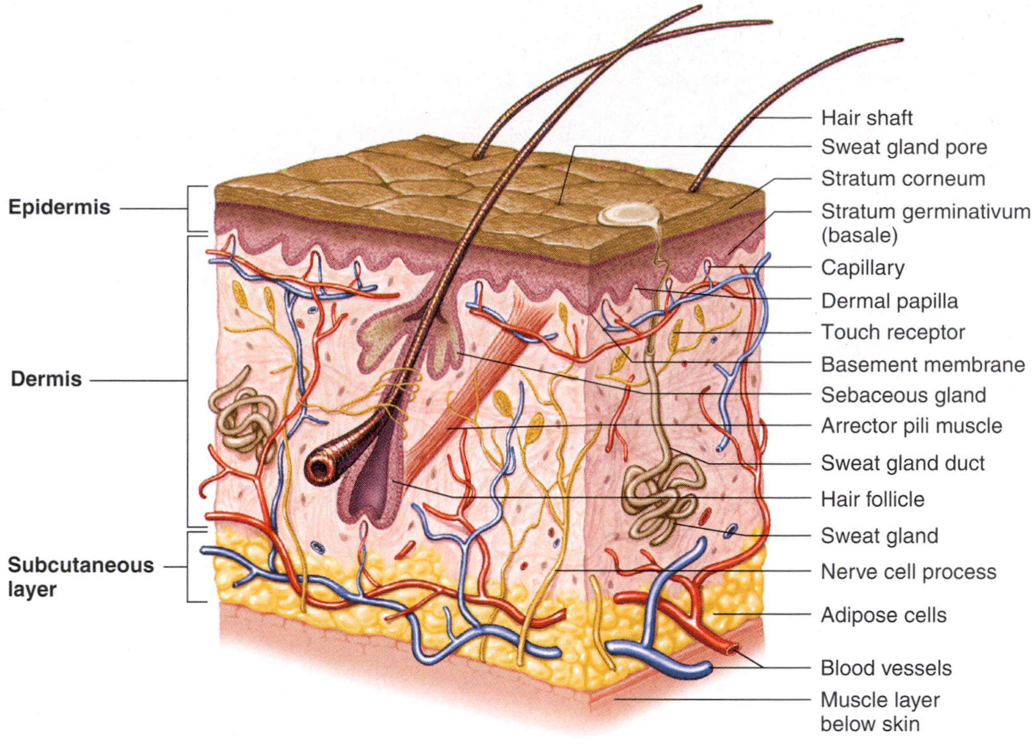

Epidermis
Dermis
Subcutaneous layer
Hair shaft
Sweat gland pore
Stratum corneum
Stratum germinativum (basale)
Capillary
Dermal papilla
Touch receptor
Basement membrane
Sebaceous gland
Arrector pili muscle
Sweat gland duct
Hair follicle
Sweat gland
Nerve cell process
Adipose cells
Blood vessels
Muscle layer below skin

Figure 2-1. Section of skin.

Dermis

The dermis is the deeper of the two skin layers and is the most complex layer containing all the major tissue types, including epithelial tissue, connective tissues, muscle tissue, and nervous tissue. The dermis contains **sudoriferous** (sweat) glands, **sebaceous** (oil) glands, hair follicles, the arrector pili muscles, collagen fibers, elastic fibers, nerve fibers, and many blood vessels. The dermis binds the epidermis to the subcutaneous tissue.

Subcutaneous Layer

The subcutaneous layer of skin, or hypodermis, is largely made of adipose and loose connective tissue. This layer also contains blood vessels and nerves. The adipose or fat tissue acts as a storage facility. It also cushions and insulates the underlying structures and organs. The amount of adipose tissue varies from body region to body region, as well as from person to person.

Skin Color

The amount of melanin in the epidermis of skin is what most determines skin color. Melanin can range in color from yellowish to brownish. The more melanin a person has in the skin, the darker the skin color. All people have about the same number of melanocytes, regardless of skin color. What varies from person to person is how active the melanocytes are in producing melanin. A person with dark skin has very active melanocytes.

As we learned in Chapter 1, our inherited characteristics come from our parents. Therefore, our skin color—meaning the activity of the melanocytes—is directly related to the genes we received from our parents. As the gene pool is varied between ethnic backgrounds, it is also varied within families, which explains the differences in skin color not only among races but also within families.

Another factor that determines skin color is the amount of **oxygenated** blood in the dermis of skin. Oxygen is carried by a pigment called **hemoglobin** in the red blood cells and oxygenation refers to the amount of oxygen dissolved in the hemoglobin of the red blood cells (RBCs). Hemoglobin that is well-oxygenated is bright red in color. Hemoglobin that is not well oxygenated is a darker red color. A person with a rich supply of oxygenated blood will have skin that is a pinkish hue. When the supply of oxygen in the blood is low, the skin looks rather pale or bluish. A bluish color of skin is called **cyanosis.**

Skin Lesions

The term *skin lesion* may be generally defined as any variation in the skin (Figure 2-2). Many of us have them; even a freckle is a lesion because it is a skin variation. Other lesions, such as ulcers and tumors, are more troublesome types of lesions. Table 2-1 lists some of the more common types of skin lesions.

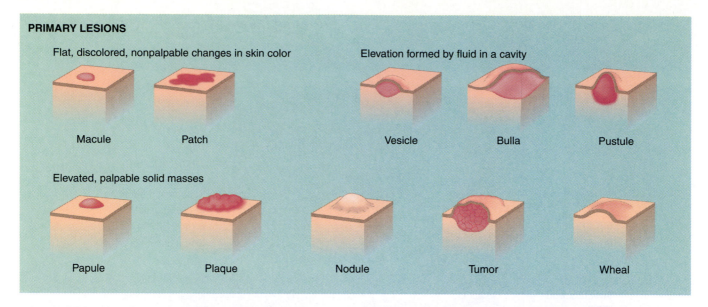

PRIMARY LESIONS

Flat, discolored, nonpalpable changes in skin color

Macule   Patch

Elevation formed by fluid in a cavity

Vesicle   Bulla   Pustule

Elevated, palpable solid masses

Papule   Plaque   Nodule   Tumor   Wheal

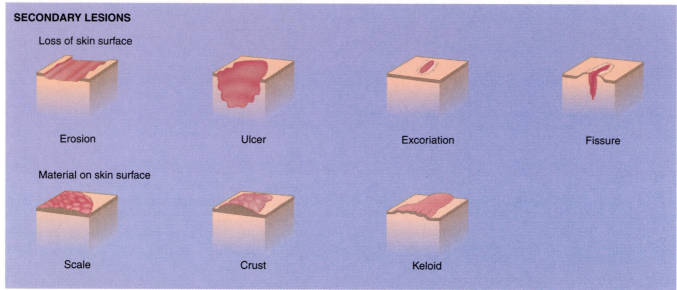

SECONDARY LESIONS

Loss of skin surface

Erosion   Ulcer   Excoriation   Fissure

Material on skin surface

Scale   Crust   Keloid

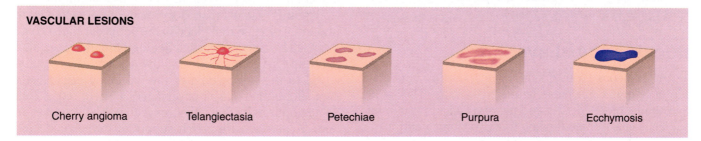

VASCULAR LESIONS

Cherry angioma   Telangiectasia   Petechiae   Purpura   Ecchymosis

Figure 2-2. Types of skin lesions.

Accessory Organs

The accessory organs of the skin include hair follicles, sebaceous (oil) glands, nails, and sudoriferous (sweat) glands. Technically, breasts are considered an accessory organ of the integumentary system, but because they are most closely associated with the female reproductive system, their makeup will be discussed in Chapter 9, *The Reproductive Systems*.

Hair Follicles

Hair **follicles** are tube-like depressions in the dermis of skin. Hair follicles are made of epithelial tissue and function

TABLE 2-1 Common Skin Lesions and Descriptions

Lesion Name	Description
Bulla	A large blister or cluster of blisters
Cicatrix	A scar, usually inside a wound or tissue
Crust	Dried blood or pus on the skin
Ecchymosis	A black and blue mark or bruise
Erosion	A shallow area of skin worn away by friction or pressure
Excoriation	A scratch; may be covered with dried blood
Fissure	A crack in the skin's surface
Keloid	An overgrowth of scar tissue
Macule	A flat skin discoloration, such as a freckle or a flat mole
Nodule	A large pimple or small node (larger than 6 cm)
Papule	An elevated mass similar to but smaller than a nodule
Petechiae	Pinpoint skin hemorrhages that result from bleeding disorders
Plaque	A small, flat scaley area of skin
Purpura	Purple-red bruises usually the result of clotting abnormalities
Pustule	An elevated (infected) lesion containing pus
Scale	Thin plaques of epithelial tissue on skin's surface
Tumor	A swelling of abnormal tissue growth
Ulcer	A wound that results from tissue loss
Vesicle	A blister
Wheal	Another term for *hive*

to generate hairs (Figure 2-3). Cells called keratinocytes make up most of the hair follicle. As hair follicles produce new keratinocytes, old ones are pushed toward the surface of skin. The old keratinocytes stick together to produce a hair. The portion of the hair embedded in skin is called the root, and the portion of the hair extending from the surface of skin is called the shaft.

Melanocytes are also found in hair follicles. They produce and distribute pigments to create hair color. A person develops gray hair when these melanocytes produce less pigment than normal.

When a hair follicle goes into a resting cycle, the hair falls out. Most of the time, the hair follicle will begin a growing cycle again and produce a new hair. However, sometimes hair follicles completely die, and **alopecia** (baldness) develops.

Arrector pili muscles are attached to most hair follicles. When a person is cold or nervous, these muscles pull on hair follicles and cause hairs to stand erect. These muscles also pull on fibers in the dermis of skin, causing goose bumps to form (see Figure 2-1).

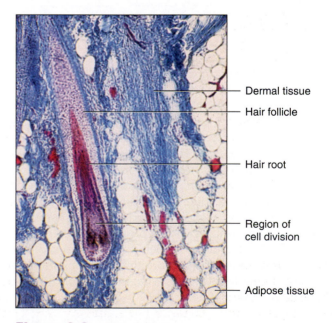

Dermal tissue

Hair follicle

Hair root

Region of cell division

Adipose tissue

Figure 2-3. Hair follicle.

Sebaceous Glands

Sebaceous glands are more commonly called oil glands. They produce an oily substance called **sebum.** Sebum is secreted onto hairs to keep them soft and pliable. Sebum eventually is deposited onto skin to keep it soft as well. Sebum also prevents bacteria from growing on skin (see Figure 2-1).

Nails

Nails function to protect the ends of the fingers and toes. They are formed by epithelial cells with hard keratin, which is more permanent than the softer keratin found in our skin. For this reason, it must be cut because it does not slough off as our skin cells do. The portion of a nail that you can see is the nail body, and the portion embedded in skin is called the nail root. The nail root contains active keratinocytes that constantly divide to produce nail growth. The white half-moon–shaped area at the base of a nail is called a **lunula.** The lunula also contains very active keratinocytes. Beneath each nail is a layer called the **nail bed.** The nail bed holds the nail down to underlying skin and provides nutrients to the nail from the blood supply under the nail bed (Figure 2-4).

Sudoriferous Glands

Most sudoriferous (sweat) glands are located in the dermis of skin. However, their ducts open onto the epidermis

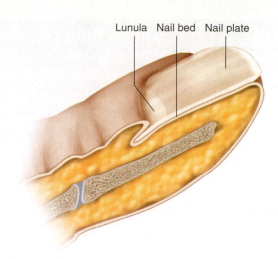

Lunula Nail bed Nail plate

Figure 2-4. Section of a nail.

of skin. There are two types of sweat glands—eccrine and apocrine.

- **Eccrine glands** are the most numerous type. They produce a watery type of sweat and are activated primarily by heat. Once sweat is deposited onto skin, it evaporates and carries heat away from the body. Eccrine sweat glands are most concentrated on the forehead, neck, and back.
- **Apocrine glands** produce a thicker type of sweat that contains more proteins than the type of sweat

Educating the Patient

Preventing Acne

Acne vulgaris, commonly known simply as acne, is an inflammatory condition of the skin follicles and sebaceous glands. It results in comedos (blackheads and whiteheads), as well as papules and pustules. They occur mainly on the face, but they can also occur on the neck, back, and chest. Acne often appears in adolescence from the surge of sex hormones that increase the amount of sebum produced by the sebaceous glands. Excess sebum and dead skin cells clog the pores where bacteria then accumulates, causing the pimples. These pimples may rupture or leak, and as the bacteria then infect the adjacent skin areas, they cause the characteristic skin inflammation. Patients may find the following instructions helpful in controlling their acne.

- Use skin-care products that are *noncomedogenic,* meaning that they will not clog pores
- Wash the face twice a day
- Keep hands away from the face
- Remove all makeup daily
- Use makeup or lotion that contains sunscreen
- Wash hair frequently because oils from hair can end up on the face
- Seek a dermatologist for severe cases; these cases may require oral antibiotics (tetracycline) or other prescription medications (retinol)

produced by eccrine sweat glands. Apocrine glands are most concentrated in areas of skin with course hair, such as the armpit and groin areas. They are primarily activated by nervousness or stress but can also be activated by heat. These are the glands responsible for producing a cold sweat. Bacteria often break down the proteins in the sweat produced by apocrine glands. As the proteins are digested, the bacteria release a foul-smelling waste product that is responsible for the smell of body odor.

Skin Healing

When skin is injured, it becomes inflamed. An inflamed area looks red because nearby blood vessels dilate. The inflamed area also swells because the dilated blood vessels "leak" and fluids seep into spaces between cells. Inflamed areas are often painful because the excess fluid activates pain receptors. However, inflammation promotes healing because more blood is delivered to the area. The extra blood carries more nutrients needed for skin repair. It also carries defensive cells to clear up the cause of inflammation.

When structures and blood vessels of the dermis are injured, a blood clot initially forms. The blood clot is eventually replaced by a scab, which is basically clotted blood and other dried tissue fluids. The scab is normally replaced by collagen fibers that bind the edges of the wound together. Collagen fibers are whitish and the major component of scars. Sometimes skin scars are replaced with new skin, but if the wound is extensive, a scar will persist. Scars cannot carry out most functions of skin, so their formation leads to the loss of certain functions.

Skin and Aging

As we all know, as the body ages, wrinkles appear. The skin loses its firmness and youthful glow. This loss occurs as a result of the loss of the elastic and collagen fibers of the dermis. It also results from the loss and shifting of the underlying adipose tissues. The dermis also becomes thinner and seems transparent in elderly patients. A decrease in circulation results in a paler skin tone.

Melanocytes decrease in number, and those still present gather in locations, causing the brown "age" or "liver" spots. This decrease in melanin also occurs in the hair, leading to gray or white hair. The hair of the scalp as well as the rest of the body becomes thinner.

Lastly, as you may have noticed with elderly friends and relatives, there is a reduced ability to tolerate temperature changes. Sudoriferous glands decrease in number and, with less perspiration, high temperatures are more difficult to adjust to. At the same time, the loss of adipose tissue and decreased circulation results in a lessened ability to retain heat, which increases sensitivity to cold.

Pathophysiology

Burns

The second leading cause of accidental death in the United States, after motor vehicle accidents, is burn injuries. There are more than 200 special burn care centers in the United States. More than 2 million burn injuries are reported each year, and more than 11,000 patients die annually from burn injuries. This year, about 1 million people will suffer a burn injury that causes a significant or permanent disability.

The extent of the affected body surface area and the severity (degree) of a burn are the most important factors in predicting the risk of death associated with burn injuries. The rule of nines is a quick way to estimate the extent of body surface area affected by burns. This method divides the body into 11 areas, each accounting for 9% of the total body surface. The genital area accounts for 1% (Figure 2-5).

Rule of Nines

The 11 body areas of the rule of nines with their percentages are as follows:

- Head — 9% (front and back, 4.5% each)
- Right arm — 9% (front and back, 4.5% each)
- Left arm — 9% (front and back, 4.5% each)
- Front of right leg — 9%
- Front of left leg — 9%
- Back of right leg — 9%
- Back of left leg — 9%
- Front of body trunk is two areas — 18% (both areas)
- Back of body trunk is two areas — 18% (both areas)
- Genital area — 1%

Total body area = 100%

continued ⟶

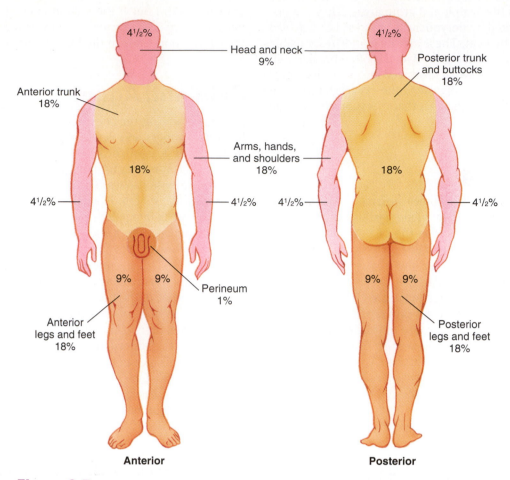

Figure 2-5. Using the rule of nines aids in estimating the extent of burns.

Burn Severity

The severity of burns indicates the thickness of the injury (Figure 2-6). The following terms are used to report burn severity:

- *Superficial (first-degree).* These burns involve only the epidermis and are characterized by pain, redness, and swelling. Unless they are extensive, they do not require medical attention and usually heal well.
- *Partial-thickness (second-degree).* These burns involve the epidermis and dermis. Pain, redness, swelling, and blisters characterize them. Medical staff should treat any partial-thickness burn that affects 1% or more of the body surface. A body surface area of 1% is about the size of a person's hand. Shock is likely to develop in partial-thickness burn injuries that affect 9% or more of the body surface. These burns can be life-threatening, depending on their extent.
- *Full-thickness.* These burns involve all layers of skin and often underlying structures such as muscles and bones. The skin often looks black or charred, which is known as eschar. Full-thickness burns always require medical attention regardless of the extent or the size of the burn area.

General Guidelines for Treating Burns

- Anything sticking to the burn should be left in place.
- Butter, lotions, or ointments should not be applied to the burn. Only ointments prescribed by a doctor or recommended by a pharmacist should be used.
- The burn should be cooled with large amounts of cool water. Ice or extremely cold water should be avoided.
- The burn should be covered with a sterile sheet or plastic bag. Burns to the face, however, should not be covered.
- Emergency medical personnel should be contacted for serious burns.
- In burns to the mouth and throat, the airways should be checked to see if there is any swelling. Burns to the head are always more serious than burns to other body parts. They almost always require emergency medical treatment.

continued ⟶

Burns (concluded)

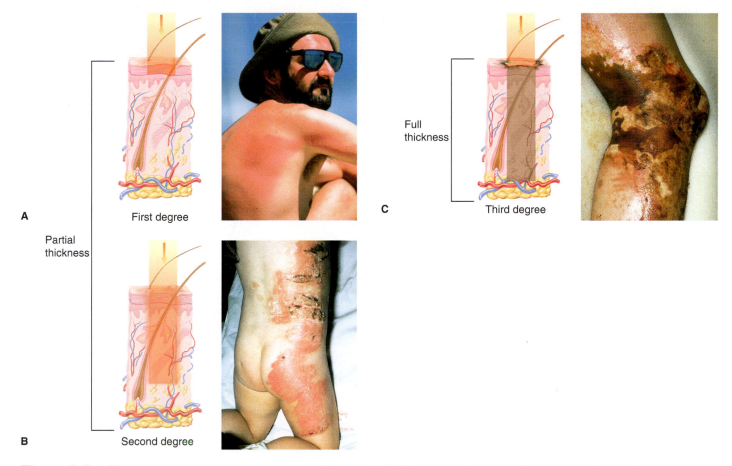

A First degree

Partial thickness

B Second degree

Full thickness

C Third degree

Figure 2-6. The degrees of burn severity include (A) superficial (first-degree) burns, (B) partial-thickness (second-degree) burns, and (C) full-thickness (third-degree) burns.

Pathophysiology

Skin Cancer and Common Skin Disorders

Skin is vulnerable to many disorders because it is the most exposed of all body organs.

Skin Cancer

Skin cancer develops from cells in the epidermis of skin. It is more common in people who have light-colored skin and who have had excessive exposure to sunlight. It can occur anywhere on the body but is most likely to appear on skin that is readily exposed to sunlight. The two most common types of skin cancer are basal cell carcinoma and squamous cell carcinoma, but the most deadly type is malignant melanoma (Figure 2-7).

Basal cell carcinoma accounts for approximately 90% of all skin cancers in the United States. Fortunately, it progresses slowly and rarely spreads to other body parts.

It is derived from cells of the stratum basale of the epidermis.

- **Signs and symptoms.** Signs and symptoms include changes on the skin and a new growth or sore on the skin that does not heal. Its appearance may be waxy, smooth, red, pale, flat, or lumpy, and it may or may not bleed.
- **Treatment.** Several forms of treatment are available:
  - Curettage and electrodessication. In curettage, a sharp instrument is used to scoop out the cancerous spot. Electrodessication uses electrical currents to minimize bleeding as well as to kill any remaining cancer cells.
  - Mohs' surgery. The cancerous spot is shaved off one layer at a time.
  - Cryosurgery. Freezing is used to kill cancer cells.
  - Laser Therapy. A beam of light destroys cancer cells.

continued →

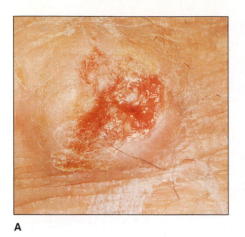
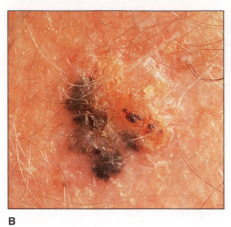
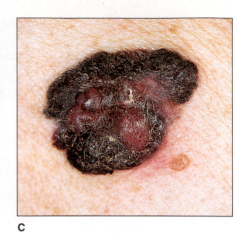

A   B   C

Figure 2-7. Types of skin cancer: (A) squamous cell carcinoma, (B) basal cell carcinoma, and (C) malignant melanoma.

Squamous cell carcinoma is much less common than basal cell carcinoma but is more likely to spread to surrounding tissues. It arises from flat cells of the epidermis and is most likely to appear on the face, lips, ears, and the backs of the hands. The signs and symptoms and the treatments for this type of cancer are the same as for basal cell carcinoma.

Malignant melanoma is the most aggressive of the skin cancers. It is also the fastest growing skin cancer, with rates increasing 5% to 7% per year with a lifetime incidence presently at 1/75. It appears to be more prevalent in females, but males, when diagnosed, seem to have a poorer prognosis. Melanoma can occur anywhere on the body but most often appears on the trunk, head, and neck in men and on the arms and legs in women. Melanoma is cancer that arises from melanocytes.

- **Signs and symptoms.** A mole that itches or bleeds is a common symptom. New moles may develop near it. It may change to have any sign of the ABCD rule:
  - *Asymmetry.* The mole should not become asymmetrical. It should look equal in size from side to side.
  - *Border.* The border of the mole should not become irregular. The edges should not blur into nearby normal tissue.
  - *Color.* The mole should be even. It should not darken or lighten or contain a mixture of colors.
  - *Diameter.* The mole should not grow larger than 6 mm, approximately the diameter of a pencil eraser.
- **Treatment.** The treatment will depend on the staging of this cancer. Available treatments include the following:
  - Surgery to remove the melanoma
  - Lymph node biopsy to determine if the cancer has spread
  - Removal of cancerous lymph nodes

- Chemotherapy for advanced stages of cancer
- Radiation therapy for advanced stages of cancer
- Immunotherapy to boost the patient's immune system

Stages of melanoma. Melanoma has five different stages, which are described from the least to the most serious:

- Stage 0. Malignancy is found only in the epidermis.
- Stage I. Malignancy has spread to the epidermis and dermis, and has a thickness of 1 to 2 millimeters.
- Stage II. Malignancy has a thickness of 2 to 4 millimeters and may have ulceration.
- Stage III. Malignancy has spread to one or more nearby lymph nodes.
- Stage IV. Malignancy has spread to other body organs or other lymph nodes far away from the original melanoma site.

Common Skin and Hair Disorders

Alopecia is a disorder that specifically targets hair. This disorder results in hair loss.

- **Causes.** Most of the time, alopecia is inherited. Other common causes include hormonal changes, chemotherapy, stress, burns, and fungal infections of the skin.
- **Signs and symptoms.** Alopecia is more commonly called baldness, but it may occur on all areas of skin including the scalp.
- **Treatment.** If a result of heredity, this disorder is not curable. Hair transplants and some drugs, such as Rogaine, may slow down hair loss. Hair loss caused by other factors, as with chemotherapy, is often temporary, but the hair may grow back a different color or texture.

continued ⟶

Skin Cancer and Common Skin Disorders *(continued)*

Cellulitis is an inflammation of connective tissues in skin and primarily occurs on the face and legs.

- **Causes.** This skin disease is caused by staphylococcal and streptococcal bacteria.
- **Signs and symptoms.** Skin appears red and tight and is often painful. The inflammation may trigger a fever.
- **Treatment.** Treatment is with oral and topical antibiotics. In serious cases, intravenous (IV) antibiotics and hospitalization may be indicated.

Dermatitis is a general term defined as inflammation of skin or a rash. It has many causes and is a sign of many types of skin disorders.

Eczema is one type of chronic dermatitis that has acute phases. Eczema often appears in childhood, but is seen equally commonly in adults.

- **Causes.** Causes of eczema are mostly unknown, but it is thought to be a type of allergy or the result of an often unknown underlying inflammatory condition. Environmental irritants, stress, diet, and medications can bring about exacerbations of this disease.
- **Signs and symptoms.** The rashes of eczema are red, scaly and itchy.
- **Treatment.** Treatments include steroids and other types of anti-inflammatory drugs. Antibiotics may be needed for any secondary infections that may develop. Avoiding known factors that trigger eczema, such as stress, are also helpful.

Folliculitis, sometimes called "swimmer's rash," is an inflammation of hair follicles.

- **Causes.** This disorder usually results from shaving or excess rubbing of skin areas. It may also be caused by bacteria and fungi, which may develop from prolonged wearing of wet swimwear or under-treated hot tubs.
- **Signs and symptoms.** Follicles become red and itchy and often look like pimples.
- **Treatment.** Treatments include regular cleansing of skin, topical antibiotics, and the use of electric razors instead of razor blades. Wearing wet swimwear for prolonged periods of time should also be avoided.

Herpes simplex types 1 and 2 are the most common types of herpes simplex.

- **Causes.** Herpes simplex types 1 and 2 are both caused by a virus. Herpes simplex type 1 causes cold sores. It is very contagious and is spread through saliva. Herpes simplex type 2, known as genital herpes, is sexually transmitted.
- **Signs and symptoms.** Herpes simplex type 1 causes painful sores on the lips, mouth, and face. Herpes simplex type 2 normally causes painful sores on genital areas.

- **Treatment.** There is no cure for herpes simplex, and its skin lesions usually recur throughout life. However, antiviral drugs such as Acyclovir prevent frequent outbreaks. Patients should also be instructed to get adequate rest and nutrition, and control stress as much as possible.

Herpes zoster is a disorder commonly known as shingles.

- **Causes.** Herpes zoster is caused by the *Varicella* virus, the same one that causes chickenpox. After a person has chickenpox, the virus becomes dormant in the spine's dorsal nerve root, but can become active again later in life to cause shingles.
- **Signs and symptoms.** Herpes zoster causes a painful blistering rash of the **dermatome,** the skin area along the pathway of the affected nerve root.
- **Treatment.** Some antiviral medications, such as Zovirax, shorten the duration of the disease, and pain medications assist with pain control. Recovery is usually complete, but recurrences of the disease do occur. Some patients do suffer from the complication known as *post-herpetic pain* syndrome, where nerve pain continues even though the rash is no longer present. It is uncertain whether the chickenpox vaccine prevents herpes zoster.

Impetigo causes the formation of oozing skin lesions that eventually crust over. It is highly contagious for those who come in contact with the lesions or the exudates from them.

- **Causes.** This disease is caused by staphylococcal and streptococcal bacteria.
- **Signs and symptoms.** The skin develops itchy, oozing lesions that eventually crust over with a distinctive honey-colored crust from the drying exudates.
- **Treatment.** This condition is treated with antibiotics. Instructing the patient to wash the lesions 2 to 3 times a day with soap and water will help remove the exudates and decrease the spread to other skin areas.

Pediculosis is more commonly known as lice and comes in three forms: head lice (*pediculosis capitis*), body lice (*pediculosis corporis*), and pubic lice (*pediculosis pubis*).

- **Causes.** All forms are caused by parasitic lice and are associated with overcrowded conditions and often with poor hygiene. Pubic lice are also spread by sexual contact.
- **Signs and symptoms.** Skin itches and can become irritated from scratching. Head lice are also identifiable by the dandruff-like nits that cannot be shaken off.
- **Treatment.** Prescription medications and shampoos are often necessary. For head lice, some patients find equal success with over-the-counter (OTC) treatments such as *Nix*.

continued ⟶

Skin Cancer and Common Skin Disorders *(concluded)*

Psoriasis is a common chronic, inflammatory skin condition.

- **Causes.** This skin disorder is most likely an inherited autoimmune disorder.
- **Signs and symptoms.** Patients with psoriasis have recurring episodes of itching and redness with outbreaks of distinctive silvery, scaly skin lesions. Some people also have joint pain with this condition.
- **Treatment.** Mild cases are treated with anti-inflammatory drugs and therapeutic ointments such as creams with vitamins A and D, hydrocortisone creams, and retinoids. Some patients also experience relief with controlled UV ray treatments. Severe cases may require hospitalization.

Ringworm is a fungal skin infection, commonly occurring in three forms: *tinea corporis* (body), *tinea capitis* (scalp), and *tinea pedis* (feet), which is commonly known as athlete's foot.

- **Causes.** All forms of ringworm are caused by fungi called dermatophytes.
- **Signs and symptoms.** Flat, circular lesions that may be dry and scaly or moist and crusty are the hallmarks of ringworm. Tinea capitis is characterized by small papules that may cause small, patchy areas of baldness.
- **Treatments.** Topical and oral antifungal agents are used to treat all forms. The spread is contained by not sharing sheets, towels, and other personal care items.

Rosacea is a skin disorder that commonly appears as facial redness, predominantly over the cheeks and nose.

- **Causes.** Rosacea results from dilation of small facial blood vessels, but the cause of this dilation is unknown. It occurs most frequently in fair-skinned people.
- **Signs and symptoms.** Redness and acne-like symptoms on the face are the most common symptoms.
- **Treatment.** Although it is not curable, rosacea is usually managed well with topical cortisone creams. In severe cases, electrolysis may be useful in destroying large or dilated blood vessels.

Scabies is a highly contagious skin condition.

- **Causes.** Scabies is caused by the itch mite that burrows beneath skin. Sometimes the burrows of the mites, which look like red pencil marks, can be seen.
- **Signs and symptoms.** Redness and severe itching, especially at night, are usually the only symptoms of scabies.
- **Treatment.** Most cases are easily treated with prescription medications such as Elamite, which is left on the skin for 6 to 10 hours and followed by a bath. Antipyretic (anti-itching) or steroid creams may control the itching. Because scabies is contagious, it is wise to treat an entire family if one member is infected.

Warts (verrucae) are harmless skin growths that can appear almost anywhere on the body surface but most commonly occur on the hands, feet, and face.

- **Causes.** These growths are caused by a virus.
- **Signs and symptoms.** Warts vary greatly in appearance; they can be smooth, flat, rough, raised, dark, small, or large.
- **Treatment.** Warts are often removed with OTC medications but can also be treated through surgery, lasers, freezing, or burning.

Educating the Patient

Cancer Warning Signs

The thought of a diagnosis of cancer is scary to everyone. Awareness of the warning signs can help patients know when to seek medical care. Always stress to patients the importance of *preventative medicine* and regular physical examinations. The American Cancer Society has put together seven cancer warning signs for adults, using the acronym *CAUTION*:

- **C** —Change in bowel or bladder habits
- **A** —A sore that will not heal
- **U** —Unusual bleeding or discharge
- **T** —Thickening or lump in the breast or elsewhere
- **I** —Indigestion or difficulty with swallowing
- **O** —Obvious change in a wart or mole
- **N** —Nagging cough or hoarseness

Summary

The integumentary system is the first line of defense for the body. The skin covers the surface of the body, protecting it from invading organisms, chemicals, UV light, and water loss. Hair, nails, and oil glands also serve as protective barriers. In addition, the skin helps regulate body temperature via body hair and sweat glands. Because the skin is so important in protecting the body, thorough understanding of lesions, including burns that disrupt this protective function, is essential for medical assistants. Diagnostic testing including allergy testing and tuberculosis screening is performed through the integumentary system, as are therapeutic procedures such as injections and intravenous infusions. Understanding this system, its layers, and the contents of those layers can help you be more effective in your role as a medical assistant.

REVIEW

CHAPTER 2

CASE STUDY QUESTIONS

Now that you have completed this chapter, review the case study at the beginning of the chapter and answer the following questions:

1. Using the rule of nines, estimate the total percentage of the patient's body surface that was affected by this burn.
2. What percentage of his body was affected by partial-thickness (second-degree) burns? What percentage was affected by full-thickness (third-degree) burns?
3. What layers of skin have been affected by each of the burn types?
4. What functions of the skin are lost by each of these injuries?
5. What types of treatments does each burn require?

Discussion Questions

1. Explain why people with darker skin tones have a lower incidence of skin cancer than those who have lighter complexions.
2. Name the two layers of the epidermis and tell how they differ.
3. Name two types of sweat glands. Where is each located and how do their secretions differ?

Critical Thinking Questions

1. What are skin lesions? Why are even simple abrasions or foot blisters possible problems for diabetics and other patients with other healing disorders?
2. With extensive full-thickness (third-degree) burns, patients may have no feeling in the burned area. How is this possible?
3. Albinos lack melanin. What body structures are affected by this? What precautions must an albino take that nonalbinos do not have to worry about?

Application Activities

1. Describe the functions of the following cell types of the epidermis:
   a. Keratinocyte
   b. Melanocyte

2. Explain the role of skin in the following functions:
   a. Protection
   b. Sensation
   c. Body temperature regulation
   d. Excretion
   e. Vitamin D synthesis
3. Describe how the following accessory organs assist in protecting the body:
   a. Nails
   b. Hair
   c. Sebaceous glands
   d. Sudoriferous glands

Virtual Fieldtrip

Visit the McGraw-Hill Higher Education Medical Assisting website at www.mhhe.com/medicalassisting3 to complete the following activity:

Use the People Living with Cancer website and search the following topics, answering questions and providing information as requested.

- In the Search box, type *Skin Cancer* and click *Go*. What month is Melanoma/Skin Cancer Detection and Prevention Month?
- Choose the topic *Skin Cancer rate up for women greater than age 40*.
  1. What two types of skin cancer are up in this age group?
  2. What activity is being blamed for this increase?
  3. What is the rate of increase for these cancers since the 1970s?
- Next, choose the topic *Teens not learning lessons from Mom's skin cancer*.
  1. If a parent has had basal or squamous cell cancer, what is increased risk to the teen?
  2. What about the increased risk if the parent has melanoma?
  3. Do these teens tend to be more careful regarding sun exposure and protecting themselves?
- Finally, choose one of the *Focus on Melanoma and Skin Cancer* links. At the bottom of the page, choose the link for the National Council on Skin Cancer Prevention. Using the *Tip* tab, choose one of the topics in the drop-down box. Write a 1- to 2-page paper on the programs available to medical assistants so that you can help your patients prevent or limit their chances of developing skin cancer.

Open the CD and complete this chapter's practice activities, play the games, listen to the key terms, and test yourself with the interactive review. E-mail, print, and/or save your results to document your proficiency.

The Skeletal System

CHAPTER OUTLINE

- Bone Structure
- Functions of Bones
- Bone Growth
- Bony Structures
- The Skull
- The Spinal Column
- The Rib Cage
- Bones of the Shoulders, Arms, and Hands
- Bones of the Hips, Legs, and Feet
- Joints

LEARNING OUTCOMES

After completing Chapter 3, you will be able to:

3.1 Describe the parts of a long bone.
3.2 List the substances that make up bone tissue.
3.3 List the functions of bones.
3.4 Identify bones by their classifications.
3.5 Describe how long bones grow.

KEY TERMS (Concluded)

hyoid	nasal	radius
ilium	occipital	sacrum
interphalangeal	ossification	scapula
intramembranous	osteoblast	scoliosis
ischium	osteoclast	sella turcica
lacunae	osteocyte	sphenoid
lamella	osteon	sternum
ligament	osteoporosis	suture
mandible	osteosarcoma	synovial
marrow	palatine	tarsal
mastoid process	parietal	temporal
maxillae	patella	tibia
medullary cavity	pectoral girdle	ulna
metacarpal	pelvic girdle	vomer
metacarpophalangeal	periosteum	xiphoid process
metatarsal	phalanges	zygomatic
metatarsophalangeal	pubis	

KEY TERMS

- acetabulum
- appendicular
- arthritis
- articular cartilage
- articulations
- atlas
- axial
- axis
- bursitis
- calcaneus
- canaliculi
- cancellous
- carpal
- carpal tunnel syndrome
- clavicle
- coccyx
- condyle
- costal
- coxal
- diaphysis
- ear ossicle
- endochondral
- endosteum
- epiphyseal disk
- epiphysis
- ethmoid
- femur
- fibula
- fontanel
- foramen magnum
- frontal
- gout
- growth plate
- hematopoiesis
- humerus

Introduction

Bones provide the body with structure and support. In this chapter you will learn about the bones of the body, their structure, and how the joints of the body work. The skeletal system is composed of 206 bones as well as joints and related connective tissues. The skeleton has two major divisions—the **axial** skeleton and the **appendicular** skeleton. The axial skeleton contains 80 bones. It includes the bones of the skull, vertebral column, and rib cage. It func-tions to support the head, neck, and trunk and protects the brain, spinal cord, and the organs in the thorax. The **hyoid** bone, which anchors the tongue, is also included in the axial skeleton. The other 126 bones of the body belong to the appendicular skeleton and include the bones of the arms, the legs, the **pectoral girdle,** and the **pelvic girdle.** The pectoral girdle attaches the arms to the axial skeleton, and the pelvic girdle attaches the legs to the axial skeleton (Figure 3-1).

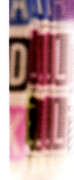

CASE STUDY

Yesterday afternoon, 13-year-old Carla was brought in by her mother. Her mother states that Carla has been increasingly complaining of a low backache. Recently, she and her mother have noted that Carla's skirts and dresses seem to hang unevenly. The physician assistant feels a brace may be needed so that Carla's condition does not worsen.

As you read this chapter, consider the following questions:

1. What could be wrong with Carla?
2. Will this patient need surgery?
3. Why will a brace be helpful?
4. What else may help Carla?

Bone Structure

Bones contain various kinds of tissues, including osseous tissue, blood vessels, and nerves. Osseous tissue can appear compact or spongy (Figure 3-2). At the microscopic level, spongy or **cancellous** bone has more spaces within it than compact bone does. These spaces are filled with red bone marrow. Compact bone looks solid; however, the following structures can be observed with a microscope:

- Osteons. **Osteons,** also known as the Haversian system, are elongated cylinders that run up and down the long axis of the bone. Each osteon has a central canal that contains blood vessels and nerves.
- Bone matrix. The matrix is the substance between bone cells. Bone cells are called **osteocytes.** Matrix is made of inorganic salts, collagen fibers, and proteins. The primary salt of the matrix is calcium phosphate. This salt makes bone matrix very hard.

- Lamella. **Lamella** are layers of bone surrounding the canals of osteons.
- Lacunae. **Lacunae** are holes in the matrix of bone that hold osteocytes.
- **Canaliculi.** These tiny canals connect lacunae to each other. They allow osteocytes to spread nutrients to each other.

All bones are made up of both compact and cancellous bone. They are classified according to their shape (Figure 3-3):

- Long bones. Long bones are located primarily in the arms and legs. Examples include the **femur** (thighbone, Figure 3-4) and the **humerus** (upper arm bone). Long bones have the following parts (Figure 3-5):
  - **Diaphysis**—the shaft of a long bone. It is tubular and consists of a thick collar of compact bone that surrounds the central medullary cavity.

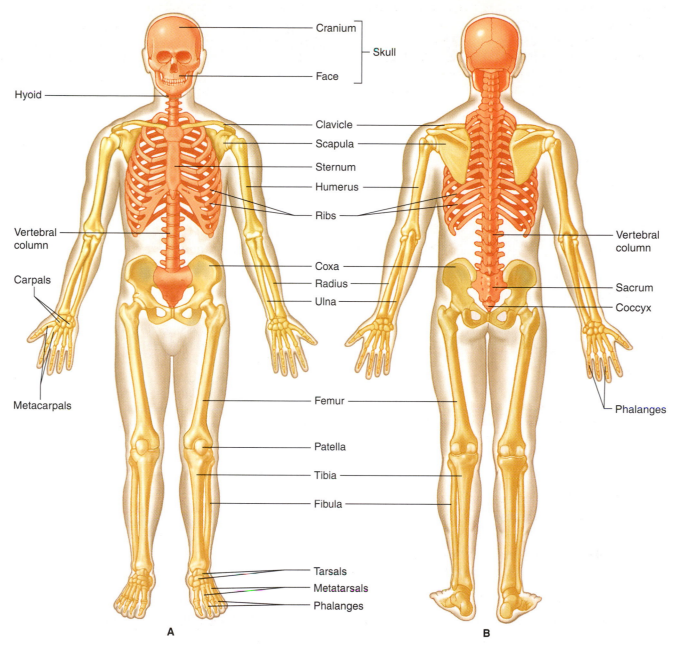

Figure 3-1. Major bones of the skeleton: (A) anterior view and (B) posterior view. The axial skeleton is shown in orange and the appendicular skeleton is shown in yellow.

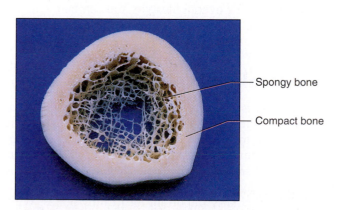

Figure 3-2. Cross-section of bone showing compact and cancellous (spongy) bone tissue.

- **Epiphysis**—the expanded end of a long bone. It consists of a thin layer of compact bone surrounding cancellous bone. Long bones have an epiphysis at both ends.
- **Articular cartilage**—the cartilage that covers the epiphyses of long bones. It functions to cushion bones and absorb stress during bone movements.
- **Medullary cavity**—the canal that runs through the center of the diaphysis. In adults it contains yellow bone **marrow,** which is mostly fat.
- **Periosteum**—a membrane that surrounds the diaphysis. It contains bone-forming cells, dense fibrous connective tissue, nerves, and blood vessels.

The Skeletal System   **37**

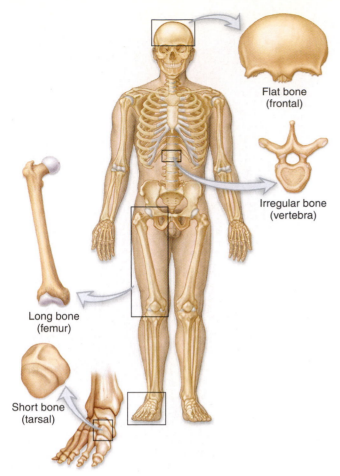

Figure 3-3. Classification of bone by shape: Four different classes of bone are recognized according to shape—long, short, flat, and irregular.

- **Endosteum**—a membrane that lines the medullary cavity and the holes of cancellous bone. It contains bone-forming cells.
- Short bones. The short bones are located in the wrists and ankles. Examples include the **carpals** (wrist bones) and some of the **tarsals** (ankle bones).
- Flat bones. Flat bones are primarily located in the skull and rib cage. Examples include the ribs and frontal bone.
- Irregular bones. Irregular bones include the vertebrae and the bones of the pelvic girdle.

Gender Differences in Skeletal Structure

You may wonder how physicians, pathologists, and instructors can tell if a skeleton is male or female. Table 3-1 outlines some of the skeletal differences between the sexes.

Functions of Bones

Bones have many functions. They give shape to body parts such as the head, legs, arms, and trunk. Bones also support and protect soft structures in the body. For example, the skull protects the brain. Bones also function in body movement because skeletal muscles attach to them, allowing us to create willful or voluntary movements.

The red marrow within cancellous bone produces new blood cells in a process called **hematopoiesis.** Bones also store calcium for the body. Every cell in the body needs calcium, so the body must have a large supply readily available.

Bone Growth

Bones grow through a process called **ossification.** There are two types of ossification: intramembranous and endochondral.

In **intramembranous** ossification, bones begin as tough, fibrous membranes. Eventually, bone-forming cells called **osteoblasts** turn the membrane to bone. Intramembranous bones are found in the skull, except for the lower jawbone.

In **endochondral** ossification, bones start out as cartilage models. Eventually, the osteoblasts form a bone collar around the diaphysis of the cartilage model. Then bone is formed in the diaphysis of the bone. This area is called the primary ossification center. Later, the epiphyses turn to bone (secondary ossification centers), and the medullary cavity and spaces in cancellous bone are formed. The cells that form holes in bone are called **osteoclasts.** As long as a bone contains some cartilage between an epiphysis and the diaphysis, it can continue to grow in length. This plate of cartilage is called an **epiphyseal disk** or **growth plate.** Once the cartilage is gone, bone growth stops. For most people, bone growth stops between the ages of 18 and 25.

Even after bone growth stops, osteoclasts and osteoblasts continually remodel bone tissue. Throughout life, osteoclasts break down bone when the body needs more calcium in the blood, and osteoblasts replace the bone when there is excess calcium in the blood.

Building Better Bones

Many factors influence bone health, including diet, exercise, and a person's overall lifestyle. You can help patients improve or maintain their bone health by teaching them about behaviors that will support bone health.

Bone-Healthy Diet

Good nutrition is essential for proper bone growth during childhood and the teen years. It is equally important in adulthood in order to maintain healthy bones. Bone-building nutrients are found in dairy products, broccoli, kale, spinach, salmon, sardines, egg yolks, whole grains, and fruits—especially bananas and oranges. Calcium and vitamin D are particularly important for healthy bones. Without vitamin D, the bloodstream cannot absorb calcium from the digestive tract. Without calcium, bone tissue will

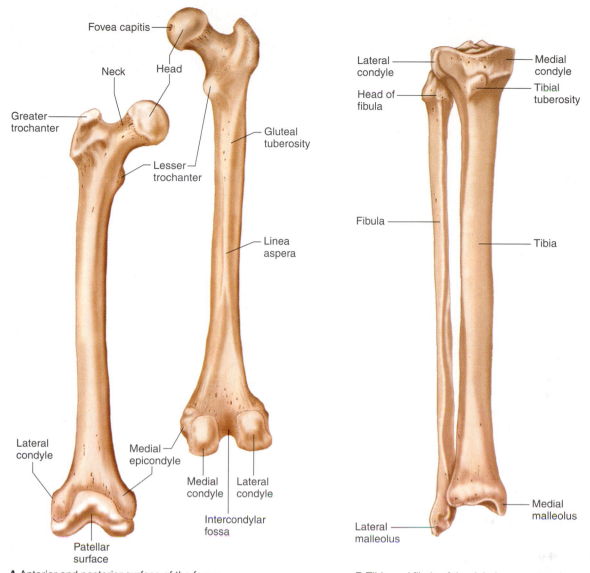

A Anterior and posterior surface of the femur.

B Tibia and fibula of the right leg, anterior view.

Figure 3-4. Bone structures: (A) bone structures of the femur and (B) bone structures of the tibia and fibula.

slowly wear away. Supplements can always be taken if a person's diet does not include adequate amounts of calcium and vitamin D.

Bone-Healthy Exercises

Weight-bearing and strength-training exercises are best for bone health. When your muscles contract, they pull on your bones. This tension stimulates bones to thicken and strengthen. Lifting weights is an effective way to increase the tension on bones. Other activities such as jogging, walking briskly, or playing a sport regularly will also stimulate bones to increase in density.

Bone-Healthy Lifestyle

A person with a bone-healthy lifestyle avoids smoking and alcohol. Smoking rids the body of calcium, which is

necessary for bone growth. Alcohol prevents calcium absorption in the digestive tract. People who smoke are almost twice as likely to develop osteoporosis as nonsmokers.

Bone Tests

Bone-density tests and bone scans are currently the most useful tools to determine bone health. Bone-density tests are painless procedures used to determine the density of a person's bones. Because osteoporosis shows no symptoms in early stages, these tests are important to have done when your doctor recommends them. Bone scans help diagnose the causes of bone pain, arthritis, bone infections, and bone cancers. These scans use radioactive dyes that are injected into the patient and that concentrate in bone tissue.

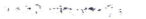

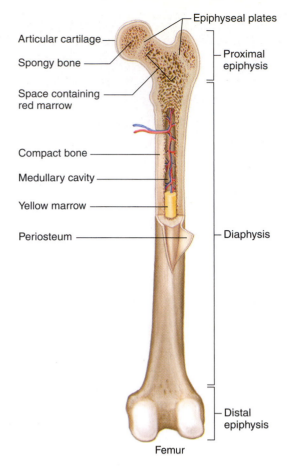

Figure 3-5. Parts of a long bone.

Bony Structures

The skeletal bones act as the rigid foundation of our bodies. By design, they are not perfectly smooth or perfectly rounded. For muscle and ligament attachment, there are projections and processes. For bones to come together at joints or **articulations,** there are depressions and hollows. In addition, blood vessels and nerves need openings within bones for entrances and exits. Each of these structures has a specific name and design. Table 3-2 lists some of these common structures and directs you to the appropriate figures throughout this chapter.

The Skull

Skull bones are divided into two types: cranial and facial bones. Cranial bones form the top, sides, and back of the skull (Figure 3-6). Facial bones form the face (Figure 3-7). The skull bones of an infant are not completely formed. The "soft spots" felt on an infant's skull are actually **fontanels,** which are tough membranes that connect the incompletely developed bones. These structures allow the infant's skull to be somewhat moldable to assist with delivery through the birth canal. As the fontanels close, the sutures of the skull are formed.

The major cranial bones are the following:

- The **frontal** bone forms the anterior portion of the cranium. It is also called the forehead bone.
- **Parietal** bones form most of the top and sides of the skull.
- The **occipital** bone forms the back of the skull. The large hole at the base of the occipital bone is called the **foramen magnum.** It allows the spinal cord to connect to the brain. Two bumps called occipital **condyles** are on either side of the foramen magnum. They sit on top of the first vertebra. When you nod your head, your occipital condyles are rocking back and forth on the first vertebra of the spinal column.
- Two **temporal** bones form the lower sides of the skull.
- A canal called the external auditory meatus runs through each temporal bone. This canal is commonly called the ear canal. A large bump called the **mastoid**

TABLE 3-1	Differences Between the Male and Female Skeletons
Part	**Differences**
Skull	Male skull is larger and heavier, with more conspicuous muscular attachments. Male forehead is shorter, facial area is less round, jaw is larger, and mastoid processes are more prominent than those of a female.
Pelvis	Male pelvic bones are heavier and thicker, and have more obvious muscular attachments. The obturator foramina and the acetabula are larger and closer together than those of a female.
Pelvic cavity	Male pelvic cavity is narrower in all diameters, and is longer, less roomy, and more funnel-shaped. The distances between the ischial spines and between the ischial tuberosities are less than in a female.
Sacrum	Male sacrum is narrower, sacral promontory projects forward to a greater degree, and sacral curvature is bent less sharply posteriorly than in a female.
Coccyx	Male coccyx is less movable than that of a female.

TABLE 3-2   Terms Used to Describe Skeletal Structures

Term	Definition	Examples
Condyle	A rounded process that usually articulates with another bone	Medial and lateral condyles of the femur (refer to Figure 3-4A)
Crest	A narrow, ridge-like projection	Iliac crest of the ilium (refer to Figure 3-11)
Epicondyle	A projection situated above a condyle	Medial epicondyle of the femur (refer to Figure 3-4A)
Foramen	An opening through a bone that is usually a passageway for blood vessels, nerves, or ligaments	Mental foramen of the mandible (refer to Figure 3-7)
Fossa	A relatively deep pit or depression	Olecrannon fossa of the humerus (refer to Figure 3-10D)
Head	An enlargement on the end of a bone	Head of the femur (refer to Figure 3-4A)
Process	A prominent projection on a bone	Mastoid process of the temporal bone (refer to Figure 3-6)
Suture	An interlocking line of union between bones	Lambdoidal suture between the occipital and parietal bones (refer to Figure 3-6)
Trochanter	A relatively large process	Greater trochanter of the femur (refer to Figure 3-4A)
Tubercle	A small, knoblike process	Greater tubercle of the humerus (refer to Figure 3-10B)
Tuberosity	A knoblike process usually larger than a tubercle	Tibial tuberosity of the tibia (refer to Figure 3-4B)

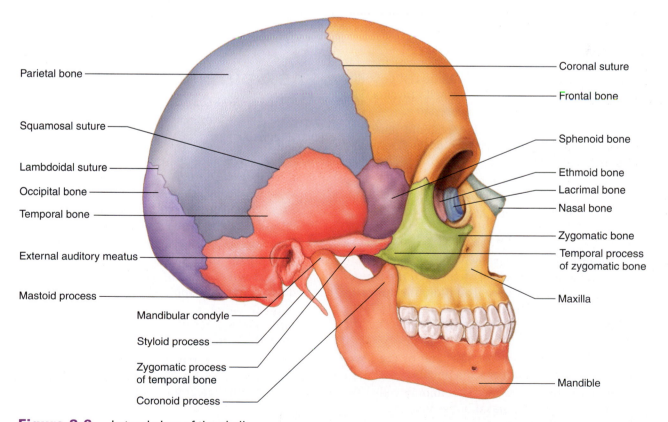

Figure 3-6. Lateral view of the skull.

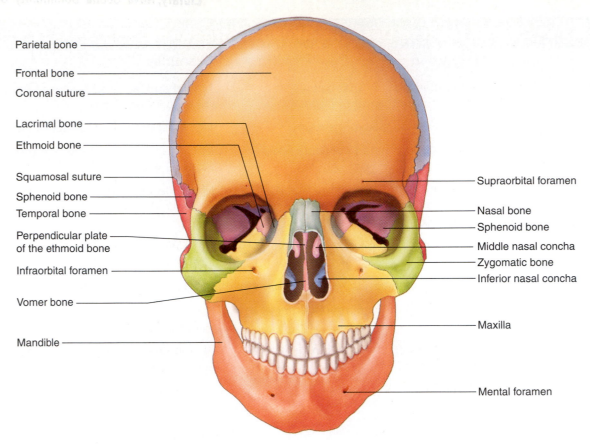

Parietal bone
Frontal bone
Coronal suture
Lacrimal bone
Ethmoid bone
Squamosal suture
Sphenoid bone
Temporal bone
Perpendicular plate of the ethmoid bone
Infraorbital foramen
Vomer bone
Mandible

Supraorbital foramen
Nasal bone
Sphenoid bone
Middle nasal concha
Zygomatic bone
Inferior nasal concha
Maxilla
Mental foramen

Figure 3-7. Anterior view of the skull.

process is located on each temporal bone just behind each ear. Mastoid processes are where major neck muscles attach to your skull.

- A **sphenoid** bone forms part of the floor of the cranium. It is shaped like a butterfly. In the center of this bone is a deep depression called the **sella turcica.** The pituitary gland sits in this deep depression.
- **Ethmoid** bones are between the sphenoid bone and the nasal bones. They also form part of the floor of the cranium.
- **Ear ossicles** are the smallest bones of the body. They are the malleus, incus, and stapes and are in the middle ear cavities of the temporal bones.

The following are major facial bones:

- The **mandible** is the lower jawbone and is the only moveable bone in the skull. It attaches to the temporal bone in front of the external auditory meatus in an area known as the temporal mandibular joint (TMJ). The mandible anchors the lower teeth and forms the chin.
- The **maxillae** form the upper jawbone of the facial skeleton, to which the upper teeth anchor.
- The **zygomatic** bones are more commonly called the cheekbones. Several thin **nasal** bones fuse together to form the bridge of the nose.

- **Palatine** bones form the hard palate, which is the roof of the mouth.
- The **vomer** is a thin bone that divides the nasal cavity.

The Spinal Column

The spinal column consists of 7 cervical vertebrae, 12 thoracic vertebrae, 5 lumbar vertebrae, a sacrum, and a coccyx (Figure 3-8):

- Cervical vertebrae, which are located in the neck, are the smallest and lightest vertebrae. The first cervical vertebra is called the **atlas** and the second is called the **axis.** When you turn your head from side to side, your atlas is pivoting around your axis.
- Thoracic vertebrae are the posterior attachment for the 12 pairs of ribs. They have long, sharp, spinous processes that you can feel when you run your finger down someone's spine.
- Lumbar vertebrae are very sturdy structures. They form the small of the back and bear the most weight of all the vertebrae.
- The **sacrum** is a triangular-shaped bone that consists of five fused vertebrae. The **coccyx** is a small, triangular-shaped bone made up of three to five fused vertebrae and is considered unnecessary. It is more commonly called the tailbone.

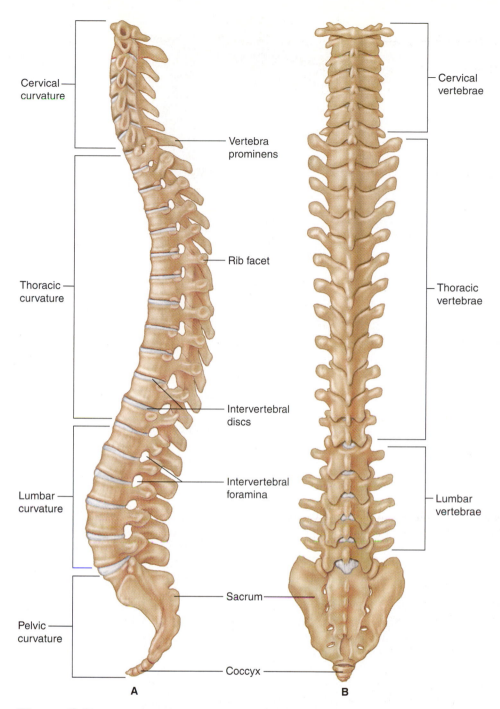

Cervical curvature

Vertebra prominens

Rib facet

Thoracic curvature

Intervertebral discs

Intervertebral foramina

Lumbar curvature

Sacrum

Pelvic curvature

Coccyx

Cervical vertebrae

Thoracic vertebrae

Lumbar vertebrae

A

B

Figure 3-8. Vertebral column: (A) lateral view and (B) posterior view.

The Rib Cage

The rib cage is made of 12 pairs of ribs and the **sternum** (Figure 3-9). The sternum forms the front, middle portion of the rib cage. It is often called the breastplate. The cartilaginous tip of the sternum is known as the **xiphoid process.** The sternum joins with the clavicles and most ribs. All 12 pairs of ribs are attached posteriorly to thoracic vertebrae. The ribs themselves are classified in three groups based on their anterior attachment:

- True. The first seven pairs of ribs are true ribs. They attach directly to the sternum through pieces of cartilage called **costal** cartilage.
- False. Rib pairs 8, 9, and 10 are called false ribs. They do not attach directly to the sternum by individual cartilage, but instead attach to the costal cartilage of rib pair number 7.
- Floating. Rib pairs 11 and 12 are called floating ribs because they do not attach anteriorly to the sternum or to any other structure.

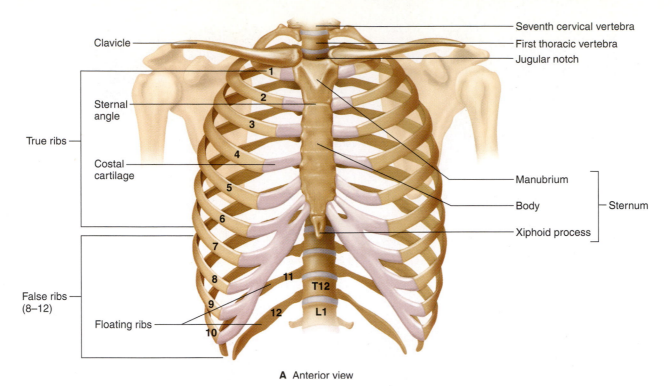

A Anterior view

Figure 3-9. Thoracic rib cage showing pectoral girdle attachment of upper extremities.

Bones of the Shoulders, Arms, and Hands

The bones of the shoulders are called the pectoral girdle and include the clavicles and the scapulae (Figure 3-10). They function to attach the arms to the axial skeleton.

- The **clavicles** are commonly known as the collarbones. They are slender in shape and each joins with the sternum and a scapula.
- **Scapulae** are thin, triangular-shaped flat bones. They are also called shoulder blades and are located on the dorsal surface of the rib cage. Each scapula joins with the head of a humerus and a clavicle.

The upper limb, or arm, bones include the humerus, radius, and ulna:

- The humerus is located in the upper part of the arm. Its proximal end joins with the scapula, and its distal end attaches at the radius and the ulna.
- The **radius** is the lateral bone of the forearm. It is on the same side of the arm as your thumb. Proximally, it joins with the humerus and the ulna, and distally with the carpal (wrist) bones.
- The **ulna** is the medial bone of the lower arm. The proximal end of the ulna joins with the humerus to form the elbow joint. Distally, it also joins with the radius and some of the carpal bones of the wrist.

The bones of the hand include carpals, metacarpals, and phalanges:

- Carpals are wrist bones. Each wrist contains eight marble-sized carpal bones.

- **Metacarpals** form the palms of the hands. Each hand has five metacarpals.
- **Phalanges** are the bones of the fingers. There are 14 phalanges in each hand—three for each finger and two per thumb.
- The joints between the phalangeal bones are the proximal and distal **interphalangeal** (PIP and DIP) joints.
- The joints that join the phalanges to the metacarpals are called the **metacarpophalangeal** (MCP) joints. You probably know these joints as the knuckles.

Refer to Figure 3-10 for the bones of the shoulders, arms, and hands.

Bones of the Hips, Legs, and Feet

The hipbones are also called **coxal** bones. They attach the legs to the axial skeleton. They also protect pelvic organs. Each coxal bone has three parts: the ilium, the ischium, and the pubis.

- The **ilium** is the most superior part of a coxal bone. When you put your hands on your hips, you are touching the ilium. The hip projection or ridge is the iliac crest.
- The **ischium** forms the lower part of a coxal bone and the pubis forms the front.
- The **pubis** bones of each coxal bone join together to form the pubic symphysis, which is also referred to as the pelvic girdle (Figure 3-11).

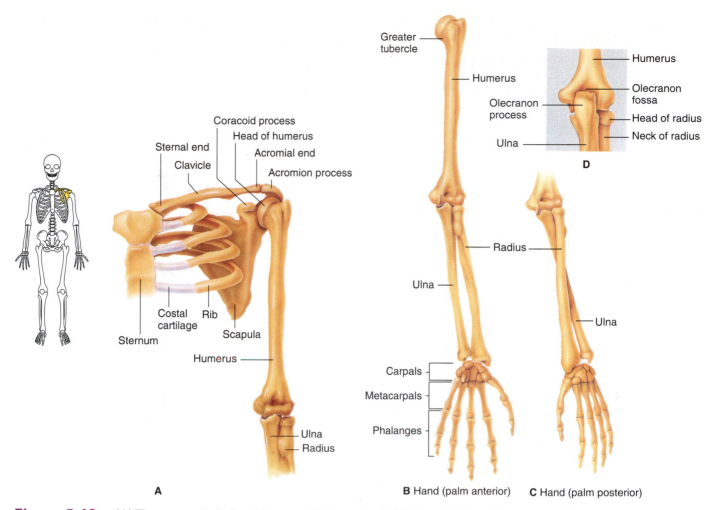

Figure 3-10.   (A) The pectoral girdle with upper limb attached. (B) Frontal view of upper limb (palm anterior). (C) Frontal view of upper limb (palm posterior). (D) Posterior view of right elbow.

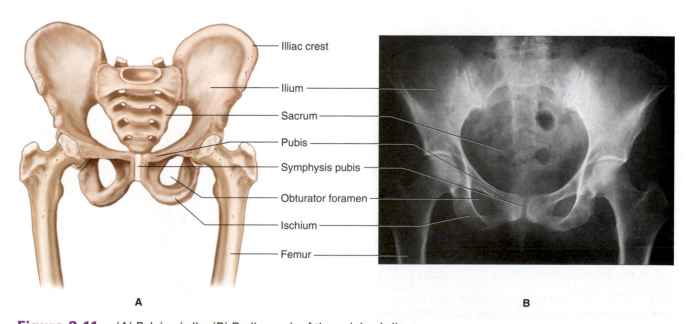

Figure 3-11.   (A) Pelvic girdle. (B) Radiograph of the pelvic girdle.

The bones of the lower limb, or leg, include the femur, the patella, the tibia, and the fibula:

- The femur is the thigh bone and the largest bone in the body. Its proximal end joins with the hipbone at the **acetabulum,** more commonly known as the hip socket, and is held in place there by ligaments and muscles.
- The distal end of the femur attaches to the tibia and the **patella** (kneecap).
- The **tibia** is the medial bone of the lower leg. It is commonly called the shinbone. Its proximal end joins with the femur and fibula, and distally to the ankle bones.
- The **fibula** is the lateral bone of the lower leg. It is much thinner than the tibia. It joins with the ankle bones at its distal end. Figure 3-12 illustrates the bones of the lower extremity.

The bones of the foot include the tarsals, the metatarsals, and the phalanges:

- The tarsal bones form the back of the foot. The **calcaneus,** or heel bone, is the largest tarsal bone. There are seven tarsal bones per foot.
- **Metatarsals** are bones that form the front of the foot. There are five metatarsals per foot.
- The bones of the toes are called phalanges. Each foot contains 14—two for each big toe and three in all the other toes. The joints between these "lower" phalanges are also interphalangeal joints just like those of the fingers.
- The joints that join the toes to the foot are called **metatarsophalangeal** (MTP) joints.

Joints

Joints are the junctions between bones. Based on their structure, joints can be classified as fibrous, cartilaginous, or synovial.

- The bones of fibrous joints are connected together with short fibers. Therefore, the bones of this type of joint do not normally move against each other. Most fibrous joints are found between cranial bones and facial bones. Fibrous joints in the skull are called **sutures.**
- The bones of cartilaginous joints are connected together with a disc of cartilage. This type of joint is slightly moveable. The joints between vertebrae are cartilaginous joints.
- The bones of **synovial** joints are covered with hyaline cartilage and are held together by a fibrous joint capsule (Figure 3-13). The joint capsule is lined with a synovial membrane. The membrane secretes a slippery fluid called synovial fluid, which allows the bones to move easily against each other. Bones are also held together through tough, cord-like structures called **ligaments.** Synovial joints are freely moveable. Examples of synovial joints are the elbows, knees, shoulders, and knuckles.

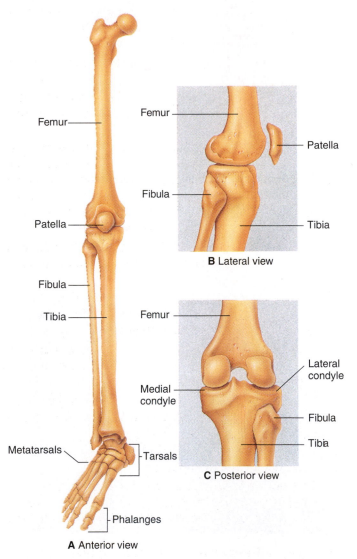

Femur

Femur

Patella

Fibula

Patella

Tibia

B Lateral view

Fibula

Tibia

Femur

Lateral condyle

Medial condyle

Fibula

Tibia

C Posterior view

Metatarsals

Tarsals

Phalanges

A Anterior view

Figure 3-12. (A) Anterior view of the right lower limb. (B) Lateral view of the right knee. (C) Posterior view of the right knee.

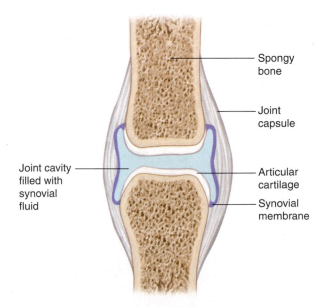

Spongy bone

Joint capsule

Joint cavity filled with synovial fluid

Articular cartilage

Synovial membrane

Figure 3-13. Structure of a synovial joint.

Pathophysiology

Common Diseases and Disorders of the Skeletal System

Arthritis is a general term meaning joint inflammation. Although there are more than 100 types of arthritis, we will discuss the two most common types.

Osteoarthritis, which is also known as degenerative joint disease (DJD), primarily affects the weight-bearing joints of the hips and knees. The cartilage between the bones and the bones themselves begin to break down.

- **Causes.** Research points to inflammatory processes or metabolic disorders as the etiology of DJD.
- **Signs and symptoms.** These include joint stiffness, and aching and pain, especially with weather changes. There is often fluid around the joint and grating noises with joint movement.
- **Treatment.** Anti-inflammatory drugs, including aspirin and NSAIDS (nonsteroidal anti-inflammatory drugs) such as naproxen and Feldene, may be used. Intra-articular steroid injections may be tried for severe cases. In some cases, a series of injections of medications containing hyaluronic acid are used when other treatments do not work. These injections serve as joint fluid replacement. Some success has been found with transplanting harvested cartilage cells from the patient's healthy knee cartilage, which are then grown in the lab and reinjected into the patient's diseased joint. Surgical scraping of the joint may also be done to remove deteriorated bone fragments. As a last resort, joint replacement may be recommended.

Rheumatoid arthritis (RA) is a chronic systemic inflammatory disease that attacks the smaller joints, typically of the hands and feet, as well as the surrounding tissues of those joints. There may be flares or attacks of pain and inflammation followed by periods of remission. RA is much more common in women than in men.

- **Causes.** RA is believed to be autoimmune in nature, triggering the joint inflammation.
- **Signs and symptoms.** In this disease, the synovial membrane is attacked, causing edema and congestion. Tissue becomes granular and thick, eventually destroying the joint capsule and bone. Scar tissue forms, bones atrophy, and visible deformities become apparent due to the bone malalignment and immobility. Patients also have moderate to severe pain in the affected joints.
- **Treatment.** Treatment includes anti-inflammatory drugs, exercise, heat or cold treatments, and cortisone injections. Researchers are working with genetic techniques to block the immune system reaction. Low-impact aerobic exercise may be helpful and some patients find warm water exercises beneficial as well.

Bursitis is inflammation of a bursa, which is a fluid-filled sac that cushions tendons. It occurs most commonly in the elbow, knee, shoulder, and hip.

- **Causes.** Overuse of, and trauma to, joints are the most common causes of this condition. Bacterial infections can also cause bursitis.
- **Signs and symptoms.** Signs and symptoms include joint pain and swelling as well as tenderness in the structures surrounding the joint.
- **Treatment.** The most common treatments are bed rest, pain medications, steroid injections, aspiration of excess fluid from the bursa, and antibiotics.

Carpal tunnel syndrome occurs when the median nerve in the wrist is excessively compressed. Typists, assembly-line workers, painters, and people who play sports such as racquetball are most likely to develop carpal tunnel syndrome.

- **Causes.** Overuse of the wrist is a common cause of this syndrome.
- **Signs and symptoms.** Weakness and numbness in the hand, and pain in the wrist, hand, or elbow are common symptoms.
- **Treatment.** This condition can be treated with wrist splints, pain medications, and steroid injections and by having the patient change work habits to better position and support the wrists. If these treatments do not improve the patient's condition, surgery to reduce the pressure on the nerves may be needed.

Ewing's family of tumors (EFT) is a group of tumors that affect different tissue types. However, the tumors primarily affect bone.

- **Causes.** Causes of EFT are not clear, but it most often affects Caucasians, the long bones of the body, and people between the ages of 10 and 20.
- **Signs and symptoms.** Fever, pain in the tumor location, fractures, and bruises in the tumor location are the primary symptoms.
- **Treatment.** Treatment options include surgery, chemotherapy, radiation therapy, a bone marrow transplant, or a stem cell transplant.

Gout, also known as gouty arthritis, is a type of arthritis that usually occurs more frequently with age.

- **Causes.** Gout is caused by deposits of uric acid crystals in the joints. People with gout cannot break down uric acid properly and remove it from their bloodstream.
- **Signs and symptoms.** Symptoms include sudden or chronic joint pain, commonly in the great toe, joint swelling and stiffness, and fever.

continued ⟶

Common Diseases and Disorders of the Skeletal System *(continued)*

- **Treatment.** The most common treatments are pain medications and changes to the patient's diet. Patients should eliminate from their diet certain foods that cause the formation of uric acid (meats, fish, beer, or wine).

Kyphosis is an abnormal curvature of the spine, most often at the thoracic level. This condition is often referred to as "humpback."

- **Causes.** Adolescent kyphosis may result from growth retardation or improper development of the epiphyses as a result of rapid growth. Poor posture may exacerbate this condition. The adult form of kyphosis is most often the result of aging and degenerative disc disease of the intervertebral discs and actual vertebral fracture from underlying osteoporosis.
- **Signs and symptoms.** In adolescent kyphosis, there may be no symptoms other than the visible back curvature. There may be mild pain, tiredness, or tenderness or stiffness of the thoracic spine. In adult kyphosis, the upper back is rounded and there may be pain, back weakness, and fatigue.
- **Treatment.** Childhood kyphosis can be treated with exercise, a firm mattress, and a back brace if needed until growth is completed to keep the spine in alignment. Spinal fusion or grafting may be needed in rare cases of neurological damage or disabling pain. Harrington rods may also be used to keep the vertebrae aligned.

Lordosis is an exaggerated inward (convex) curvature of the lumbar spine. Sometimes this condition is called swayback.

- **Cause.** Wearing high heels is a frequent cause. The positioning of the feet with the elevated heel height causes an inward positioning of the back as a counterbalancing measure.
- **Signs and symptoms.** The main sign is visual inward curvature of the lower back. There may be mild pain with this exaggerated curvature.
- **Treatment.** Prevention is best by avoiding excessive heel height. Once the condition begins, exercise and appropriate footwear will at least keep the condition stable.

Osteogenesis imperfecta is more commonly called brittle-bone disease. People with this disease have decreased amounts of collagen in their bones, which leads to very fragile bones. There are four types of this disease: type 1 is the most common, and type 2 is the most severe.

- **Causes.** The disorder is hereditary and very often runs in families.
- **Signs and symptoms.** Signs and symptoms include fractures (all types), blue sclera (type 1), dental problems (types 1 and 4), hearing loss (type 1), a triangular face (type 1), abnormal spinal curves (types 1 and 4), very small stature (types 2 and 3), a small chest (type 2), a barrel-shaped chest (type 3), fractures at birth (type 3), loose joints (types 3 and 4), and small muscles (type 3).
- **Treatment.** Because there are many symptoms of this disease, the list of treatments is extensive and includes the following: fracture repair, surgery to strengthen bones by inserting metal rods into them, dental procedures, physical therapy, braces to prevent bone deformities, wheelchairs and other supportive aids, medications, and counseling. Other surgeries may be required to treat lung and heart problems that sometimes occur with this disease.

Osteoporosis is a condition in which bones thin (become more porous) over time. It is a very common disorder in the United States and affects women more than men and Caucasians more than any other race. This condition occurs because of hypocalcemia, so bone is broken down to release calcium and is not replaced in sufficient amounts, so bone density decreases.

- **Causes.** The causes include hormone deficiencies (estrogen in women and testosterone in men), a sedentary lifestyle, a lack of calcium and vitamin D in the diet, bone cancers, corticosteroid excess (usually as a result of endocrine diseases), smoking, excess alcohol consumption, and the use of steroids.
- **Signs and symptoms.** There are usually no symptoms in the early stages of this disease. Patients at high risk, especially those with a family history of osteoporosis, should request bone densitometry studies to catch the disease before symptoms begin. Patients in later stages of the disease may experience fractures (usually of the spine, wrists, or hips), back and neck pain, a loss of height over time, and an abnormal curving of the spine (kyphosis).
- **Treatment.** The most common treatments include medications to prevent bone loss and relieve bone pain, hormone replacement therapy, lifestyle changes to prevent bone loss (including regular exercise and diets or supplements that include calcium, phosphorous, and vitamin D), moderation in use of alcohol, and stopping smoking.

Osteosarcoma is a type of bone cancer that originates from osteoblasts, the cells that make bony tissue. It occurs most often in children, teens, and young adults and more often in males than females. Usually this type of cancer affects bones of the legs.

- **Causes.** The etiology of this type of cancer is unclear.
- **Signs and symptoms.** Primary symptoms include pain in affected bones (usually the legs), swelling around affected bones, and an increase in pain with movement of the affected bones.

continued ⟶

Common Diseases and Disorders of the Skeletal System *(concluded)*

- **Treatment.** Treatments include surgery, chemotherapy, and radiation therapy. Amputation of the affected limb, followed by a prosthesis fitting, may be needed in some cases to prevent metastasis.

Paget's disease causes bones to enlarge and become deformed and weak. It usually affects people older than the age of 40.

- **Causes.** This disease may be caused by a virus or various hereditary factors.
- **Signs and symptoms.** Bone pain, deformed bones, and fractures are common symptoms. Patients may experience headaches and hearing loss if the disease affects skull bones.
- **Treatment.** Treatments include surgery to remodel bones, hip replacements, medications to prevent bone weakening, and physical therapy.

Scoliosis is an abnormal, S-shaped curvature of the thoracic or lumbar spine.

- **Causes.** This disorder can develop prenatally when vertebrae do not fuse together. It can also result from diseases that cause weakness of the muscles that hold vertebrae together. Other causes of scoliosis are unknown but they may be genetic.
- **Signs and symptoms.** A patient with scoliosis usually has a spine that looks bent to one side, with one shoulder or hip appearing to be higher than the other. Patients often experience back pain.
- **Treatment.** Treatment includes different types of back braces, surgery to correct spinal curves, and physical therapy to strengthen the muscles of the back and abdomen.

Summary

The bones of the skeletal system are divided into two major divisions: the axial and the appendicular skeletons. Bone growth takes place through a process known as ossification and the "soft spots" within an infant's skull to allow for molding of the skull during birth and growth in infancy are called fontanels. In addition to bones, the skeletal system consists of cartilage, tendons, and ligaments. The skeletal system provides support for the body, protects internal organs, serves as attachments for muscles to produce movement, stores minerals such as calcium, and produces new blood cells in a process called hematopoiesis. Bones are joined to other bones by three different types of joints, which allow various amounts of movement. Bones are used as landmarks for procedures such as injections, EKGs, and x-rays. It is important for medical assistants to have knowledge of the skeletal system when it is healthy as well as during illness in order to effectively perform their duties that relate to this body system.

REVIEW

CHAPTER 3

CASE STUDY QUESTIONS

Now that you have completed this chapter, review the case study at the beginning of the chapter and answer the following questions:

1. What could be wrong with Carla?
2. Will this patient need surgery?
3. Why will a brace be helpful?
4. What else may help Carla?

Discussion Questions

1. List and describe the functions of bone.
2. Describe how joints are classified. Give examples of each classification.
3. Describe the basic differences in bone structure between the male and female skeleton.
4. Explain the basic differences between rheumatoid arthritis and osteoarthritis.

Critical Thinking Questions

1. Your 50-year-old female patient complains that she is "shrinking." After comparing her present height to that of 3 years ago, you find she has indeed "lost" almost 1 inch. What is the likely diagnosis? What assistance can you offer this patient?
2. If a physician needed a red bone marrow sample from a patient, from where is he likely to get the sample?
3. Tarsal bones are often called ankle bones. Why is this term not entirely correct?

Application Activities

1. State whether each of the following is a bone of the axial or appendicular skeleton and give its location.
   a. Humerus
   b. Femur
   c. Clavicle
   d. Parietal bone
   e. Zygomatic bones
   f. Metacarpals
2. Name the bone that forms the following:
   a. Forehead
   b. Chin
   c. Palms of the hands
   d. Fingers
   e. Hip
   f. Cheekbone
3. Name a location of each of the following bone structures:
   a. Foramen
   b. Head
   c. Fossa
   d. Crest
   e. Process

Virtual Fieldtrip

Visit the McGraw-Hill Higher Education Medical Assisting Website at www.mhhe.com/medicalassisting3 to complete the following activity:

Choose either bone cancer or one of the bone disorders listed to the left of the home page at the website chosen. Answer the following questions related to your topic:

- Is there a known cause for the disease and, if so, what is it?
- What are the risk factors for this condition?
- What are some of the treatment options?
- What is the patient's prognosis?

 Open the CD and complete this chapter's practice activities, play the games, listen to the key terms, and test yourself with the interactive review. E-mail, print, and/or save your results to document your proficiency.

The Muscular System

CHAPTER OUTLINE

- Functions of Muscle
- Types of Muscle Tissue
- Production of Energy for Muscle
- Structure of Skeletal Muscles
- Attachments and Actions of Skeletal Muscles
- Major Skeletal Muscles

LEARNING OUTCOMES

After completing Chapter 4, you will be able to:

4.1 List the functions of muscle.

4.2 List the three types of muscle tissue and describe the locations and characteristics of each.

4.3 Describe how visceral (smooth) muscle produces peristalsis.

4.4 Explain how muscle tissue generates energy.

4.5 Describe the structure of a skeletal muscle.

4.6 Define the terms *origin* and *insertion*.

4.7 List and define the various types of body movements produced by skeletal muscles.

4.8 List and identify the major skeletal muscles of the body, giving the action of each.

4.9 Explain the differences between strain and sprain injuries.

4.10 Describe the changes that occur to the muscular system as a person ages.

4.11 Describe the causes, signs and symptoms, and treatments of various diseases and disorders of the muscular system.

KEY TERMS

abduction
acetylcholine
acetylcholinesterase
adduction
aerobic respiration
agonist
antagonist
aponeurosis
botulism
circumduction
creatine phosphate
depression
dorsiflexion
elevation
endomysium
epimysium
eversion
extension
fascia
fascicle
fibromyalgia
flexion
hyperextension
insertion
intercalated disc
inversion
Krebs cycle
lactic acid
multiunit smooth muscle
muscle fatigue
muscle fiber
muscular dystrophy
myasthenia gravis
myocytes
myofibrils

KEY TERMS *(Concluded)*

myoglobin	protraction	supination
norepinephrine	retraction	synergist
origin	rhabdomyolysis	tendon
oxygen debt	rotation	tendonitis
perimysium	sarcolemma	tetanus
peristalsis	sarcoplasm	torticollis
plantar flexion	sarcoplasmic reticulum	trichinosis
prime mover	sphincter	visceral smooth
pronation	striations	muscle

Introduction

Bones and joints do not themselves produce movement. By alternating between contraction and relaxation, muscles cause bones and supported structures to move. The human body has more than 600 individual muscles. Although each muscle is a distinct structure, muscles act in groups to perform particular movements. This chapter focuses on the differences among three muscle tissue types, the structure of skeletal muscles, muscle actions, and the names of skeletal muscles.

CASE STUDY

Five days ago, a 40-year-old woman came to the doctor's office where you work as a medical assistant. She complained about pain in her back and right leg. Because this patient had a history of disc damage in her spine, she was sent home with pain medication and an order for bed rest for a 24-hour period. Two days later, she returned to the office with nausea, a severe headache, muscle twitching in her legs and arms, severe back pain, and tightness in her chest. The doctor once more asked the patient to elaborate on her activities the day before she fell ill. He was told that she had sprayed her furniture and carpets with an organophosphate insecticide to get rid of fleas in her house. She had also dipped her cats and dogs with the same insecticide. The doctor explained that organophosphates block acetylcholinesterase and immediately transferred her to the hospital for respiratory therapy and medicine to combat the insecticide poisoning.

As you read this chapter, consider the following questions:
1. What is the function of acetylcholinesterase?
2. Why does this patient exhibit muscle twitching and back pain?
3. What type of respiratory therapy will this patient require?
4. What precautions should a person take when using insecticides that contain organophosphates?
5. Why is it important for patients to give their doctor a complete account of their activities prior to an illness?

Functions of Muscle

Muscle tissue is unique because it has the ability to contract. It is this contraction that allows muscles to perform various functions. In addition to allowing the human body to move, muscles provide stability, the control of body openings and passages, and warming of the body.

Movement

Skeletal muscles are attached to bones by tendons. Because skeletal muscles cross joints, when these muscles contract, the bones they attach to move. This allows for various body motions, such as walking or waving your hand. Facial muscles are attached to the skin of the face, so when they contract, different facial expressions are produced, such as smiling or frowning. Smooth muscle is found in the walls of various organs, such as the stomach, intestines, and uterus. The contraction of smooth muscle in these organs produces the movement of their contents, such as the movement of food material through the intestine or the birth of a child being pushed from the mother's uterus. Cardiac muscle of the heart produces the atrial and ventricular contractions that pump blood into the blood vessels.

Stability

You rarely think about it, but muscles are holding your bones tightly together so that your joints remain stable. There are also very small muscles holding your vertebrae together to make your spinal column stable.

Control of Body Openings and Passages

Muscles also form valve-like structures called **sphincters** around various body openings and passages. These sphincters control the movement of substances into and out of these passages. For example, a urethral sphincter prevents urination until you relax it to permit urination.

Heat Production

When muscles contract, heat is released, which helps the body maintain a normal temperature. This is why moving your body can make you warmer if you are cold.

Types of Muscle Tissue

There are three types of muscle tissue: skeletal, smooth, and cardiac. Study Table 4-1 to review their locations and features.

Muscle cells or **myocytes** are called **muscle fibers** because of their long lengths. The cell membrane of a muscle fiber is called a **sarcolemma.** The cytoplasm of this cell type is called **sarcoplasm,** and the endoplasmic reticulum is called **sarcoplasmic reticulum.** Most of the sarcoplasm is filled with long structures called **myofibrils.** The arrangement of filaments in myofibrils produce the **striations** observed in skeletal and cardiac muscle cells. Muscle fibers are controlled by motor neurons that release neurotransmitters onto the fibers. See Figure 4-1 for an illustration of the structure of a skeletal muscle.

Skeletal Muscle

Skeletal muscle fibers respond only to the neurotransmitter **acetylcholine.** Acetylcholine causes skeletal muscle to contract. Once contraction has occurred, skeletal muscles release an enzyme called **acetylcholinesterase,** which breaks down acetylcholine. This allows the muscle to relax.

Smooth Muscle

There are two types of smooth muscle—multiunit and visceral. **Multiunit smooth muscle** is found in the iris of the eye and the walls of blood vessels. This muscle type contracts in response to neurotransmitters and hormones. **Visceral smooth muscle** contains sheets of muscle cells that closely contact each other. It is found in the walls of hollow organs such as the stomach, intestines, bladder, and uterus. Muscle fibers in visceral smooth muscle respond to neurotransmitters, but they also stimulate each other to contract; therefore, the muscle fibers tend to contract and relax together. This type of muscle produces an action called peristalsis. **Peristalsis** is a rhythmic contraction that pushes substances through tubes of the body, such as in the lower two-thirds of the esophagus, where

peristalsis moves the food bolus, or in the Fallopian tubes, where these muscle movements propel the ovum or egg through the tubes to the uterus.

Two neurotransmitters are involved in smooth muscle contraction—acetylcholine and **norepinephrine.** Depending on the smooth muscle type, these neurotransmitters cause or inhibit contractions.

Cardiac Muscle

Groups of cardiac muscle are connected to each other through **intercalated discs.** These discs allow the fibers in that group to contact and relax together. This design allows the heart to work as a pump. First the atria (holding chambers) contract and relax together, then the ventricles (pumping chambers) contract to send blood to the lungs and body, after which they relax and the cycle starts again. Cardiac muscle is also self-exciting, which means that it does not need nerve stimulation to contract. Nerves only speed up or slow down the contraction of the heart. Like smooth muscle, cardiac muscle responds to two neurotransmitters—acetylcholine and norepinephrine. Acetylcholine slows the heart rate, and norepinephrine speeds it up.

Production of Energy for Muscle

Because a lot of ATP (adenosine triphosphate), which is a type of chemical energy, is needed for sustained or repeated muscle contractions, a muscle cell must have multiple ways to store or make this substance. There are three ways through which muscle cells make this energy:

1. **Creatine phosphate** production. Creatine phosphate production is a rapid way for a muscle to produce energy. When ATP is used during muscle contraction, it loses a phosphate and, therefore, energy. Creatine phosphate "donates" a phosphate group, restoring energy potential. This is a very rapid way for muscles to produce energy.

TABLE 4-1	Types of Muscle Tissue					
Muscle Group	Major Location	Major Function	Striated (Yes/No)	Mode of Control	Rate of Contraction	Intercalated Discs
Skeletal muscle	Attached to bones and skin of the face	Produces body movements and facial expressions	Yes	Voluntary	Fast to contract and relax	No
Smooth muscle	Walls of hollow organs, blood vessels, and iris	Moves contents through organs; vasoconstriction	No	Involuntary	Slow to contract and relax	No
Cardiac muscle	Wall of the heart	Pumps blood through heart	Yes	Involuntary	Groups of muscle fibers contract as a unit	Yes

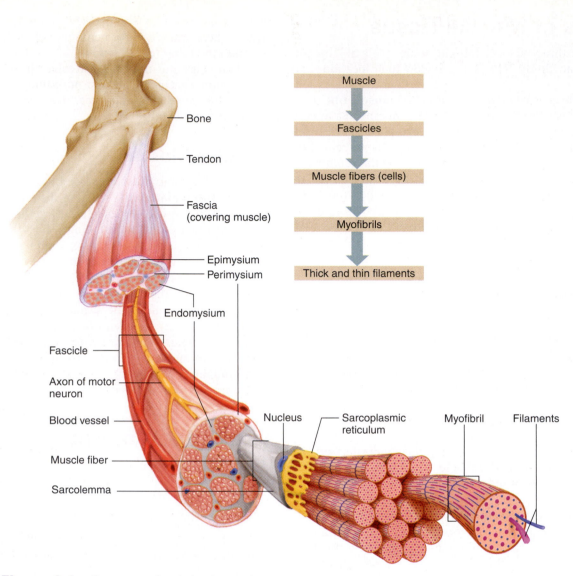

Figure 4-1. Structure of a skeletal muscle.

Muscle

Fascicles

Muscle fibers (cells)

Myofibrils

Thick and thin filaments

2. **Aerobic respiration** uses the body's store of glucose to make ATP. A cell breaks down glucose into pyruvic acid using oxygen (hence the term *aerobic*). The pyruvic acid is further converted into acetyl coenzyme A, which begins a series of reactions known as the **Krebs cycle** or the citric acid cycle. The oxygen needed for this method is stored in the muscle pigment called **myoglobin,** which also gives muscle its pinkish color.

3. **Lactic acid** production occurs when a cell is low in oxygen and must convert pyruvic acid to lactic acid. This conversion produces a small amount of ATP for the cell, but because lactic acid is a waste product, it must then be released from the cell.

Oxygen Debt

Oxygen debt occurs when skeletal muscle is used strenuously for several minutes. When pyruvic acid is converted to lactic acid for energy production, the lactic acid builds up and causes muscle fatigue. The lactic acid is brought to the liver via the bloodstream to be converted back into glucose, which requires more energy. The amount of oxygen the liver cells need to make enough ATP for this conversion results in the oxygen debt. This process explains why your body still burns energy even after you are done exercising.

Muscle Fatigue

Muscle fatigue is a condition in which a muscle has lost its ability to contract. It usually develops because of an accumulation of lactic acid. It can also occur if the blood supply to a muscle is interrupted or if a motor neuron loses its ability to release acetylcholine onto muscle fibers. Cramps—which are painful, involuntary contractions of muscles—can accompany muscle fatigue.

Structure of Skeletal Muscles

Skeletal muscles are the major organs that make up the muscular system. A skeletal muscle consists of connective tissues, skeletal muscle tissue, blood vessels, and nerves. When you see marbling in a steak, you are actually viewing connective tissues in the steak. The red portion of the steak is the muscle tissue.

The following connective tissue coverings are associated with skeletal muscles (see Figure 4-1):

- **Fascia.** This structure covers entire skeletal muscles and separates them from each other.
- **Tendon.** This tough, cord-like structure is made of fibrous connective tissue that connects muscles to bones.
- **Aponeurosis.** This tough, sheet-like structure is made of fibrous connective tissue. It typically attaches muscles to other muscles.
- **Epimysium.** This tissue is a thin covering that is just deep to the fascia of a muscle. It surrounds the entire muscle.
- **Perimysium.** This connective tissue divides a muscle into sections called **fascicles.**
- **Endomysium.** This covering of connective tissue surrounds individual muscle cells.

Attachments and Actions of Skeletal Muscles

The actions of skeletal muscles depend largely on what the skeletal muscles are attached to. Insertions and origins are sites of attachments for skeletal muscles. The attachment sites for skeletal muscles are known as origins and insertions. An **origin** is an attachment site for the less moveable bone during muscle contraction. An **insertion** is an attachment site for the more moveable bone during muscle contraction. For example, the biceps brachii (the muscle on the anterior upper arm) attaches to two places on the scapula and to one site on the radius. When the biceps brachii contracts, the radius moves and the arm bends at the elbow. Therefore, the origin of the biceps brachii is where it attaches to the scapula. The insertion site of the biceps brachii is its attachment site on the radius (Figure 4-2).

Most of the time, body movement is not produced by only one muscle, but by a group of muscles. However, one muscle is responsible for most of the movement, and this muscle is called the **prime mover.** Other muscles help the prime mover by stabilizing joints, and these muscles are called **synergists.** An **antagonist,** also referred to as an **agonist,** is a muscle that produces a movement opposite to the prime mover. When the prime mover contracts, the antagonist must relax in order to produce a smooth body movement. For example, when you bend your arm at the elbow, the prime mover is the biceps brachii. The synergist muscles are the brachialis and brachioradialis. The antagonist or agonist is the triceps brachii because its action is to extend the arm at the elbow. While the prime mover and

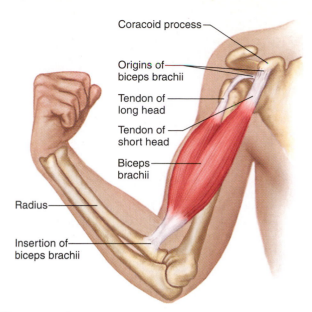

Figure 4-2. Origins and insertion of biceps brachii.

synergists contract, the agonist relaxes; when the agonist contracts, the prime mover and synergists relax.

The body movements produced by skeletal muscles include the following:

- **Flexion**—bending a body part or decreasing the angle of a joint
- **Extension**—straightening a body part or increasing the angle of a joint
- **Hyperextension**—extending a body part past the normal anatomical position
- **Dorsiflexion**—pointing the toes up
- **Plantar flexion**—pointing the toes down
- **Abduction**—moving a body part away from the midline of the body
- **Adduction**—moving a body part toward the midline of the body
- **Rotation**—twisting a body part; for example, turning your head from side to side
- **Circumduction**—moving a body part in a circle; for example, moving your arm in a circular motion
- **Pronation**—turning the palm of the hand down or lying face down
- **Supination**—turning the palm of the hand up or lying face up
- **Inversion**—turning the sole of the foot medially
- **Eversion**—turning the sole of the foot laterally
- **Retraction**—moving a body part posteriorly
- **Protraction**—moving a body part anteriorly
- **Elevation**—lifting a body part; for example, elevating your shoulders as in a shrugging expression
- **Depression**—lowering a body part; for example, lowering your shoulders

See Figures 4-3, 4-4, and 4-5 for illustrations of these types of movements. It is important for medical assistants

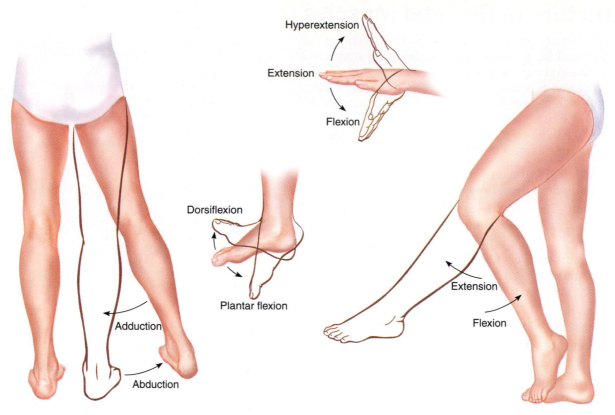

Figure 4-3. Adduction, abduction, dorsiflexion, plantar flexion, hyperextension, extension, and flexion.

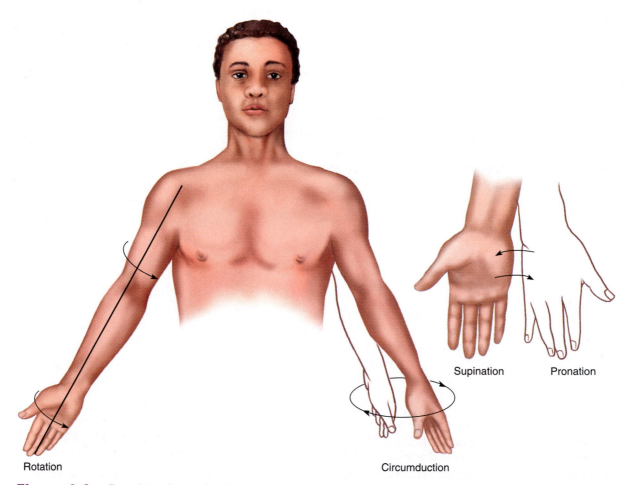

Figure 4-4. Rotation, circumduction, supination, and pronation.

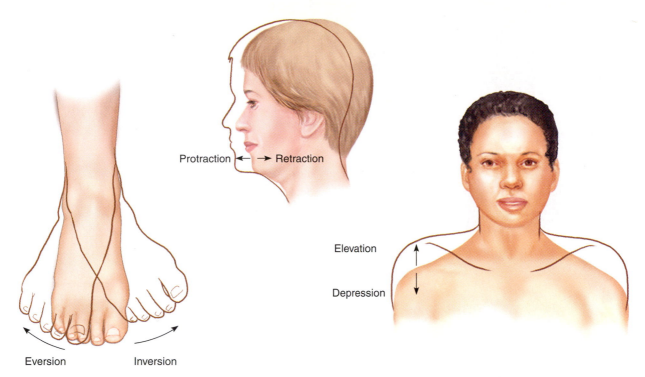

Figure 4-5. Eversion, inversion, protraction, retraction, elevation, and depression.

to understand these movements to assist with judging and measuring your patients' abilities to perform range of motion (ROM) exercises when assessing injuries and illnesses.

Major Skeletal Muscles

The name of a skeletal muscle often describes it in some way. Usually the name indicates the location, size, action, shape, or number of attachments of the muscle. For example, the pectoralis major is named for its large size (major) and its location (pectoral, or chest, region). The sterno-cleidomastoid is named for its attachment sites—*sterno* (sternum), *cleido* (clavicle), and *mastoid* (the mastoid process of the temporal bone, located behind the ear). As you study muscles, you will find it easier to remember them if you think about what the name describes.

Muscles of the Head

The muscles of the head include those that move the head, provide facial expression, and move the jaw. See Figures 4-6 and 4-7 for illustrations of the various muscles. Hints to assist you with remembering the locations for some of these muscles are found in parentheses.

Muscles that move the head include the following:

- Sternocleidomastoid. This muscle pulls the head to one side and also pulls the head to the chest. (sterno = sternum, cleido = clavicle, mastoid = mastoid)
- Splenius capitis. This muscle rotates the head and allows it to bend to the side. (capit = head)

Muscles of facial expression include the following:

- Frontalis. This muscle raises the eyebrows. (frontal = pertaining to the front)
- Orbicularis oris. This muscle allows the lips to pucker. (oris = oro or mouth)
- Orbicularis oculi. This muscle allows the eyes to close. (oculi = eye)
- Zygomaticus. This muscle pulls the corners of the mouth up. (zygomat = cheekbone)
- Platysma. This muscle pulls the corners of the mouth down.

The muscles of the jaw allow for mastication (chewing) and include the following:

- Masseter and temporalis. These muscles close the jaw. (masseter as in mastication or chewing; temporo = temple)

Arm Muscles

Muscles that move the arm include muscles of the arm and forearm (see Figures 4-6, 4-7, and 4-8). The muscles that move the arm include the following:

- Pectoralis major. This muscle pulls the arm across the chest; it also rotates and adducts the arms. (pectoro = chest)
- Latissimus dorsi. This muscle acts to extend, adduct, and rotate the arm inwardly. (latissimus = butterfly, dorsi = back)
- Deltoid. This muscle acts to abduct and extend the arm at the shoulder.

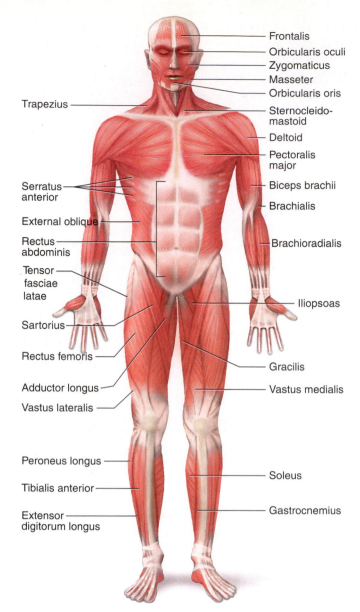

Figure 4-6. Anterior view of superficial skeletal muscles.

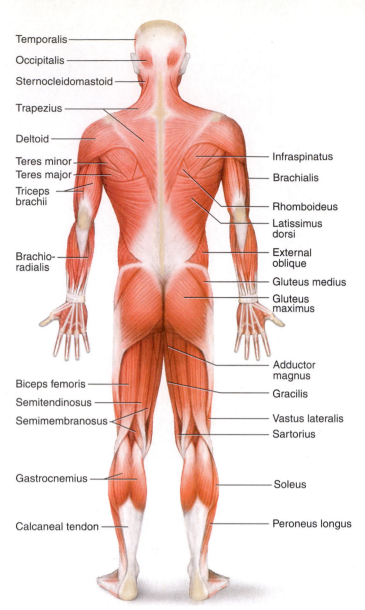

Figure 4-7. Posterior view of superficial skeletal muscles.

- Subscapularis. This muscle rotates the arm medially. (sub = below, scapulo = shoulder blade)
- Infraspinatus. This muscle rotates the arm laterally. (infra = below, spinat = spine)

Muscles that move the forearm include the following:

- Biceps brachii. This muscle flexes the arm at the elbow and rotates the hand laterally. (bi = two, ceps = insertion, brachii = arm)
- Brachialis. This muscle flexes the arm at the elbow. (brachii = arm)
- Brachioradialis. This muscle flexes the forearm at the elbow.(brachii = arm, radio = radius)
- Triceps brachii. This muscle extends the arm at the elbow. (tri = three, ceps = insertion, brachii = arm)

- Supinator. This muscle rotates the forearm laterally (supination). (supine = palm up)
- Pronator teres. This muscle rotates the forearm medially (pronation). (prone = palm down)

Muscles of the Wrist, Hand, and Fingers

Muscles that move the wrist, hand, and fingers can be seen in Figures 4-6, 4-7, and 4-8. These muscles include the following:

- Flexor carpi radialis and flexor carpi ulnaris. These muscles flex and abduct the wrist. (radio = radius, ulna = ulna)
- Palmaris longus. This muscle flexes the wrist.

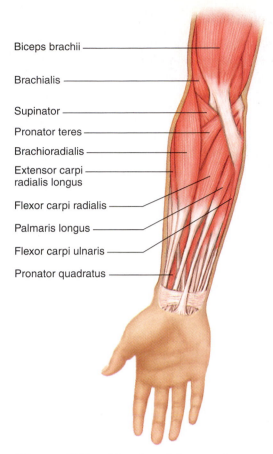

Biceps brachii

Brachialis

Supinator

Pronator teres

Brachioradialis

Extensor carpi
radialis longus

Flexor carpi radialis

Palmaris longus

Flexor carpi ulnaris

Pronator quadratus

Figure 4-8. Muscles of the anterior forearm.

- Flexor digitorum profundus. This muscle flexes the distal joints of the fingers but not the thumb. (digits = fingers)
- Extensor carpi radialis longus and brevis. These muscles extend the wrist and abduct the hand. (carpo = wrist, radio = radius, long = long, brev = brief or short)
- Extensor carpi ulnaris. This muscle extends the wrist. (carpo = wrist, ulna = ulna)
- Extensor digitorum. This muscle extends the fingers but not the thumb. (digit = finger)

Respiratory Muscles

The muscles of respiration include the following:

- Diaphragm. This muscle separates the thoracic cavity from the abdominal cavity; its contraction causes inspiration.
- External and internal intercostals. The contraction of these muscles expands and lowers the ribs during breathing. See Figure 4-9 for an illustration of the internal intercostal muscle. (inter = between, costo = rib)

Abdominal Muscles

The muscles of the abdominal wall include the following:

- External and internal obliques. These muscles compress the abdominal wall. (oblique = diagonal)

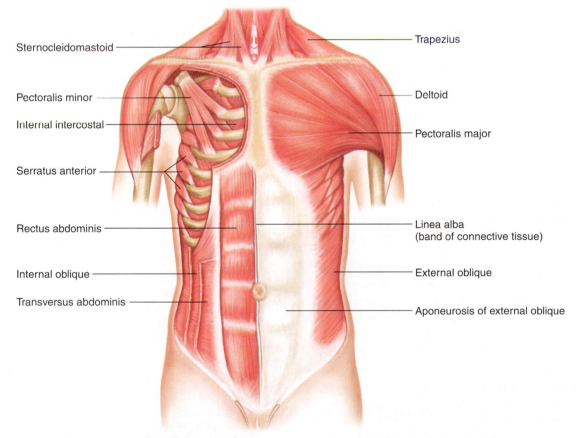

Sternocleidomastoid

Pectoralis minor

Internal intercostal

Serratus anterior

Rectus abdominis

Internal oblique

Transversus abdominis

Trapezius

Deltoid

Pectoralis major

Linea alba
(band of connective tissue)

External oblique

Aponeurosis of external oblique

Figure 4-9. Muscles of the anterior chest and abdominal wall.

- Transverse abdominis. This muscle also compresses the abdominal wall. (transverse = across)
- Rectus abdominis. This muscle acts to flex the vertebral column and compress the abdominal wall. (rectus = erect)

See Figures 4-6, 4-7, and 4-9 for illustrations of these muscles.

Muscles of the Pectoral Girdle

The muscles that move the pectoral girdle (shoulder) include these muscles:

- Trapezius. This muscle raises the arms and pulls the shoulders downward. (trapezius = trapezoid)
- Pectoralis minor. This muscle pulls the scapula downward and raises the ribs. (pectoro = chest, minor = smaller)

See Figures 4-6, 4-7, and 4-9 for illustrations of these muscles.

Leg Muscles

The leg muscles include muscles of the thigh and lower leg (see Figures 4-6 and 4-7). Muscles that move the thigh include the following:

- Iliopsoas major. This muscle flexes the thigh.
- Gluteus maximus. This muscle extends the thigh.
- Gluteus medius and minimus. These muscles abduct the thighs and rotate them medially.
- Adductor longus and magnus. These muscles adduct the thighs and rotate them laterally. (adduct = toward the midline)
- Biceps femoris, semitendinosus, and semimembranosus. These three muscles are known as the *hamstring group*. They act to flex the leg at the knee and extend the leg at the thigh.
- Rectus femoris, vastus lateralis, vastus medialis, and vastus intermedius. These four muscles are known as the *quadriceps group;* they act to extend the leg at the knee.

Educating the Patient

Muscle Strains and Sprains

Strains are injuries that excessively stretch muscles or tendons. Sprains are more serious injuries that result in tears to tendons, ligaments, and/or the cartilage of joints. You can teach patients to prevent these types of injuries by doing the following:

- Warm up. Warming up muscles for just a few minutes before an intense activity raises muscle temperature. This increase in temperature prevents injuries by making muscle tissue more pliable.
- Stretch. Stretching improves muscle performance and should always be done after the warm-up or after exercising. A person should never stretch further than he can hold for 10 seconds.
- Cool down. Slowing down the exercise before completely stopping prevents dizziness and fainting. If a person suddenly stops exercising, blood can pool in the legs and is prevented from reaching the brain. Cooling down also helps to remove lactic acid from muscles.

If sprains or strains do occur, immediate RICE treatment is recommended:

- R is for rest. Resting minimizes bleeding, further injury, and swelling.

- I is for ice. Ice minimizes swelling and pain. A bag that is filled with crushed ice conforms better to a body part than one filled with ice cubes. A bag full of frozen peas or other small vegetables can also be used. The ice should be applied for 10 minutes and then removed for 10 minutes. This should be kept up for about an hour and repeated several times during a 24-hour period. Ice can be applied for a shorter period of time if blood vessels dilate during its application.
- C is for compression, which minimizes swelling. A bandage should be loosely wrapped around the injured area and the bag of ice. Compression should be applied and removed along with the ice.
- E is for elevation. The injured muscle should be elevated, which minimizes swelling, and elevation should be continued as long as swelling is present.

If the patient does not feel that his or her symptoms have improved in several days' to a week's time, a physician should be contacted to rule out a more serious injury, such as a torn ligament or muscle, or even a bone fracture.

Educating the Patient

Aging and the Musculoskeletal System

Although the aging of the skeletal system causes more obvious difficulties for patients with diseases and conditions such as arthritis, fractures, and osteoporosis, the muscular decline often goes hand-in-hand with these changes. Aging causes a decline in the speed and strength of muscle contractions even though the actual endurance of muscle fibers changes very little. Elderly patients often have increasing difficulty with dexterity and gripping ability. Mobility may decrease related to the combined decline of the musculoskeletal system. The diet and exercise history of the patient, as well as his or her family history, also has a direct impact on the patient's mobility and activity level as the patient ages.

Assistive devices such as railings, tub and shower seats, and gripping devices can assist patients who are experiencing difficulties. Exercise routines, particularly pool exercises such as swimming and physical therapy, are often helpful in maintaining strength and mobility.

- Sartorius. This muscle flexes the leg at the knee and thigh. It also abducts the thigh, rotating the thigh laterally but rotating the lower leg medially; it carries out the act of sitting cross-legged.

Muscles of the Ankle, Foot, and Toes

Muscles that move the ankle, foot, and toes include the following:

- Tibialis anterior. This muscle inverts the foot and points the foot up (dorsiflexion).

- Extensor digitorum longus. This muscle extends the toes and points the foot up.
- Gastrocnemius. This muscle flexes the foot and flexes the leg at the knee. It is more commonly referred to as the calf muscle.
- Soleus. This muscle also flexes the foot.
- Flexor digitorum longus. This muscle flexes the foot and toes.

See Figures 4-6 and 4-7 for illustrations of these muscles.

Pathophysiology

Common Diseases and Disorders of the Muscular System

Botulism is usually thought of as a disease that affects the gastrointestinal tract, but it can also affect various muscle groups. This disease most commonly affects infants. Although a person can survive this disease, its effects may be long-lasting.

- **Causes.** This disease is a rare but very serious disorder caused by the bacterium *Clostridium botulinum*, which normally lives in soil and water. If this bacterium gets on food, it produces a toxin that can lead to a type of food poisoning. The foods most likely to contain *Clostridium botulinum* are canned vegetables, cured pork, raw fish, honey, and corn syrup. A person can also acquire this bacterium through open wounds that are not cleaned properly.
- **Signs and symptoms.** This disease causes many symptoms, including dysphagia (difficulty swallowing), paralysis, muscle weakness, nausea and vomiting, abdominal cramps, double vision, dyspnea (difficulty breathing), poor feeding and suckling in infants, the inability to urinate, the absence of reflexes, and constipation. The signs and symptoms usually appear 8 to 40 hours after the toxin is ingested. The diagnosis is usually made by either a blood test to identify the toxin or an analysis of the suspected food.

- **Treatment.** Treatment includes emergency hospitalization, intubation to open airways, mechanical ventilation if respiratory muscles are impaired, intravenous fluids or nasogastric feeding if swallowing is impaired, and the administration of an antitoxin.
- **Prevention tips.** You can instruct patients to prevent botulism by observing the following guidelines:
  - Never give honey or corn syrup to infants.
  - Sterilize home-canned foods properly (250°F for 35 minutes).
  - Do not use foods from bent or bulging cans.
  - Never eat foods that smell as if they may have spoiled.
  - Cook and store foods properly.

Fibromyalgia is a fairly common condition that results in chronic pain primarily in joints, muscles, and tendons. It most commonly affects women between the ages of 20 and 50.

continued →

Common Diseases and Disorders of the Muscular System (continued)

- **Causes.** The causes of this disorder are poorly understood. Fibromyalgia may be caused by sleep disturbance, emotional distress, decreased blood flow to muscles, a virus, or any combination of these factors.
- **Signs and symptoms.** Symptoms include fatigue, tenderness in different areas of the body, sleep disturbances, and chronic facial pain. The diagnosis is usually made by ruling out other possible diseases. It is not normally diagnosed unless a person has muscle and joint pain for at least 3 months in certain body areas.
- **Treatment.** Treatment is varied and includes antidepressants, anti-inflammatory medications, physical therapy, lifestyle changes to reduce stress, counseling to improve coping skills, reduction or elimination of caffeine to improve sleeping, and diet supplements to improve nutrition.

Muscular dystrophy (MD) is a group of inherited disorders characterized by muscle weakness and a loss of muscle tissue. There are at least seven types of muscular dystrophy, and they are distinguished from each other by types of symptoms, the age at when symptoms appeared, and the cause.

- **Causes.** The causes of this disorder are primarily hereditary. Genetic fetal testing is available.
- **Signs and symptoms.** The signs and symptoms vary widely and depend on the type of muscular dystrophy. The symptoms of Duchenne muscular dystrophy, which is the most common and widely known type, progress steadily and are eventually fatal. Other types cause mild symptoms, and patients usually have normal life expectancies. Specific signs and symptoms include muscle weakness in various muscle groups, depending on the type of dystrophy; difficulty walking; drooling; a delayed development of motor skills; frequent falls; mental retardation in some types; a curved spine; the formation of a claw hand or clubfoot; a loss of muscle mass; the accumulation of fat or fibrous connective tissue in muscles; and arrhythmias in some types. The progression of the muscular weakness may also include eventual paralysis of the affected muscle groups. The diagnosis is primarily made through a muscle biopsy. Other tests include deoxyribonucleic acid (DNA) testing; an EMG (electromyography) test, which tests muscle weakness; or an ECG (electrocardiogram), which tests cardiac function.
- **Treatment.** Treatment includes physical therapy to maintain muscle function, the use of braces and wheelchairs, various medications based on the type of MD, and spinal surgery.

Myasthenia gravis is a condition in which affected persons experience muscle weakness. In this autoimmune condition, a person produces antibodies that prevent muscles from receiving neurotransmitters from neurons. It most commonly affects young women and older men, especially if they have other autoimmune disorders.

- **Causes.** This disease is usually considered an autoimmune disorder.
- **Signs and symptoms.** The signs and symptoms usually get better with rest and worsen with activity. They include double vision; muscle weakness; dysphagia (difficulty swallowing), difficulty talking, chewing, lifting, or walking; fatigue; drooling; and difficulty breathing. The diagnosis may be difficult, but a single-fiber EMG test is often useful. This test measures the response of a muscle fiber to nervous stimulation. Other tests include acetylcholine receptors antibody tests and the Tensilon test. In a positive Tensilon test, muscle activity increases after medication is given that blocks the breakdown of acetylcholine.
- **Treatment.** Treatments include lifestyle changes to avoid excessive stress, getting adequate rest and heat, the use of an eye patch to treat double vision, medications to improve communication between nerves and muscles, medications to suppress the immune system, plasmapheresis to remove harmful antibodies from blood, and removal of the thymus.

Rhabdomyolysis is a condition in which the kidneys have been damaged in relation to serious muscle injuries.

- **Causes.** Kidneys become damaged because of toxins released from muscle cells. When muscles are damaged, excessive amounts of the pigment myoglobin are released, which is then broken down into harmful chemicals. Muscles are most often damaged through trauma; excessive use (for example, marathon running); overdoses of cocaine, heroine, and other drugs; alcoholism; and a blockage of the blood supply to the muscles.
- **Signs and symptoms.** Symptoms include dark urine, muscle tenderness, muscle weakness, muscle stiffness, seizures, joint pain, and fatigue. The diagnosis includes urinalysis for the presence of myoglobin, creatine phosphokinase (CPK), and creatinine; blood is also tested for the presence of myoglobin, CPK, or high levels of potassium. CPK is an enzyme released into the blood when muscles are damaged. Creatinine is a protein released by the breakdown of muscle tissue.
- **Treatment.** Treatment includes hydration to rapidly eliminate toxins from the kidneys, diuretics to help flush toxins from the body, medications to flush excess potassium from the body, and therapy for kidney failure.

Tendonitis is described as the painful inflammation of a tendon as well as of the tendon-muscle attachment to a bone. The most common locations for tendonitis are the shoulder, hip, heel, and hamstrings. Tendonitis may also be associated with bursitis, the inflammation of the bursa located in synovial joints such as the shoulder, elbow, and knee.

continued ⟶

Common Diseases and Disorders of the Muscular System (concluded)

- **Causes.** Tendonitis usually occurs after a sports-related activity that results in injury to the muscle tendon or tendon-to-bone attachment. Other musculoskeletal disorders may also cause or exacerbate this condition.
- **Signs and symptoms.** Pain at the joint or muscle attachment that results in limited range of motion (ROM) of the affected area.
- **Treatment.** For the initial injury, ice should be used for the first 12 to 24 hours to minimize inflammation. After this initial time period, heat application will assist with joint and muscle pain. If calcium deposits are found in the tendon, which can be confirmed by x-ray, heat will aggravate the condition, whereas continued use of ice packs will be helpful for the discomfort. Resting the affected area and oral analgesics will also be helpful to control pain.

Tetanus is commonly called lockjaw. This disease has a high mortality rate, especially in infants. Immediate treatment is necessary to prevent death or long-lasting effects. However, this disease is completely preventable through regular vaccinations.

- **Causes.** A toxin produced by the bacterium *Clostridium tetani*, which lives naturally in soil and water, causes this disease. People most commonly acquire this bacterium through open wounds caused by objects contaminated with soil.
- **Signs and symptoms.** Symptoms usually appear between 5 and 10 days after infection. Muscle spasms in the jaw, neck, and facial muscles are usually the first signs. Other signs and symptoms include worsening of the muscle spasms that spread to other body locations and may cause bone fractures; dyspnea (breathing difficulties); irritability; fever; profuse sweating; and drooling. The diagnosis is usually based on the type of wound and the characteristic signs and symptoms of the disease. Tetanus antibody tests can also be used in diagnosis, but cultures of the wound site often produce false-negative findings.
- **Treatment.** Administering antitoxin and antibiotics is a key treatment. Others include wound cleaning, muscle relaxants, sedation, and bed rest. The insertion of an endotracheal tube and mechanical ventilation may be needed for patients with severe breathing difficulties.

Torticollis is also known as wry neck. This disease is a cervical deformity in which the head bends toward the affected side while the chin rotates to the opposite side.

- **Causes.** Torticollis may be acquired or congenital. It is caused by spasm or shortening of the sternocleidomastoid muscle. Breech or other difficult birth is often the cause of the congenital form as a result of the previously noted malpositioning, or from injury or scar tissue from ruptured muscle fibers before or during the birth process. The acquired form is the result of underlying disease, cervical spine injury, or chronic muscle spasms.
- **Signs and Symptoms.** There is obvious malpositioning of the head and neck in an affected individual.
- **Treatment.** For the congenital form, passive exercises to stretch the muscles as well as corrected head positioning during sleep (to maintain the straightening accomplished through the exercises) may be helpful. The treatment for acquired torticollis should consist of treating the underlying disease if possible. Otherwise, heat, cervical traction, a neck brace, exercise, massage, and psychotherapy to assist the patient in dealing with the psychological and emotional effects related to the deformity are all treatment options.

Trichinosis is an infection caused by parasites (worms).

- **Causes.** This disease is caused by worms that are usually ingested by eating undercooked meat. Once ingested, the worms can leave the digestive tract and infect skeletal muscles, the heart, the lungs, and the brain. This disease is preventable by not eating meat from wild animals. Proper cooking will also prevent trichinosis. There is no cure for this disease once the worms leave the digestive tract and infect other tissues.
- **Signs and symptoms.** Common symptoms include abdominal pain, diarrhea, muscle pain, fever, and pneumonia. In more serious cases, arrhythmias (irregular heart rhythms), heart failure, and encephalitis (swelling of the brain) can result. The diagnosis is usually based on the symptoms, a blood test to determine if there is an increase in eosinophils in blood, or a muscle biopsy that reveals the presence of the worms.
- **Treatment.** Patients with this disease are treated with medications to kill worms in the digestive tract and with anti-inflammatory drugs to reduce muscle pain and swelling.

Summary

Skeletal muscle works in conjunction with the skeletal system to produce movement. This movement is accomplished voluntarily. In addition, skeletal muscles help stabilize joints and are important in heat production. Muscles under involuntary control include smooth and cardiac muscle. Smooth muscles control body openings and passages. Cardiac muscle is responsible for the pumping action of the heart. Medical assistants should understand the muscular system in order to give muscular injections, prepare patients for massage therapy, demonstrate ambulatory techniques, and assist in the care (and prevention) of sprains and strains, as well as other muscular disorders.

REVIEW

CHAPTER 4

CASE STUDY QUESTIONS

Now that you have completed this chapter, review the case study at the beginning of the chapter and answer the following questions:

1. What is the function of acetylcholinesterase?
2. Why does this patient exhibit muscle twitching and back pain?
3. What type of respiratory therapy will this patient require?
4. What precautions should a person take when using insecticides that contain organophosphates?
5. Why is it important for patients to give their doctor a complete account of their activities prior to an illness?

Discussion Questions

1. List the four types of muscle function, explaining how each of these functions is essential to body functioning.
2. How are muscles named? Give an example for each method of naming a muscle.
3. Name the three muscle types, giving the location of each and briefly explaining how contraction occurs for each muscle type.
4. What is oxygen debt, and how does it develop?

Critical Thinking Questions

1. Why is it important to do warm-up activities before participating in sporting events?
2. Explain why physical therapy and massage are prescribed for patients in wheelchairs, who are bed bound, or even for those in a coma.
3. Using the acronym *RICE*, explain how a patient should care for a sprained ankle.
4. Elderly patients often have stability issues and loss of muscle strength. Explain why this occurs.

Application Activities

1. Define the following terms related to muscle structure:
   a. Fascia
   b. Epimysium
   c. Fascicle
   d. Perimysium
   e. Aponeurosis
   f. Tendon
2. Describe the following actions:
   a. Flexion
   b. Extension
   c. Pronation
   d. Supination
   e. Abduction
   f. Adduction
   g. Dorsiflexion
   h. Plantarflexion
3. Briefly describe the signs and symptoms of the following muscular diseases:
   a. Botulism
   b. Fibromyalgia
   c. Muscular dystrophy
   d. Myasthenia gravis
   e. Tetanus
   f. Trichinosis
   g. Tendonitis
4. Give the locations for the following muscles:
   a. Sternocleidomastoid
   b. Orbicularis oris
   c. Pectoralis major
   d. Latissimus dorsi
   e. Triceps brachii
   f. Gluteus maximus
   g. Gastrocnemius

Virtual Fieldtrip

Visit the McGraw-Hill Higher Education Medical Assisting website at www.mhhe.com/medicalassisting3 to complete the following activity:

Pick one of the following muscular diseases that interests you: myasthenia gravis, muscular dystrophy, fibromyalgia, rhabdomyolysis, tetanus, or botulism. Using the alphabetic grid at the top of the Medline Health Topics page, locate the site for your chosen topic and answer the following questions regarding this condition:

- The cause of the disease or condition
- Diagnostic tests done to confirm the disease
- Conventional treatments for patients as well as alternatives, if given
- Social/psychological effects on the patient and his or her family and/or caregivers
- Preventative measures that may be taken, if any
- The patient's prognosis

When your research is completed, create an informational poster, computer slide show, or pamphlet to share your information with others. The object of this assignment is to really get to understand your disease and the patients who have it that you may encounter. Consider "interviewing" a patient with this condition or check out other websites to further your understanding.

Open the CD and complete this chapter's practice activities, play the games, listen to the key terms, and test yourself with the interactive review. E-mail, print, and/or save your results to document your proficiency.

CHAPTER 5

The Cardiovascular System

KEY TERMS

agglutination
agranulocyte
albumins
anemia
aneurysm
aortic semilunar valve
arrhythmia
atherosclerosis
atria
atrioventricular node
atrioventricular septum
baroreceptors
basophil
bicuspid valve
bilirubin
biliverdin
bundle of His
capillary
carboxyhemoglobin
carditis
cerebrovascular accident
chordae tendineae
chylomicron
coagulation
coronary sinus
deoxyhemoglobin
diapedesis
diastolic pressure
embolus
endocardium
eosinophil
epicardium
erythroblastosis fetalis
erythrocyte
erythropoietin

CHAPTER OUTLINE

- The Heart
- Blood Vessels
- Blood Pressure
- Circulation
- Blood

LEARNING OUTCOMES

After completing Chapter 5, you will be able to:

5.1 Describe the structure of the heart and the function of each part.
5.2 Trace the flow of blood through the heart.
5.3 List the most common heart sounds and what events produce them.
5.4 Explain how heart rate is controlled by the electrical conduction system of the heart.
5.5 List the different types of blood vessels and describe the functions of each.
5.6 Define blood pressure and tell how it is controlled.
5.7 Trace the flow of blood through the pulmonary and systemic circulation.
5.8 List the major arteries and veins of the body and describe their locations.

KEY TERMS *(Concluded)*

fibrinogen	lymphocyte	Rh antigen
globulins	megakaryocytes	RhoGAM
granulocyte	mitral valve	serum
hematocrit	monocyte	sinoatrial node
hemocytoblast	murmur	systemic circuit
hemolytic anemia	myocardial infarction	systolic pressure
hemostasis	myocardium	thalassemia
hepatic portal system	neutrophil	thrombocytes
hypertension	oxyhemoglobin	thrombophlebitis
interatrial septum	parietal pericardium	thrombus
interventricular septum	pericardium	tricuspid valve
leukemia	platelets	varicose veins
leukocyte	pulmonary circuit	vasoconstriction
leukocytosis	pulmonary semilunar valve	vasodilation
leukopenia	pulmonary trunk	ventricle
lipoprotein	Purkinje fibers	visceral pericardium

5.9 List and describe the components of blood.

5.10 Give the functions of red blood cells, the different types of white blood cells, and platelets.

5.11 List the substances normally found in plasma.

5.12 Explain how bleeding is controlled.

5.13 Explain the differences among blood types A, B, AB, and O.

5.14 Explain the difference between Rh-positive blood and Rh-negative blood.

5.15 Explain the importance of blood typing and tell which blood types are compatible.

5.16 Describe the causes, signs and symptoms, and treatments of various diseases and disorders of the cardiovascular system.

Introduction

The cardiovascular system consists of the heart and blood vessels. It is responsible for sending blood to the lungs to pick up oxygen and to the digestive system to pick up nutrients in order to deliver oxygen and nutrients to all the organ systems in the body. This system also circulates waste products to certain organ systems so that these wastes can be removed from the blood.

CASE STUDY

A 42-year-old man was referred to the cardiologist's office for an evaluation. The patient had recently started an exercise program for weight loss. For the last 3 weeks, following exercise, he had noticed radiating chest pain (angina pectoris) that stopped after rest. This condition had worsened in the last week. The cardiologist ordered a stress echocardiogram (a test that visualizes the heart during increasing stress). The echocardiogram results suggested that the patient had coronary artery disease (CAD). The patient was scheduled for a cardiac catheterization the next morning. It was noted in the patient's chart that he smoked two packs of cigarettes per day.

As you read this chapter, consider the following questions:

1. What symptoms suggest that this patient is suffering from coronary artery disease and not some other disorder?
2. Why is it important to test the heart under stress rather than obtaining a resting echocardiogram?
3. What lifestyle changes should this patient make to prevent future heart attacks?
4. Why is a cardiac catheterization needed in addition to the stress echocardiogram?
5. What are the treatment options for this patient?

The Heart

Structures of the Heart

The heart is a cone-shaped organ about the size of a loose fist. It is located within the mediastinum and extends from the level of the second rib to about the level of the sixth rib. Although many people think that the heart is found in the left side of the chest, the heart is located only slightly left of the midline of the body. The heart is bordered laterally by the lungs, posteriorly by the vertebral column, and anteriorly by the sternum. Inferiorly, the heart rests on the diaphragm.

Cardiac Membranes. A membrane called the **pericardium** covers the heart and the large blood vessels attached to it (Figure 5-1). The pericardium consists of an outer fibrous layer that covers two inner layers. The innermost layer is called the **visceral pericardium,** and it lies directly on top of the heart. The layer on top of the visceral pericardium is called the **parietal pericardium.** The fibrous pericardium and the parietal pericardium form the pericardial sac. The space between the parietal pericardium and visceral pericardium is called the pericardial cavity. The pericardial cavity contains a slippery, serous fluid called pericardial fluid. Pericardial fluid reduces friction between the membranes when the heart contracts.

The Heart Wall. The wall of the heart (Figure 5-2) is made of the following three layers:

- **Epicardium.** This outermost layer is also known as the visceral pericardium and contains fat, which helps to cushion the heart.

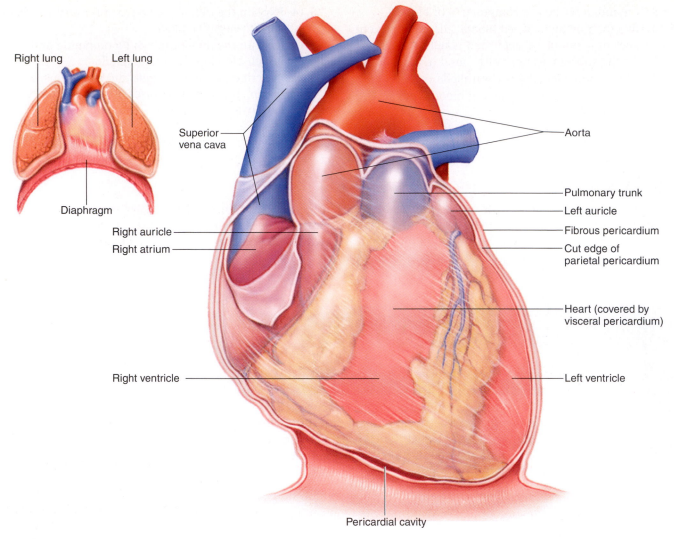

Right lung   Left lung

Superior
vena cava

Diaphragm

Right auricle

Right atrium

Right ventricle

Aorta

Pulmonary trunk

Left auricle

Fibrous pericardium

Cut edge of
parietal pericardium

Heart (covered by
visceral pericardium)

Left ventricle

Pericardial cavity

Figure 5-1. Location and membranes of the heart.

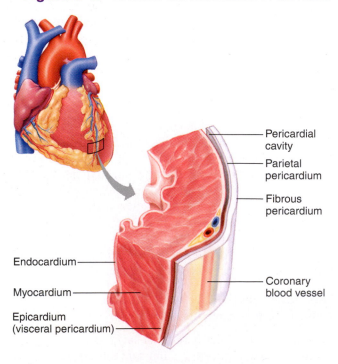

Pericardial
cavity

Parietal
pericardium

Fibrous
pericardium

Endocardium

Myocardium

Epicardium
(visceral pericardium)

Coronary
blood vessel

Figure 5-2. Layers of the wall of the heart.

• **Myocardium.** This middle layer is the thickest layer of the wall and is made primarily of cardiac muscle.

• **Endocardium.** This innermost layer is thin and very smooth, and stretches as the heart pumps blood. This layer contains the Purkinje fibers, part of the cardiac electrical conduction system, which is discussed later in this chapter.

Heart Chambers and Valves. The heart contains four hollow chambers, two on the left and two on the right (Figure 5-3). The upper chambers of the heart are called **atria** (the singular form is *atrium*). They have thin walls and function to receive blood returning to the heart from the lungs and the body. The atria are separated from each other by a walled membrane known as the **interatrial septum.** The bottom chambers of the heart are called **ventricles.** The septum separating the ventricles is the **interventricular septum.** The ventricles function to pump blood into the arteries, which send the blood to the lungs and the body. The **atrioventricular septum** is the wall that separates the atria from the ventricles. The four valves within the heart that keep blood flowing in one direction are the tricuspid and the bicuspid (mitral) valves located

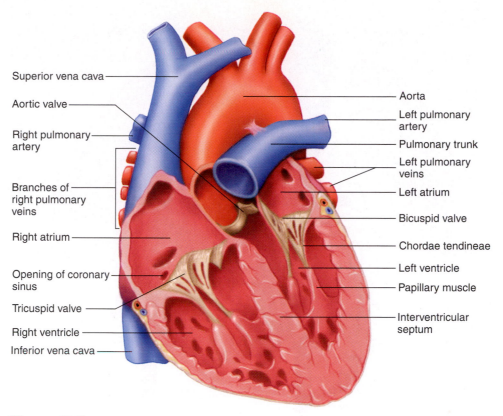

Figure 5-3. Coronal section of the heart.

Labels on figure:
Superior vena cava
Aortic valve
Right pulmonary artery
Branches of right pulmonary veins
Right atrium
Opening of coronary sinus
Tricuspid valve
Right ventricle
Inferior vena cava
Aorta
Left pulmonary artery
Pulmonary trunk
Left pulmonary veins
Left atrium
Bicuspid valve
Chordae tendineae
Left ventricle
Papillary muscle
Interventricular septum

between the atria and ventricles, and the pulmonary semilunar and aortic semilunar valves, which are located between the ventricles and their arteries.

Tricuspid Valve. The **tricuspid valve** has three cusps and is situated between the right atrium and the right ventricle. It prevents blood from flowing back into the right atrium when the right ventricle contracts. This valve is also called the right AV (atrioventricular) valve. The cusps of this valve are anchored by cordlike structures called **chordae tendineae** to bumps of cardiac muscle called papillary muscles. These muscles contract when the ventricles contract to close the valve.

Bicuspid Valve. The **bicuspid valve** has two cusps and is located between the left atrium and the left ventricle. It prevents blood from flowing back into the left atrium when the left ventricle contracts. This valve is also known as the **mitral valve** and the left AV valve. Like the tricuspid valve, the bicuspid valve also has chordae tendineae attached to papillary muscles.

Pulmonary Semilunar Valve. The **pulmonary semilunar valve** is situated between the right ventricle and the trunk of the pulmonary arteries. It prevents blood from flowing back into the right ventricle. Because its cusps are shaped like a half moon, this valve is called a semilunar valve.

Aortic Semilunar Valve. The **aortic semilunar valve** is situated between the left ventricle and the aorta. It prevents blood from flowing back into the left ventricle and is also known as a semilunar valve because of the shape of its cusps.

Blood Flow Through the Heart

Blood that is low in oxygen (deoxygenated) and rich in carbon dioxide enters the right atrium of the heart through large veins called the inferior and superior venae cavae. From the right atrium, the blood flows through the tricuspid valve into the right ventricle. When the right ventricle contracts, blood is pushed through the pulmonary semilunar valve into a larger artery called the **pulmonary trunk.** The pulmonary trunk branches into the left and right pulmonary arteries, which carry blood to the lungs. In the lungs, blood picks up oxygen and gets rid of carbon dioxide. Blood rich in oxygen and low in carbon dioxide then returns to the heart through the four pulmonary veins. The pulmonary veins empty the oxygenated blood into the left atrium. Cardiac circulation up until this point is often referred to as *pulmonary circulation.* From the left atrium, blood flows through the bicuspid (mitral) valve into the left ventricle. When the left ventricle contracts, blood is pushed through the aortic semilunar valve into the aorta. The aorta distributes blood into its branches and throughout the body. Because blood now enters all of the body's blood vessels, this left heart circulation is known as *systemic circulation.*

In the body, the blood gives oxygen to cells and picks up carbon dioxide. Veins of the body pick up the oxygen-poor blood and empty it into the vena cavae, and the whole circuit starts all over again. Note that arteries carry blood away from the heart and veins carry blood to the heart (Figure 5-4).

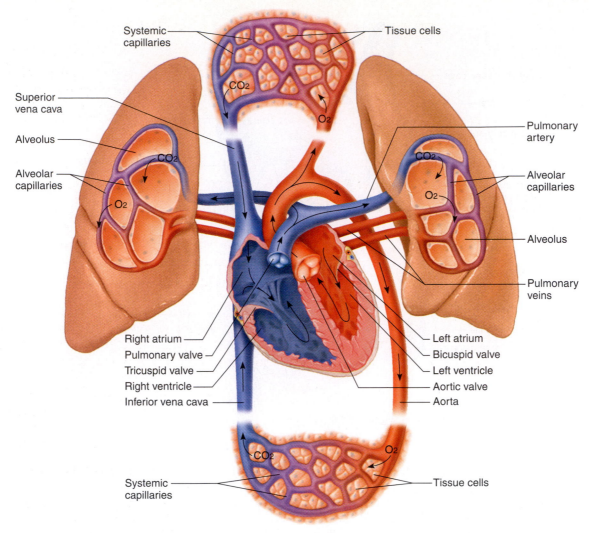

Figure 5-4. Pathway of blood through the heart and lungs and on to other body parts. The right side of the heart delivers blood to the lungs and the left side delivers blood to all other body parts.

Cardiac Cycle

One heartbeat makes up one cardiac cycle. In one cardiac cycle, the top chambers (atria) of the heart contract and relax together and then the bottom chambers (ventricles) of the heart contract and relax together. In other words, a cardiac cycle consists of one complete cardiac contraction and one complete cardiac relaxation. When the right atrium contracts, the tricuspid valve opens and blood flows into the right ventricle. Likewise, when the left atrium contracts, the bicuspid valve opens and blood flows into the left ventricle. When the right ventricle contracts, the tricuspid valve must close, the pulmonary semilunar valve opens, and blood is pushed into the trunk of the pulmonary artery. When the left ventricle contracts, the bicuspid valve must close, the aortic semilunar valve opens, and blood is pushed into the aorta.

The following factors influence the cardiac cycle:

- Exercise. Strenuous exercise increases the heart rate because skeletal muscles need more oxygen.

- Parasympathetic nerves. The parasympathetic nerve to the heart is the vagus nerve, and it generally keeps the heart rate relatively low.

- Sympathetic nerves. The sympathetic nerves increase the heart rate during times of stress.

- Cardiac control center. This center is located in the medulla oblongata. When blood pressure rises, this control center sends impulses to decrease the heart rate. When blood pressure falls, it sends impulses to increase the heart rate.

- Body temperature. An increase in body temperature usually increases the heart rate. This explains the high heart rate when a person runs a fever.

- Potassium ions. Low concentrations of potassium ions in the blood decrease the heart rate, but a high concentration causes an arrhythmia (abnormal heart rate).

- Calcium ions. Low concentrations of calcium ions in the blood depress heart actions, but high concentrations cause heart contractions called titanic contractions, which are longer than normal heart contractions.

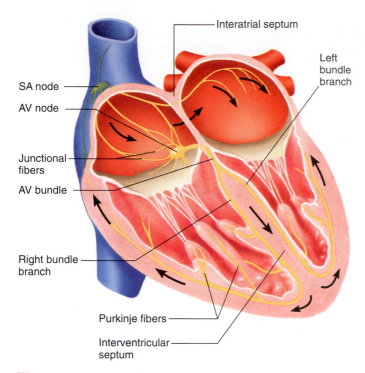

Figure 5-5. Cardiac conduction system.

Heart Sounds

During one cardiac cycle you can hear two heart sounds. The sounds are called *lubb* and *dubb*. These sounds are generated when valves in the heart snap shut. Lubb is the first heart sound and occurs when the ventricles contract and the tricuspid and bicuspid valves snap shut. Dubb is the second heart sound and occurs when the atria contract and the pulmonary and aortic semilunar valves snap shut.

Physicians will listen to heart sounds in order to diagnose certain conditions. For example, if AV valves (tricuspid or bicuspid) are damaged, they will not close completely. This allows blood to leak back into atria when the ventricles contract and produces an abnormal heart sound called a **murmur.** Murmurs may indicate serious heart conditions, although many times heart murmurs are harmless.

Cardiac Conduction System

The cardiac conduction system consists of a group of structures that send electrical impulses through the heart. When cardiac muscle receives an electrical impulse, it contracts (Figure 5-5). The components of the cardiac conduction system are as follows:

- **Sinoatrial node** (SA node). This node is located in the wall of the right atrium and generates an impulse that flows to the atrioventricular node. The SA node is also called the natural pacemaker of the heart because it generates the heart's rhythmic contractions.
- **Atrioventricular node** (AV node). This node is located between the atria, just above the ventricles. After the impulse reaches the AV node, the atria contract and the impulse is sent to the bundle of His.
- **bundle of His** (also known as the atrioventricular or AV bundle) This structure is located between the ventricles and splits into two branches, forming the left and right *bundle branches,* before sending the electrical impulse to the Purkinje fibers.
- **Purkinje fibers.** These fibers are located in the lateral walls of the ventricles. After the impulse flows through the Purkinje fibers, the ventricles contract and the SA node will start the flow of a new impulse.

Physicians use a test called an electrocardiogram (ECG or EKG) to tell if the cardiac conduction system is working properly. In a normal ECG, three waves are produced (Figure 5-6). The first wave (P wave) indicates that an electrical impulse was sent through the atria, which causes them to contract (depolarization). The second wave (the QRS wave) is the largest of the three and indicates that an electrical impulse was sent through the ventricles, which causes them to contract. The third wave (T wave) indicates electrical changes that are occurring in the ventricles as they relax (repolarization).

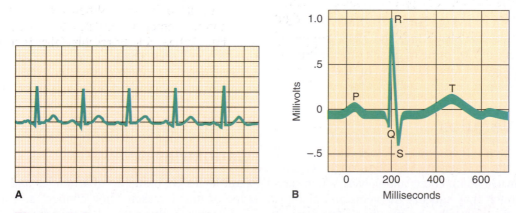

Figure 5-6. Electrocardiogram: (A) a normal ECG and (B) waves of a normal ECG pattern.

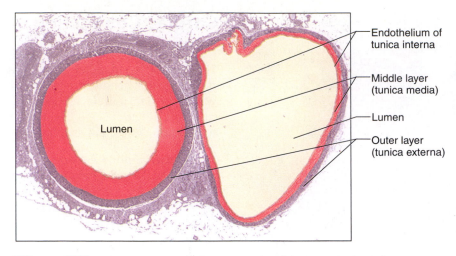

Figure 5-7. Cross-sections of an artery (left) and a vein (right).

Blood Vessels

Blood vessels form a closed pathway that carries blood from the heart to cells and back again. These vessels include arteries, arterioles, veins, venules, and capillaries.

Arteries and Arterioles

Arteries are the strongest of the blood vessels. The muscular layer of arteries contains smooth muscle and is thicker than the muscular layer of other types of blood vessels (Figure 5-7). Arteries, the largest of which is the aorta, carry blood away from the heart and are under high pressure, which is the main reason they need to have thick walls. The muscular wall of an artery can constrict (**vasoconstriction**) to increase blood pressure or it can dilate (**vasodilation**) to decrease blood pressure. Small branches of arteries are called arterioles.

The tissues of the heart receive their blood supply through coronary arteries. Branches of the coronary arteries eventually give rise to very small blood vessels called capillaries. The capillaries of the heart are in the myocardium and allow oxygen to diffuse into the cardiac muscle cells. Blood leaving capillaries in the heart go to cardiac veins. Cardiac veins eventually deliver the oxygen-poor blood to a large vein called the **coronary sinus**. The coronary sinus empties the blood into the right atrium. A myocardial infarction (MI) or heart attack often occurs as a result of blockage of one or more of the coronary arteries.

Veins and Venules

Blood is under no pressure in veins and does not move very easily. Therefore, the movement of blood through veins requires skeletal muscle contractions and valves. When skeletal muscles contract, they squeeze the veins and blood is pushed through them, much like the way toothpaste is pushed out of a tube. The valves in veins prevent blood

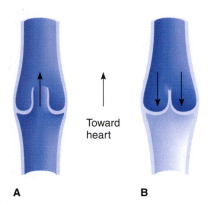

Figure 5-8. Venous valve: (A) valve opens when blood is flowing toward the heart and (B) valve closes to prevent blood from flowing away from the heart.

from flowing backward (Figure 5-8). **Varicose veins** occur when valves are destroyed and blood pools in veins, causing them to become dilated or expanded.

The sympathetic nervous system also influences the flow of blood through veins. The sympathetic nervous system causes vein walls to constrict, which forces blood through the veins. This only happens if blood pressure gets abnormally low in arteries.

Venules are very small blood vessels that are formed when capillaries merge together (Figure 5-9). Venules merge together to make veins, the largest of which are the superior and inferior venae cavae. Veins carry blood toward the heart. The muscular layer in the walls of veins is thinner than the layer found in arteries.

Capillaries

Capillaries are branches of arterioles and are the smallest type of blood vessel. They connect arterioles to venules and have very thin walls that are only about one cell layer thick. These thin walls allow substances to pass into and

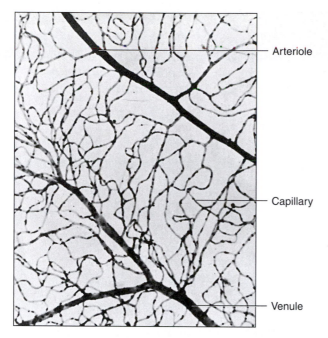

Figure 5-9. Light micrograph of a capillary network.

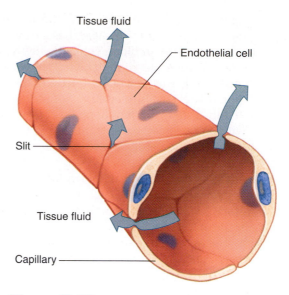

Figure 5-10. Structure of a capillary wall.

out of capillaries (Figures 5-9 and 5-10). For example, oxygen and nutrients can pass out of a capillary into a body cell, and carbon dioxide and other waste products can pass out of a body cell into a capillary. In fact, capillaries are often referred to as exchange vessels, because they are the only type of blood vessels that allow substances to move in and out of the blood.

Tissues that require a lot of oxygen, such as muscle and nervous tissues, will have a lot of capillaries. Capillary openings have precapillary sphincters that control the amount of blood that flows into them. When the sphincter relaxes, more blood flows into the capillary.

The substances that move through the capillary wall (oxygen, carbon dioxide, nutrients, water, and metabolic wastes) do so through diffusion, filtration, and osmosis (review Chapter 1). When blood first enters a capillary, it has high concentrations of oxygen and nutrients. The body cells surrounding the capillary usually have low concentrations of oxygen and nutrients but high concentrations of carbon dioxide and other waste products. Substances naturally diffuse from an area of high concentration to an area of low concentration. Therefore, oxygen and nutrients diffuse out of the capillary and into body cells. At the same time, carbon dioxide and waste products diffuse out of the body cells and into the capillary.

Because blood is under pressure as it enters the capillary, water is forced through the capillary wall via filtration. This allows water to enter a body cell. By the time blood leaves a capillary, it has a high solid concentration and a low water concentration; water therefore moves back into the capillary through osmosis. Water always moves toward the greater concentration of solids, if possible. For a review of diffusion, filtration, and osmosis, see Chapter 1, which provides more detailed explanations about these processes.

Blood Pressure

Blood pressure is defined as the force that blood exerts on the inner walls of blood vessels. Blood pressure is highest in arteries and lowest in veins. In the clinical setting, blood pressure refers to the pressure in arteries.

Arterial blood pressure rises and falls as the ventricles of the heart contract and relax. When the ventricles contract, blood pressure is greatest in the arteries. This pressure is called the **systolic pressure** or systole. When the ventricles relax, blood pressure in arteries is at its lowest. This pressure is called the **diastolic pressure** or diastole. Blood pressure is usually reported as the systolic number over the diastolic number. For example, in the blood pressure reading 120/80, 120 denotes the systolic pressure and 80 refers to the diastolic pressure.

You can feel the surge of blood through arteries when you take a pulse. The pulse is created as the artery expands when pressure increases and then subsequently relaxes as blood pressure decreases. Common places to feel a pulse are the carotid and radial arteries.

Many factors affect blood pressure, the most common being cardiac output, blood volume, vasoconstriction, and blood viscosity (thickness). Cardiac output is the total amount of blood pumped out of the heart in one minute. As cardiac output increases and decreases, blood pressure increases and decreases. When a person loses a large amount of blood, his blood pressure significantly decreases. If blood pressure falls too low, vasoconstriction, which is the tightening of blood vessel walls, helps to raise blood pressure. In contrast, if blood pressure is too high, vasodilation, which is the widening of blood vessels, decreases the blood pressure. Under certain circumstances, such as dehydration, blood becomes more viscous, or thicker, than normal. This also decreases blood pressure.

Blood pressure is controlled to a large extent by the amount of blood pumped out of the heart. The amount of blood entering the heart should be equal to the amount of blood pumped out of the heart. The heart has a way to ensure that this happens. When blood enters the left ventricle, the wall of the ventricle is stretched. The more the wall is stretched, the harder it will contract and the more blood it will pump out. This is referred to as *Starling's law of the heart*. If only a small amount of blood enters the left ventricle, it will not be stretched very much and therefore will not contract very forcefully. In this case, not much blood is pumped out of the heart.

Baroreceptors also help regulate blood pressure. Baroreceptors measure blood pressure and are located in the aorta and carotid arteries. If pressure increases in these blood vessels, this information is sent to the cardiac center in the medulla oblongata. The cardiac center then knows to decrease the heart rate, which lowers blood pressure. If pressure gets too low in the aorta, baroreceptors pick up this information and relay it to the cardiac center. The cardiac center then increases the heart rate to raise blood pressure.

Circulation

Pulmonary Circuit

The **pulmonary circuit** or pulmonary circulation is the route that blood takes from the heart to the lungs and back to the heart again. The function of this circuit is to oxygenate blood. It also allows carbon dioxide to leave blood and enter the lungs (see Figure 5-4). The pulmonary circuit can be summarized as follows:

right atrium → tricuspid valve → right ventricle → pulmonary semilunar valve → pulmonary (artery) trunk → pulmonary arteries → lungs → pulmonary veins → heart (left atrium)

Systemic Circuit

The **systemic circuit** or systemic circulation is the route blood takes from the heart through the body and back to the heart. The function of this circuit is to deliver oxygen and nutrients to body cells. It also picks up carbon dioxide and waste products from body cells (see Figure 5-4). The systemic circuit can be summarized as follows:

left atrium → bicuspid valve → left ventricle → aortic semilunar valve → aorta → arteries → arterioles → capillaries → venules → veins → venae cavae → heart (right atrium)

Arterial System

As stated earlier, arteries carry blood away from the heart. Most of them carry oxygen-rich blood, although pulmonary arteries carry oxygen-poor blood. Many arteries in the body are also paired, meaning that there is a left and a right artery of the same name. The aorta comes directly off the left ventricle and is the largest artery in the body. It has many branches that supply blood to various parts of the body.

TABLE 5-1	Major Arteries of the Body
Artery	**Anatomic Location or Organ Supplied**
Lingual	Tongue
Facial	Face
Occipital	Back of scalp and neck
Maxillary	Teeth, jaw, and eyelids
Ophthalmic	Eye
Axillary	Armpit area
Brachial	Upper arm
Ulnar	Forearm and hand
Radial	Forearm and hand
Intercostals	Rib area
Lumbar	Posterior abdominal wall
External iliac	Anterior abdominal wall
Common iliac	Legs, gluteal area, and pelvic organs
Femoral	Thigh
Popliteal	Posterior knee
Tibial	Lower leg and foot

Other arteries are summarized in Table 5-1. Also see Figure 5-11.

Venous System

Veins are blood vessels that carry blood toward the heart. Most veins in the body carry oxygen-poor blood, but the pulmonary veins are exceptions. Large veins often have the same names as the arteries they run next to. However, there are exceptions to this rule as well. For example, the veins next to carotid arteries are called jugular veins.

Large veins empty blood into vena cavae, which are the largest veins of the body. The superior vena cava generally collects blood from veins above the heart and the inferior vena cava collects blood from veins below the heart. The major veins of the body are summarized in Table 5-2. Also see Figure 5-12.

Veins of digestive organs carry blood from the digestive tract to the liver. The liver then processes nutrients in the blood and returns it to general circulation through hepatic veins. The collection of veins carrying blood to the liver is called the **hepatic portal system.**

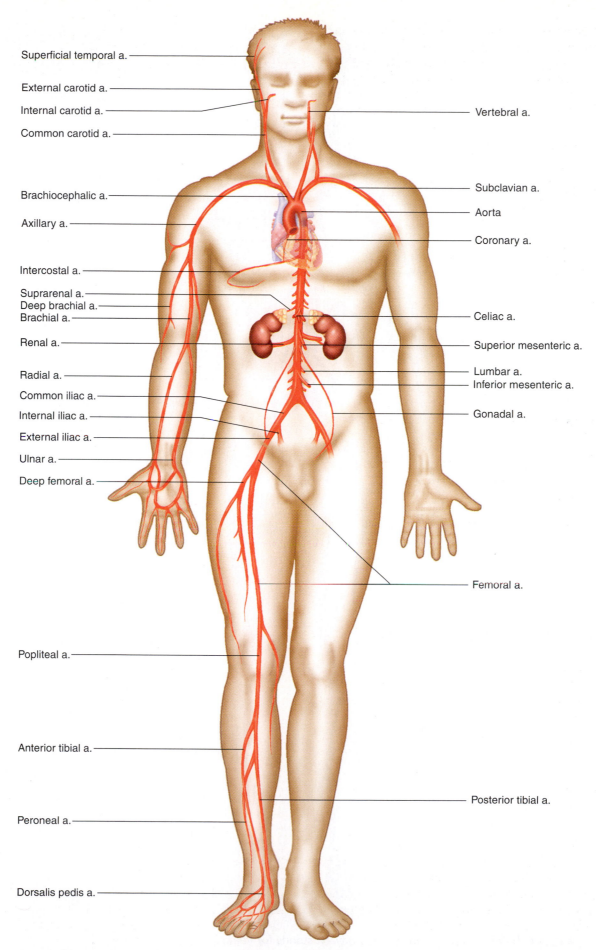

Superficial temporal a.

External carotid a.

Internal carotid a.

Common carotid a.

Brachiocephalic a.

Axillary a.

Intercostal a.

Suprarenal a.
Deep brachial a.
Brachial a.

Renal a.

Radial a.

Common iliac a.

Internal iliac a.

External iliac a.

Ulnar a.

Deep femoral a.

Popliteal a.

Anterior tibial a.

Peroneal a.

Dorsalis pedis a.

Vertebral a.

Subclavian a.

Aorta

Coronary a.

Celiac a.

Superior mesenteric a.

Lumbar a.
Inferior mesenteric a.

Gonadal a.

Femoral a.

Posterior tibial a.

Figure 5-11.   Major arteries of the body. (*a.* stands for *artery.*)

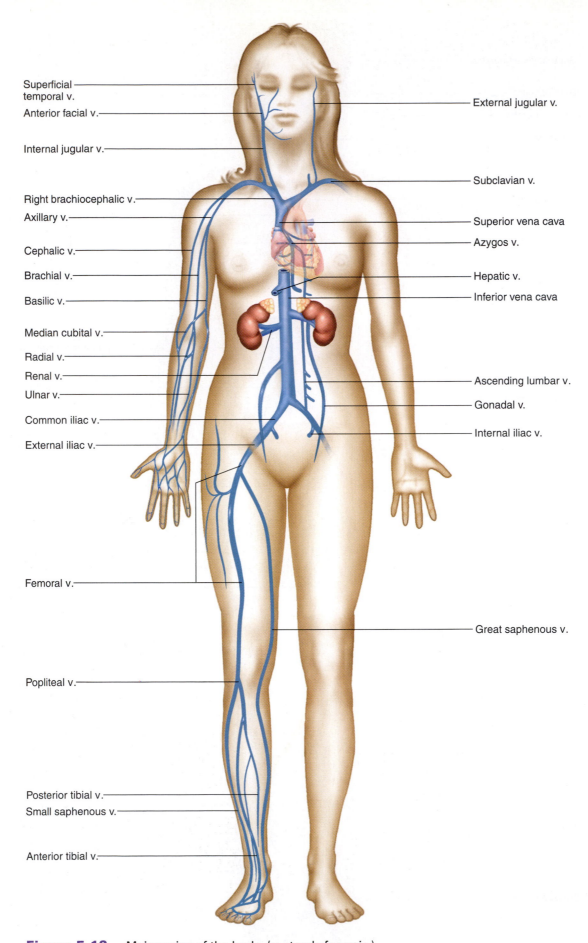

Superficial temporal v.

Anterior facial v.

Internal jugular v.

Right brachiocephalic v.

Axillary v.

Cephalic v.

Brachial v.

Basilic v.

Median cubital v.

Radial v.

Renal v.

Ulnar v.

Common iliac v.

External iliac v.

Femoral v.

Popliteal v.

Posterior tibial v.

Small saphenous v.

Anterior tibial v.

External jugular v.

Subclavian v.

Superior vena cava

Azygos v.

Hepatic v.

Inferior vena cava

Ascending lumbar v.

Gonadal v.

Internal iliac v.

Great saphenous v.

Figure 5-12. Major veins of the body. (*v.* stands for *vein.*)

TABLE 5-2	Major Veins of the Body	
Vein	**Anatomic Location or Organ Drained**	
Jugular	Head and neck	
Brachiocephalic	Head and neck	
Axillary	Armpit area	
Brachial	Upper Arm	
Ulnar	Lower arm and hand	
Radial	Lower arm and hand	
Intercostal	Thorax	
Azygos	Thorax and abdomen	
Gastric—part of the hepatic portal system	Stomach to the liver	
Splenic—part of the hepatic portal system	Spleen, pancreas, and stomach to the liver	
Mesenteric—part of the hepatic portal system	Intestines to the liver	
Hepatic portal—part of the hepatic portal system	Gastric, splenic, and mesenteric veins to the liver	
Hepatic	Liver to the inferior vena cava	
Iliac	Pelvic organs, legs, and gluteal areas	
Femoral	Thighs	
Popliteal	Knees	
Saphenous	Legs	

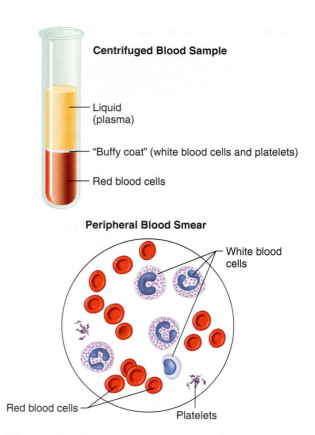

Figure 5-13. Centrifuged blood sample and peripheral blood smear showing blood components.

Blood

Blood is a type of connective tissue that is made up of multiple parts, including red and white blood cells, cell fragments called platelets, and plasma (the fluid part of the blood). An average-sized adult contains approximately 4 to 6 liters of blood. However, blood volume varies from person to person depending on the person's size, the amount of adipose tissue, and the concentrations of certain ions in the blood, with females generally having less blood volume than males.

Components of Blood

The percentage of red blood cells in a sample of blood is referred to as **hematocrit.** A healthy person normally has a hematocrit level of about 45%. Most of the cells are red blood cells, with only about 1% being white blood cells and platelets. The rest of blood (approximately 55%) is plasma (Figure 5-13).

Red Blood Cells. Red blood cells (RBCs), called **erythrocytes,** are biconcave-shaped cells that are small enough to pass through capillaries (Figure 5-14). Mature RBCs do not contain nuclei because they must lose their nuclei in order to make room for a pigment called hemoglobin. Hemoglobin's function is to carry oxygen and carbon dioxide. Hemoglobin that carries oxygen is called **oxyhemoglobin** and is bright red in color; hemoglobin that is not carrying oxygen is called **deoxyhemoglobin** and has a darker red color. Oftentimes, because the deoxyhemoglobin is now carrying carbon dioxide, it is referred to as **carboxyhemoglobin.** We now can measure the amount of carbon dioxide in the blood, just as the amount of oxygen can be measured.

An RBC count is the number of red blood cells in 1 cubic millimeter of blood (a cubic millimeter of blood is roughly 20 drops of blood). This count is normally between 4 million and 6.5 million RBCs. Because the function of an RBC is to transport oxygen throughout the body, a low count reflects a decreased ability to carry oxygen. This condition is known as **anemia.**

When RBCs age, macrophages in the liver and spleen destroy them. When an RBC is destroyed, a pigment called **biliverdin** is released from the cell. The liver usually converts biliverdin into an orange-colored pigment called **bilirubin.** Bilirubin is used to make bile, which is needed for the digestion of fats. However, sometimes bilirubin is not used to make bile; instead, it builds up in the bloodstream. This causes a person's skin to appear yellowish, which is a condition known as *jaundice.*

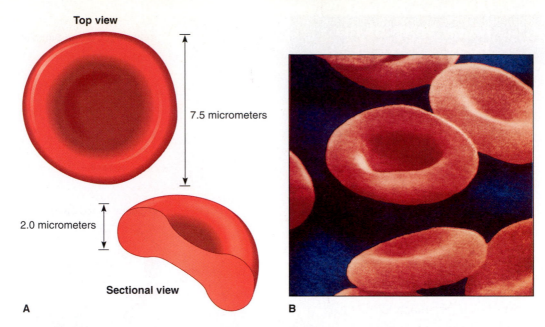

Top view

7.5 micrometers

2.0 micrometers

Sectional view

A

B

Figure 5-14. Red blood cells: (A) biconcave shape of red blood cells and (B) scanning electron micrograph of red blood cells.

During fetal development, RBCs are made in the yolk sac, the liver, and the spleen. However, once a baby is born, most blood cells are produced in red bone marrow by cells called **hemocytoblasts.** The average life span of an RBC is only about 120 days, so red bone marrow is constantly making new cells. The hormone **erythropoietin** is responsible for regulating the production of RBCs. This hormone is produced by the kidneys and stimulates the red bone marrow to produce new RBCs. The kidneys release this hormone when oxygen concentrations in the blood get low.

Vitamin B_{12} and folic acid are two dietary factors that affect RBC production. These vitamins are necessary for DNA synthesis, so any actively dividing tissue such as red bone marrow is affected when DNA cannot be produced.

Iron is also necessary to make hemoglobin. Too few RBCs or too little hemoglobin can result in anemia.

Educating the Patient

Chest Pain

Chest pain is a common reason people go to the emergency room every year. Although all chest pains should be taken seriously, they do not always indicate life-threatening heart conditions. There are two primary causes of chest pain—cardiac and noncardiac. Use the information in this box to teach patients about the conditions that cause chest pain.

The cardiac causes of chest pain include the following:

- Myocardial infarction (MI). Commonly called heart attacks, myocardial infarctions are caused by the complete blockage of coronary arteries and are life-threatening conditions. The pain associated with a heart attack is often described as pressure or fullness in the chest. Sometimes pain also occurs in the back, neck, face (especially jaw), shoulder, or arms (the left arm more than the

right). Other signs and symptoms include shortness of breath, sweating, nausea, and dizziness. Women especially are noted to have fewer of the "classic signs" of MI and should be educated about this.

- Angina. Angina is caused by a narrowing of coronary arteries and is not immediately life-threatening. However, it is an indication that the heart muscle is not receiving enough oxygen. The pain of angina is usually described as a tight feeling in the chest and is often brought about by stress or physical activity. This type of chest pain usually goes away after the stress or physical activity stops. A doctor should monitor patients with angina regularly. Most patients with angina carry sublingual nitroglycerin with them to assist with alleviating their chest pain.

continued ——➤

Educating the Patient

Chest Pain (concluded)

- Pericarditis. This condition is characterized by inflammation of the sac surrounding the heart. It usually produces a sharp and localized pain in the chest. It is not immediately life-threatening but should be treated. This condition often produces a fever.
- Coronary spasms. In this condition, coronary arteries temporarily spasm and limit blood flow to cardiac muscle tissue. The pain accompanied by coronary spasms is similar to that of angina. It should be treated as soon as possible.

The noncardiac causes of chest pain include the following:

- Heartburn. Heartburn occurs when acids from the stomach are pushed into the esophagus, and known as gastroesophageal reflux disease or GERD. Heartburn pain is described as a burning sensation. This pain usually follows a meal and gets worse if a patient bends forward or tries to lie on his or her back.
- Panic attacks. During times of intense stress or fear, chest pains can occur and are often accompanied by increased heart and breathing rates as well as excessive sweating.
- Pleurisy. This condition occurs when the membranes surrounding the lungs become inflamed. Pleurisy produces a sharp chest pain that usually feels worse when a patient coughs or inhales.
- Costochondritis. This condition occurs when the cartilage attached to ribs becomes inflamed. The chest pain associated with this condition feels much like the pain of a heart attack but generally occurs only when someone pushes on the patient's chest.
- Pulmonary embolism. This condition occurs when a blood clot blocks an artery in the lungs. The pain associated with it is severe, sharp, and increases when a patient inhales deeply or coughs. A pulmonary embolism can also produce shortness of breath, an increased heart rate, and dizziness. This condition is life-threatening.
- Sore muscles. Chest pain from sore muscles usually occurs only during body movements such as raising the arms.

- Broken ribs. Fractures of the ribs tend to produce sharp and localized chest pains.
- Inflammation of the gallbladder (cholecystitis) or pancreas (pancreatitis). Pain associated with these conditions usually begins in the abdomen and spreads to the chest.

Tests used to determine the cause of chest pain include the following:

- Electrocardiogram (ECG/EKG). This test is useful in determining if an MI is occurring or has already occurred.
- Stress tests. Stress tests are ECGs performed while a patient is exercising or has been given drugs to increase her heart rate. Stress tests are useful for determining the health of coronary blood vessels while under stress.
- Blood tests. These tests are useful in determining if a heart attack has occurred. When heart tissue is damaged, certain enzymes such as CPK and LDH are found in the blood.
- Chest x-ray. X-rays show the size and shape of the lungs and heart and can therefore indicate any serious conditions.
- Nuclear scan. These scans follow radioactive substances through the blood vessels of the heart and lungs. They can reveal narrow or obstructed arteries.
- Electron beam computerized tomography (EBCT). This procedure is much like a CT scan of the arteries. It is useful for finding narrowed arteries.
- Coronary catheterization. This procedure uses a contrast medium that is followed through coronary arteries. It can also show narrowing of the arteries.
- Echocardiogram. This procedure uses sound waves (ultrasound) to visualize the shape of the heart.
- Endoscopy. This procedure involves inserting a tube with a tiny camera down the throat and into the stomach. It helps to diagnose disorders of the stomach or esophagus that might produce chest pains.

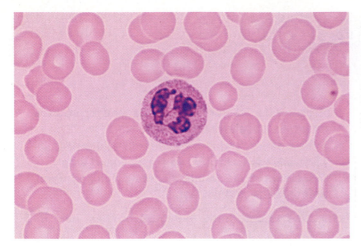

Figure 5-15. Neutrophils have distinct nuclei with many lobes.

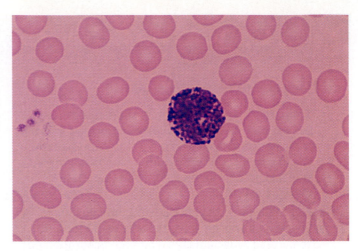

Figure 5-17. Basophils have cytoplasmic granules that stain deep blue.

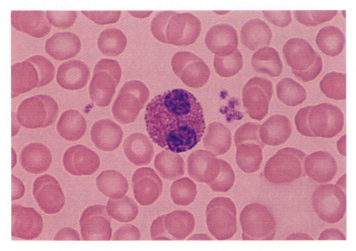

Figure 5-16. Eosinophils have cytoplasmic granules that stain red.

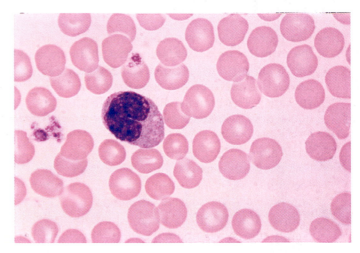

Figure 5-18. Monocytes have large kidney-shaped nuclei. They do not have cytoplasmic granules.

White Blood Cells. White blood cells (WBCs), which are called **leukocytes,** are divided into two categories: granulocytes and agranulocytes. **Granulocytes** have granules in their cytoplasm and include neutrophils, eosinophils, and basophils. **Agranulocytes** do not have granules in their cytoplasm and include monocytes and lymphocytes.

Neutrophils account for about 55% of all WBCs (Figure 5-15). As phagocytes, they are important for destroying bacteria, viruses, and toxins in the blood. **Eosinophils** account for about 3% of all WBCs and are effective in getting rid of viruses and parasitic infections such as worms (Figure 5-16). Eosinophils also help control inflammation and allergic reactions. **Basophils** account for less than 1% of all WBCs. They release substances such as histamine, which promotes inflammation, and heparin, which is an anticoagulant (Figure 5-17).

Monocytes account for about 8% of all WBCs. They are important for destroying bacteria, viruses, and toxins in the blood (Figure 5-18). **Lymphocytes** account for about 33% of all WBCs and provide immunity for the body (Figure 5-19). Lymphocytes and their specific function in the immune system will be discussed further in Chapter 10.

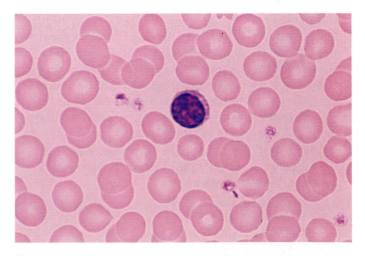

Figure 5-19. Lymphocytes have large round nuclei.

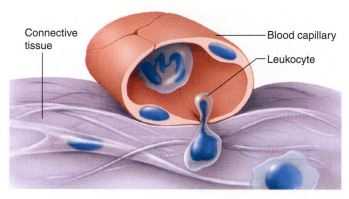

Connective tissue

Blood capillary

Leukocyte

Figure 5-20. Diapedesis of a white blood cell into surrounding tissue.

A WBC count is the number of WBCs in 1 cubic millimeter of blood. This count is normally between 5,000 and 10,000 cells. A WBC count above normal is termed **leukocytosis.** This condition often results from bacterial infections. A WBC count below normal is called **leukopenia,** which is caused by some viral infections and various other conditions.

A differential WBC count lists the percentages of the different types of leukocytes in a sample of blood. This is a useful test because the numbers of different WBCs change in certain diseases. For example, neutrophil numbers increase at the beginning of a bacterial or viral infection but monocyte numbers will not increase until about 2 weeks after a bacterial infection. Eosinophil numbers increase during viral or worm infections as well as with allergic reactions. In AIDS, lymphocyte numbers fall.

Some WBCs stay in the bloodstream to fight infections, whereas others leave the bloodstream by squeezing through blood vessel walls to reach other tissues. The squeezing of a cell through a blood vessel wall is called **diapedesis** (Figure 5-20).

Blood Platelets. **Platelets** are fragments of cells that are found in the bloodstream (see Figure 5-13). Platelets are also called **thrombocytes** and are important in the clotting process of blood. Platelets come from cells called **megakaryocytes** that are in red bone marrow. A normal platelet count is between 130,000 and 360,000 platelets per cubic millimeter of blood.

Blood Plasma. Plasma is the liquid portion of blood. It is mostly water but also contains a mixture of proteins, nutrients, gases, electrolytes, and waste products. The three major types of proteins found in plasma are albumins, globulins, and fibrinogen. **Albumins** are the smallest of the plasma proteins and are important for pulling water into the bloodstream to help maintain blood pressure. **Globulins** transport lipids and some fat-soluble vitamins in plasma. Some globulins become antibodies. **Fibrinogen** is important in the blood clotting process. The term **serum** is used for the fluid that is left when all clotting factors are removed from plasma.

Nutrients in plasma include amino acids, glucose, nucleotides, and lipids that have all been absorbed from the digestive tract. Because lipids are not water soluble and because plasma is mostly water, lipids must combine with molecules called **lipoproteins** to be transported. The different types of lipoproteins are **chylomicrons,** very low-density lipoproteins (VLDL), low-density lipoproteins (LDL), and high-density lipoproteins (HDL).

The gases dissolved in plasma include oxygen, carbon dioxide, and nitrogen. Many electrolytes are dissolved in plasma. They include sodium, potassium, calcium, magnesium, chloride, bicarbonate, phosphate, and sulfate. Molecules that contain nitrogen but are not proteins make up a group called nonprotein nitrogenous substances. They include amino acids, urea, and uric acid. Urea and uric acid are waste products produced by cells.

Bleeding Control

Hemostasis refers to the control of bleeding. This is important when blood vessels are damaged and bleeding begins. Three processes occur in hemostasis: (1) blood vessel spasm, (2) platelet plug formation, and (3) blood coagulation.

When a blood vessel breaks, the smooth muscle at the site of the damage in its wall contracts and causes the blood vessel to spasm. This spasm reduces the amount of blood lost through the vessel. Platelets also begin to stick to the broken area and to each other to form a platelet plug. The platelet plug slows or controls the bleeding temporarily (Figure 5-21).

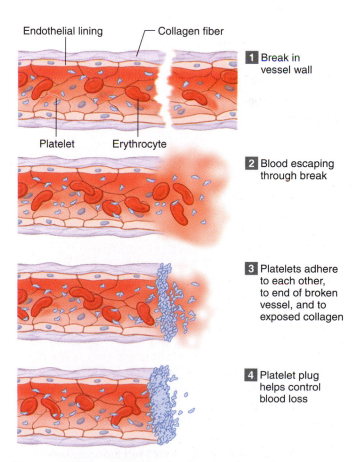

Endothelial lining — Collagen fiber

Platelet   Erythrocyte

1 Break in vessel wall

2 Blood escaping through break

3 Platelets adhere to each other, to end of broken vessel, and to exposed collagen

4 Platelet plug helps control blood loss

Figure 5-21. Steps in platelet plug formation.

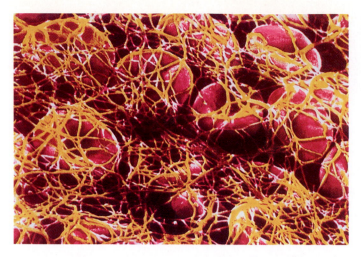

Figure 5-22. Scanning electron micrograph of a blood clot. Yellow fibrin threads are covering red blood cells.

A blood clot eventually replaces the platelet plug. The formation of a blood clot is called blood **coagulation.** In this process, the plasma protein fibrinogen is converted to fibrin. Once fibrin forms, it sticks to the damaged area of the blood vessel, creating a meshwork that entraps blood cells and platelets. The resulting mass, the blood clot, stops bleeding until the vessel has repaired itself (Figure 5-22).

When a blood vessel is injured, it is normal for a blood clot to form. However, sometimes blood clots form on the side of a blood vessel with no known injury; this abnormal blood clot is called a **thrombus.** The danger of a thrombus is that a portion of it can break off and start moving through the bloodstream. The moving portion of the thrombus is called an **embolus.** An embolus is dangerous because it will eventually block a small artery. An embolus that originates in the vein of a leg travels to the right atrium of the heart through the inferior vena cava and is pumped by the right ventricle to the lungs. Here the embolus gets stuck in a small artery and causes pulmonary embolism. If the embolus lodges in a coronary artery, an MI may develop. If the embolus blocks a cerebral artery, the result may be a **cerebrovascular accident** (CVA) or stroke. All of these are serious and possibly fatal conditions if not treated or if treatment can not be initiated quickly enough.

Blood Types

The ABO blood group consists of four different blood types: A, B, AB, and O. They are distinguished from each other in part by their antigens and antibodies.

Agglutination is the clumping of RBCs following a blood transfusion. This clumping is not desirable because it leads to severe anemia. Agglutination occurs because proteins called *antigens* on the surface of RBCs bind to antibodies in plasma (Figure 5-23). To prevent agglutination, antigens should not be mixed with antibodies that

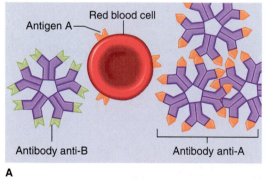

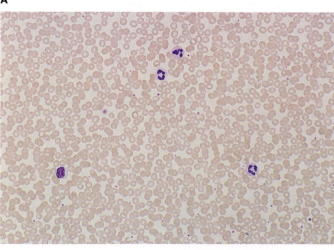

A

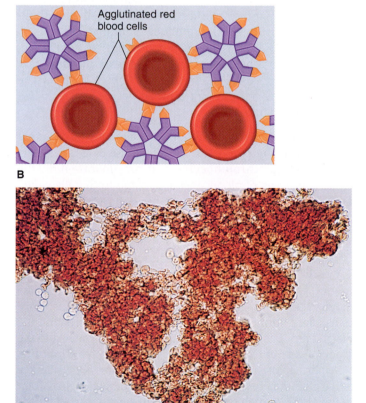

B

C

D

Figure 5-23. Agglutination: (A) red blood cells with antigen A are added to blood that contains antibody anti-A; (B) antibody anti-A reacts with antigen A, causing the agglutination of blood; (C) normal blood; and (D) agglutinated blood.

TABLE 5-3 ABO Blood Group

Blood Type	Antigen Present	Antibody Present	Blood That Can Be Received
A	A	B	A and O
B	B	A	B and O
AB	A and B	None	A, B, AB, and O
O	None	A and B	O

will bind to them. Fortunately, most antibodies do not bind to antigens on blood cells; only very specific ones bind to them.

Type A. People with type A blood have antigen A on the surface of their RBCs. They also have antibody B in their plasma. Antibody B will only bind to antigen B.

Type B. People with type B blood have antigen B on the surface of their RBCs. They also have antibody A in their plasma.

If a person with type A blood is given type B blood, then the antibody B in the recipient's blood will bind with the RBCs of the donor blood because those cells have antigen B on their surfaces. Therefore, agglutination occurs, and the donated RBCs are destroyed. This is why a person with type A blood should not be given type B blood (and vice versa).

Type AB. People with type AB blood have both antigen A and antigen B on the surface of their RBCs. They have neither antibody A nor antibody B in their plasma. People with type AB blood are called universal recipients, because most of them can receive all ABO blood types.

They can receive these blood types because they lack antibody A and antibody B in their plasma, so there is no reaction with antigens A and B of the donor blood.

Type O. People with type O blood have neither antigen A nor antigen B on the surface of their RBCs. However, they do have both antibody A and antibody B in their plasma. People with type O blood are called universal donors because their blood can be given to most people regardless of recipient's blood type. Type O blood will not agglutinate when given to other people because it does not have the antigens to bind to antibody A or antibody B. Table 5-3 summarizes the ABO blood group. Also see Figure 5-24.

The Rh Factor. The **Rh antigen** is a protein first discovered on RBCs of the Rhesus monkey, hence the name Rh. People who are Rh-positive have RBCs that contain the Rh antigen. People who are Rh-negative have RBCs that do not contain the Rh antigen. If a person who is Rh-negative is given Rh-positive blood, then the Rh-negative person's blood will make antibodies that bind to the Rh antigens. If the Rh-negative person is given Rh-positive blood a second time, the antibodies will bind to the donor cells and agglutination will occur.

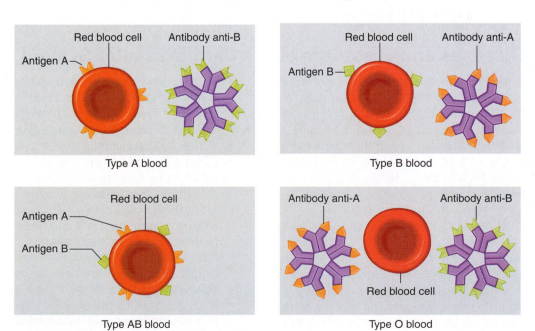

Figure 5-24. A, B, AB, and O blood types.

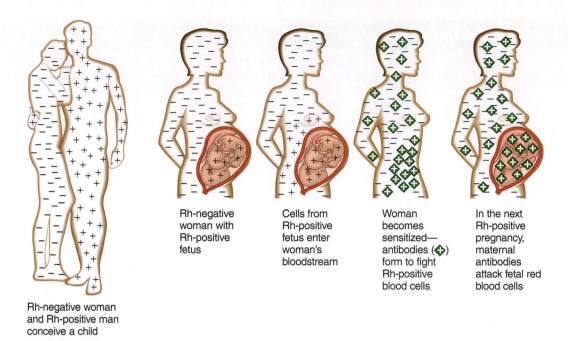

Rh-negative
woman with
Rh-positive
fetus

Cells from
Rh-positive
fetus enter
woman's
bloodstream

Woman
becomes
sensitized—
antibodies (⊕)
form to fight
Rh-positive
blood cells

In the next
Rh-positive
pregnancy,
maternal
antibodies
attack fetal red
blood cells

Rh-negative woman
and Rh-positive man
conceive a child

Figure 5-25. Development of antibodies in an Rh-negative woman in relation to the blood of her Rh-positive fetus.

Clinically, it is very important for a female to know her Rh type. If an Rh-negative female mates with an Rh-positive male, there is a fifty-fifty chance that her fetus will be Rh-positive. When the blood of an Rh-positive fetus mixes with the blood of a mother who is Rh-negative, the mother develops antibodies against the fetus's RBCs. The first Rh-positive fetus usually does not suffer from these antibodies because it takes so long for the mother's body to generate them. However, if the mother conceives a second Rh-positive fetus, the fetus's blood will be attacked by the antibodies right away. The second fetus then develops a condition called **erythroblastosis fetalis,** and the baby is born severely anemic, often needing multiple blood transfusions at birth and often several times as a neonate (Figure 5-25). Erythroblastosis fetalis is prevented by giving an Rh-negative woman the drug **RhoGAM.** RhoGAM prevents an Rh-negative mother from making antibodies against the Rh antigen.

Pathophysiology

Common Diseases and Disorders of the Cardiovascular System

Anemia is a condition in which a person does not have enough RBCs or hemoglobin in the blood to carry an adequate amount of oxygen to the body's cells. It is the most common blood disorder in the United States and can be a sign of a more serious disorder. It generally affects more women than men. Many types of anemia can be prevented through a healthy diet high in iron, vitamin B_{12}, and folic acid. Others types of anemia require medical attention for more serious, underlying conditions.

- **Causes.** The causes of this condition are many and include the following:
  - Iron deficiency. Iron deficiency is the most common cause of anemia. Iron is needed to make hemoglobin, which is the pigment that carries most oxygen in the blood. Pregnant women and women with heavy menstrual cycles are most susceptible to this type of anemia.

- Chronic blood loss. Slow blood loss can occur in conditions such as ulcers, colon polyps, or colon cancer.
- Vitamin deficiency. Vitamin B_{12} and folic acid are needed to make enough RBCs.
- Inability to absorb vitamin B_{12}. This condition is called *pernicious anemia.* Some intestinal disorders prevent the absorption of vitamin B_{12}.
- Side effect of medication. Some oral contraceptives, seizure medications, and anti-neoplastic drugs used to treat cancer can cause anemia.
- Chronic illness. Chronic diseases such as AIDS, cancer, rheumatoid arthritis, leukemia, and kidney failure can cause anemia.
- Bone marrow disorder. When the bone marrow fails to produce enough blood cells, *aplastic anemia* results. This is a life-threatening type of anemia.

continued ⟶

Common Diseases and Disorders of the Cardiovascular System *(continued)*

Toxins, chemotherapy, and radiation therapy can all destroy bone marrow.

- Destruction of RBCs. Some blood diseases, such as *sickle cell disease,* cause RBCs to be destroyed faster than they can be made. These types of anemia are called **hemolytic anemias.**

- **Signs and symptoms.** Signs and symptoms of all forms of anemia include tiredness, weakness, pallor (paleness), tachycardia, numb or cold hands and feet, dizziness, headache, and jaundice.

- **Treatment.** Injections of vitamin B$_{12}$ may be necessary. Treatment often begins with addressing the underlying causes, such as an ulcer or colon polyps. Other treatment options include administering various medications, discontinuing the use of medications that can cause anemia, and blood transfusions or bone marrow transplants if defective or diseased bone marrow is the cause.

An **aneurysm** is defined as a ballooned, weakened arterial wall. The most common locations of aneurysms are the aorta and arteries in the brain, legs, intestines, and spleen. An aortic aneurysm is a bulge in the wall of the aorta. Most aortic aneurysms occur in the abdominal aorta (abdominal aortic aneurysm) but some occur in the thoracic aorta. Most aortic aneurysms do not rupture; however, when they do, the resultant hemorrhage is a serious life-threatening emergency.

- **Causes.** Most causes are unknown. One identified risk to developing an aneurysm is **atherosclerosis,** which is a hardening of the fatty plaque deposits within the arteries, usually associated with a diet high in cholesterol. Smoking and obesity also increase the risk of atherosclerosis. Congenital conditions may cause an aneurysm—some individuals are born with weak aortic walls. A traumatic injury to the chest may also be a risk factor. The risk of developing an aneurysm can be reduced by not smoking, losing excess weight, and by having a diet low in fats and cholesterol. Periodic screening is an option for patients with a family history of aortic aneurysms.

- **Signs and symptoms.** There are usually no signs and symptoms of an aneurysm, although hypertension can be a sign. When symptoms do exist, a pulsation in the abdomen and back pain are the most commonly seen. A sudden pain in the abdomen or back, dizziness, a fast pulse, or a loss of consciousness are signs that an aneurysm has ruptured.

- **Treatment.** The primary treatment is surgery to repair the aneurysm.

Arrhythmias are abnormal heart rhythms in which the heart beats too quickly (tachycardia) or too slowly (bradycardia). The most common type of heart arrhythmia is atrial fibrillation, which is a sporadic and rapid beating of the atria. The most serious type of heart arrhythmia is ventricular fibrillation, which produces ineffective contractions of the ventricles. Most sudden cardiac deaths are caused by ventricular fibrillation.

- **Causes.** These abnormal rhythms usually result when electrical impulses of the cardiac conduction system do not flow correctly through the heart. The list of risk factors and causes is long and includes electrical shock, certain drugs, herbal supplements containing ephedra (although most have been removed from the market because of the high risk of arrhythmias), high blood pressure, previous heart attack, decreased blood flow to the heart, coronary artery disease, heart valve disorders, weakening of the heart muscle (cardiomyopathy), some genetic diseases such as Wolff-Parkison-White syndrome, thyroid conditions, diabetes mellitus, sleep apnea, electrolyte imbalances (including potassium, sodium, and calcium), excess alcohol consumption, smoking, caffeine consumption, and drugs such as amphetamines or cocaine.

- **Signs and symptoms.** Symptoms include shortness of breath, dizziness or fainting, an uncharacteristically rapid or slow heart rate, a fluttering feeling in the chest, and chest pain.

- **Treatment.** The first management of arrhythmias should be to treat the underlying cause. Other treatment options include the following:
  - Pacemakers.
  - Various medications such as beta blockers and anti-arrhythmics.
  - Cardiopulmonary resuscitation if there is no evidence of blood flow.
  - Vagal maneuvers to slow the heart rate. These include holding the breath, straining (bearing down as if the patient is having a bowel movement), or putting one's face in cool water.
  - Electrical shock (defibrillation) to reset heart rhythms.
  - Radiofrequency catheter ablation, a procedure that destroys a small amount of heart tissue in order to change the flow of the electrical current through the heart.
  - Implantation of an ICD (implantable cardioverter defibrillator), a device that regulates heart rhythms.
  - *Maze* procedure, which is an operation to form scars in the atria. These scars correct the electrical flow through the heart.
  - Surgery to correct heart defects such as narrow coronary arteries.

Carditis is an inflammation of the heart. It is more specifically referred to as *endocarditis, myocarditis,* or *pericarditis,* depending on the layer of the heart that is affected.

continued ⟶

Common Diseases and Disorders of the Cardiovascular System *(continued)*

Endocarditis is an inflammation of the innermost lining of the heart, including the heart valves.

- **Causes.** Bacterial infections are the most common cause of endocarditis. Patients are more susceptible to this condition if they have abnormal heart valves.
- **Signs and symptoms.** Common signs and symptoms include weakness, fever, excessive sweating, general body aches, difficulty breathing, and blood in the urine.
- **Treatment.** The treatment for this condition is intravenous antibiotics followed by oral antibiotics for up to 6 weeks.

Myocarditis is an inflammation of the muscular layer of the heart. It is relatively uncommon but very serious because it leads to weakening of the heart wall.

- **Causes.** The most common cause of myocarditis is a viral infection, but it may also be caused by exposure to certain chemicals, allergens, and bacteria.
- **Signs and symptoms.** Signs and symptoms include fever as well as chest pains that feel like a heart attack. Difficulty breathing, decreased urine output, fatigue, and fainting may also accompany myocarditis.
- **Treatment.** Treatment normally includes steroids to reduce inflammation, bed rest, and a low-sodium diet.

Pericarditis is inflammation of the pericardium, which is a group of membranes that surround the heart.

- **Causes.** This condition is most commonly caused by complications of viral or bacterial infections. However, heart attacks and chest injuries can also lead to pericarditis.
- **Signs and symptoms.** Symptoms include sharp, stabbing chest pains, especially during deep breaths. Fever, fatigue, and difficulty breathing while lying down are also common symptoms.
- **Treatment.** The treatment usually includes painkillers. Diuretics are used to remove excess fluids around the heart. If pericarditis is caused by bacteria, antibiotics are used. In chronic cases, surgery may be required to remove part of the membranes surrounding the heart.

Congestive heart failure is a slowly developing condition in which the heart weakens over time. Eventually, the heart is no longer able to pump enough blood to meet the body's needs.

- **Causes.** There are many risk factors for this condition, including smoking, being overweight, a diet high in cholesterol, a lack of exercise, atherosclerosis, history of MI, high blood pressure, a damaged heart valve, excessive alcohol consumption, and diabetes mellitus. Congenital heart defects (those present at birth) and drugs that weaken the heart (especially cocaine,

heroin, and some antineoplastic drugs for cancer) may also contribute to the development of this disorder. This condition may be prevented by controlling high blood pressure and high cholesterol, not smoking, maintaining a healthy diet, engaging in regular exercise, and treating any existing atherosclerosis or diabetes.

- **Signs and symptoms.** Signs and symptoms include shortness of breath; constant wheezing; prominent neck veins; fluid retention that causes swelling in the legs, feet, or abdomen; nausea; dizziness; and an irregular or rapid heartbeat.
- **Treatment.** Common treatment options include medications to slow a rapid heartbeat, diuretics to decrease edema and fluid accumulation in the lungs, and medications to reduce blood pressure. In more serious cases, surgery to repair defective heart valves or other heart defects, implantation of a cardiac pacemaker, or a heart transplant may be needed.

Coronary artery disease (CAD) is also known as atherosclerosis. It affects more Americans than any other type of heart disease. Males and African Americans are more likely to develop coronary artery disease than are women or Caucasians. However, the gap between men and women regarding heart disease is closing rapidly, with more and more women (and Caucasians) being diagnosed with CAD.

- **Causes.** This condition is characterized by the narrowing of coronary arteries. Usually the narrowing is produced by the buildup of fat, cholesterol, and calcium in the arteries. The risk factors for developing this condition include high levels of LDL cholesterol in the blood, a diet high in fat and cholesterol, smoking, high blood pressure, obesity, a lack of exercise, and diabetes mellitus. As with congestive heart failure, this condition may be prevented by controlling high blood pressure and high cholesterol, not smoking, having a healthy diet, engaging in regular exercise, and treating any existing diabetes and/or atherosclerosis.
- **Signs and symptoms.** There are often no signs or symptoms until a heart attack occurs. The most common symptoms include angina (a type of chest pain caused by a decreased blood flow to the heart), shortness of breath, tightness in the chest, fatigue, and swelling in the legs or feet (edema).
- **Treatment.** Treatment includes lipid-lowering agents such as Mevacor and Lipitor in addition to a low-fat diet and exercise, aspirin therapy, and medications to slow a rapid heartbeat. Surgery such as coronary angioplasty or, in severe cases or those not responding to angioplasty, CABG (coronary artery bypass grafting) to repair, widen, or detour around narrowed coronary arteries may be needed.

continued ⟶

Common Diseases and Disorders of the Cardiovascular System *(continued)*

Hypertension, commonly known as high blood pressure, is defined as a consistent resting blood pressure measured at 140/90 mm Hg or higher. This condition is commonly known as the "silent killer" because it increases a person's risk of heart attack, stroke, heart failure, and kidney failure, while often presenting no symptoms to the patient. African Americans are twice as likely to have high blood pressure as Caucasians are.

- **Causes.** Many of the causes are unknown. Known causes and risk factors include narrowing of the arteries, various medications such as oral contraceptives and cold medicines, kidney disease, endocrine disorders, pregnancy, drug use (especially cocaine and amphetamines), sleep apnea, obesity, smoking, a high-sodium diet, excessive alcohol consumption, stress, and diabetes.
- **Signs and symptoms.** There are usually no symptoms to hypertension. When symptoms do present, they include excessive sweating, muscle cramps, fatigue, frequent urination, headaches, dizziness and an irregular heart rate.
- **Treatment.** The first management tool of hypertension control should be to treat the underlying cause if known. Other common treatments include a diet low in sodium and cholesterol, regular exercise, various medications to slow the heart rate and dilate blood vessels, diuretics to reduce blood volume, and lifestyle changes such as managing stress and stopping smoking. Patient compliance is the key to the successful management of hypertension, which most often cannot be cured, only controlled. Because hypertension itself often has no symptoms and medications just as often have side effects, patients frequently stop their anti-hypertensive regimes because "I felt better off the medication." Be sure that they understand that medication compliance is crucial to their treatment and long-term health. They must tell the physician when a medication is not working for them because there are often many options available for treatment.

Leukemia is a condition in which the bone marrow produces a large number of WBCs that are not normal. These abnormal cells prevent normal WBCs from carrying out their defensive functions. This disorder is sometimes referred to as cancer of the WBCs. There are several different kinds of leukemia: acute lymphocytic (lymphatic) leukemia, acute myelogenous leukemia, chronic lymphocytic (lymphatic) leukemia, and chronic myelogenous leukemia.

- **Causes.** Causes include mutations (changes) in WBCs, chemotherapy for the treatment of other cancers, genetic factors (for example, the inheritance of abnormal genes), and exposure to environmental and chemical agents that cause changes in the WBCs.

- **Signs and symptoms.** The signs and symptoms are many and include fatigue, dyspnea on exertion (DOE), an enlarged liver (hepatomegaly) or spleen (splenomegaly), swollen (nontender) lymph nodes, abnormal bruising, cuts that heal slowly, frequent infections, nosebleeds, bleeding gums, chronic fever, unexplained weight loss, and excessive sweating.
- **Treatment.** Treatment options include chemotherapy, radiation therapy, medications to strengthen the immune system, antibodies to destroy mutated WBCs, bone marrow transplant, and stem cell transplant.

Murmurs are simply defined as abnormal heart sounds. Normally, heart sounds are clear, strong, and smooth as valves close completely, and blood flows over the lining of the heart with no resistance. Not all murmurs indicate a heart disorder. Murmurs are graded from 1 to 6, 1 being barely audible (and the least serious).

- **Causes.** Not all the causes of heart murmurs are known. In children, the failure of the foramen ovale or ductus arteriosis to close completely after birth can cause murmurs. Other causes include stress and defective heart valves that do not close completely.
- **Signs and symptoms.** The signs and symptoms vary considerably depending on the cause and severity of the heart murmur. Severe symptoms include weakness, pallor, edema (fluid retention), and other common signs associated with heart failure.
- **Treatment.** Many times, no treatment is required. Surgery to correct valvular defects or other heart defects may be needed in more serious cases.

A **myocardial infarction,** commonly called a heart attack, is characterized by damage to cardiac muscle because of a lack of blood supply. Historically, heart attacks have been and often still are fatal, but with new treatments, more and more people survive MIs. However, they can be left with permanent damage because cardiac muscle does not grow back once it is lost.

- **Causes.** The causes and contributing factors include blockage of coronary arteries as a result of atherosclerosis or a blood clot. Drugs such as cocaine can also cause coronary arteries to spasm. Preventing an MI includes treating or reducing the risk of atherosclerosis, including the use of lipid-lowering agents to lower cholesterol. This condition may be further prevented by controlling high blood pressure, not smoking, having a healthy diet, engaging in regular physical exercise, and avoiding the use of drugs such as cocaine.
- **Signs and symptoms.** Common symptoms include recurring, squeezing chest pain; pain in the shoulder, arm, back, teeth, or jaw; chronic pain in the upper abdomen; shortness of breath, especially on exertion; sweating (diaphoresis); dizziness or fainting; and nausea or vomiting.

continued ⟶

- **Treatment.** The first treatment, if possible, is chewing an aspirin at the onset of symptoms. In an unconscious patient without a pulse or respiration, CPR (cardiopulmonary resuscitation) should be administered. Other treatment options include the use of a defibrillator (if available) and thrombolytic drugs to destroy the blood clots that block a coronary artery. It should be noted that these drugs are only effective if begun within 3 hours of the first symptom, so time is crucial. Anti-coagulant medications, such as heparin and warfarin, should be administered to thin the blood, as well as those that slow the heart rate, such as atenalol. Surgery to replace or repair blocked coronary arteries (angioplasty or CABG) may also be necessary.

Sickle cell anemia is a condition in which abnormal hemoglobin causes RBCs to change to a sickle (crescent) shape. These sickle-shaped RBCs get stuck in capillaries. Sickle cell anemia affects about 1 in every 500 African Americans and 1 in every 1400 Hispanics born in the United States.

- **Causes.** The primary cause is hereditary. As an autosomal recessive disorder, a person with this disease must inherit a sickle cell gene from both parents. If only one sickle cell gene is inherited, the person is said to have sickle cell trait and may have only mild symptoms of the disease. However, the person with sickle cell trait may pass the trait or the disease on to his or her children. This condition may be prevented through genetic screening of the parents.
- **Signs and symptoms.** The signs and symptoms are many and include anemia, periodic episodes of pain called *crises*, chest pain, numbness in the hands or legs, fainting, fatigue, swollen hands and feet, jaundice, frequent infections, sores on the skin, delayed growth, stroke, seizures, and breathing difficulties. Retina damage, which causes visual problems, and spleen, liver, or kidney and lung damage may also be seen.
- **Treatment.** There is no cure for sickle cell disease, but treatment includes antibiotics to treat infections, blood transfusions, pain medications, bone marrow transplants, supplemental oxygen, and medications to promote the development of normal hemoglobin.

Thalassemia is an inherited form of anemia with a defective hemoglobin chain causing micocytic (small), hypochromic (pale), and short-lived RBCs.

- **Causes.** The primary cause is hereditary. Patients of Mediterranean descent are most likely to carry the defective autosomal recessive gene that causes this disease. Like sickle cell, thalassemia comes in two forms. *Thalassemia major* is the disease. Patients with *thalassemia minor* have only minimal symptoms, if any; this form is considered to be a "carrier" form of the disease. Also like sickle cell, both parents must send the defective gene to the child in order for the child to be diagnosed with this disease. Inheriting only one gene results in the carrier status.

- **Signs and symptoms.** Thalassemia major is evident in infancy with anemia, fever, failure to thrive, and splenomegaly (enlarged spleen). It is confirmed by the characteristic changes in RBCs noted on microscopic examination. As the child matures, splenomegaly may interfere with breathing. In addition, skin becomes freckled or bronzed from the iron deposits created by the rapidly destroyed RBCs. Headache, nausea, and anorexia are common signs and symptoms.
- **Treatment.** There is no cure for thalassemia. Frequent transfusions are necessary to treat the anemia caused by the destruction of the defective RBCs. A splenectomy may be recommended. Symptoms are otherwise treated as needed, including pain medication for the acute episodes known as crises, which are similar to those of sickle cell patients. Patients and their families may require counseling to assist with dealing with the day-to-day reality of this disease.

Thrombophlebitis is a condition in which a blood clot and inflammation develop in a vein. It most commonly occurs in the veins of the legs. The danger of this disorder is that the blood clot may break loose (embolism). Once it reaches the heart, it is pumped to the lungs. If it blocks a blood vessel, it will cause a pulmonary embolism (an obstruction in the lungs). If the blood clot reaches the aorta and is pumped into arterial circulation, it can block a coronary artery, causing a heart attack, or it can block a cerebral artery in the brain, causing a CVA (stroke).

- **Causes.** The causes and risk factors include prolonged inactivity, oral contraceptives, post-menopausal estrogen replacement therapy, certain types of cancer, paralysis in the arms or legs, the presence of a venous catheter, a family history of this condition, varicose veins, and trauma to veins.
- **Signs and symptoms.** The most common symptoms are tenderness and pain in the affected area; redness, swelling, and tenseness of the affected areas; fever; and a positive Homan's sign.
- **Treatment.** This disorder is most often treated by the application of heat to the affected area, elevation of the legs, anti-inflammatory drugs, anti-coagulant medications, the wearing of support stockings, and the removal of varicose veins. Surgery to remove the clot may be needed in some cases.

Varicose veins are twisted, dilated veins that are usually seen in the legs. They affect women more often than men. When varicose veins occur in the rectum, they are called *hemorrhoids*.

- **Causes.** Varicose veins may be caused by prolonged sitting or standing, damage to valves in the veins,

continued ⟶

a loss of elasticity in the veins, obesity, pregnancy, oral contraceptives, or hormone replacement therapy. Family history also seems to play a part in the development of varicose veins. In some cases, varicose veins may be prevented or at least minimized through exercise and elevation of the legs.

- **Signs and symptoms.** Signs and symptoms include discomfort in the legs, discolorations around the ankles, clusters of veins, and enlarged, dark veins that are seen through skin.

- **Treatment.** The treatment of varicose veins includes the following:
  - Sclerotherapy, which is a procedure that prevents blood from flowing through varicose veins.
  - Laser surgery to prevent blood from flowing through affected veins.
  - Vein stripping, which involves removing affected veins.
  - Insertion of a catheter in the affected veins in order to destroy them.
  - Endoscopic vein surgery to close off affected veins.

Summary

The cardiovascular system acts as the transport system for the body. It brings oxygen to tissues and carries away carbon dioxide. Nutrients are picked up from the digestive system and delivered throughout the body, whereas waste products are carried away so that certain organs may remove them. The cardiovascular system consists of the heart and blood vessels and includes arteries, veins, and capillaries.

Blood is the transport medium that is pumped throughout the body. It is a liquid tissue that consists of plasma and formed elements (RBCs, WBCs, and platelets). It is important for the medical assistant to have an understanding of this system in order to effectively perform electrocardiograms, phlebotomy, and blood tests. Additionally, the more you understand the diseases and disorders related to these body systems, the better you can assist patients in understanding the prevention and treatment for many of these conditions.

REVIEW

CHAPTER 5

CASE STUDY QUESTIONS

Now that you have completed this chapter, review the case study at the beginning of the chapter and answer the following questions:

1. What symptoms suggest that this patient is suffering from coronary artery disease and not some other disorder?
2. Why is it important to test the heart under stress rather than obtaining a resting echocardiogram?
3. What lifestyle changes should this patient make to prevent future heart attacks?
4. Why is a cardiac catheterization needed in addition to the stress echocardiogram?
5. What are the treatment options for this patient?

Discussion Questions

1. Trace the flow of blood from the superior and inferior venae cavae and back.
2. List the components of plasma and give the importance of each.
3. Explain the cardiac conduction system and relate it to the PQRS complex of an ECG reading.

Critical Thinking Questions

1. Why is it important for a woman to know her Rh blood type either before she gets pregnant or early into her pregnancy?
2. Where are the three locations in the body where an embolus is the most dangerous? What condition(s) will it cause in each location?
3. Explain the basic functions of each type of blood cell. Give the two categories of white blood cells and the names of each white blood cell type found in each of these categories.

Application Activities

1. For each blood type, give the antigen present on the RBCs and the antibody present in plasma:
   a. Type A
   b. Type B
   c. Type AB
   d. Type O
2. Give the name of the artery and vein supplying and draining each of the body areas listed below:
   a. upper arm
   b. face
   c. armpit
   d. head and neck
   e. forearm and hand
   f. abdominal organs and abdominal wall
   g. pelvic organs
   h. thigh
   i. lower leg including knee
3. Explain how two patients, one with a low RBC count and a normal hemoglobin and the other with a normal RBC count but low hemoglobin, may both be diagnosed with anemia.
4. Tell how the following affect systemic blood pressure:
   a. An increase in stroke volume
   b. A decrease in peripheral resistance
   c. A decrease in blood volume
   d. Vasoconstriction of systemic arteries

Virtual Fieldtrip

Visit the McGraw-Hill Higher Education Medical Assisting website at www.mhhe.com/medicalassisting3 to complete the following activity:

On the American Heart Association (AHA) home page, choose the link for heart attack and stroke warning signs. Answer the following questions:

- Both of these conditions are potentially deadly, but how is each ranked on the "killer" listing from the AHA?
- How do heart attack symptoms differ between men and women?
- What are the warning signs for stroke?

Open the CD and complete this chapter's practice activities, play the games, listen to the key terms, and test yourself with the interactive review. E-mail, print, and/or save your results to document your proficiency.

CHAPTER 6

The Respiratory System

CHAPTER OUTLINE

- Organs of the Respiratory System
- The Mechanisms of Breathing
- The Transport of Oxygen and Carbon Dioxide in the Blood
- Respiratory Volumes

LEARNING OUTCOMES

After completing Chapter 6, you will be able to:

6.1 Explain the functions of the respiratory system.

6.2 Explain the difference between internal respiration and external respiration.

6.3 Describe how the larynx produces voice sounds.

6.4 List the structures contained within the lungs.

6.5 Describe the coverings of the lungs and chest cavity.

6.6 Describe the events that lead to the inspiration and expiration of air.

6.7 Explain how the brain controls breathing and how normal breathing patterns can be disrupted.

6.8 Describe how oxygen is transported from the lungs to body cells.

6.9 Describe how carbon dioxide is transported from body cells to the lungs.

6.10 List and explain various respiratory volumes and tell how they are used to diagnose respiratory problems.

6.11 Describe the causes, signs and symptoms, and treatments of various diseases and disorders of the respiratory system.

KEY TERMS

allergic rhinitis
alveoli
anthracosis
asbestosis
asthma
atelectasis
bicarbonate ions
bronchi
bronchial tree
bronchioles
chronic obstructive
    pulmonary disease
    (COPD)
coryza
cricoid cartilage
diaphoresis
dyspnea
emphysema
empyema
epiglottic cartilage
epiglottis
expiration
glottis
hemoptysis
hemothorax
hydrothorax
hyperventilation
hypoxia
inspiration
larynx
nares
nasal conchae
nasal septum
orthopnea
paranasal sinuses

KEY TERMS *(Concluded)*

pharynx	respiratory volume	thyroid cartilage
pleura	severe acute respiratory	trachea
pleural effusion	syndrome (SARS)	upper respiratory (tract)
pleurisy	silicosis	infection
pleuritis	sinusitis	uvulotomy
pneumoconiosis	surfactant	ventilation
pneumothorax	thoracocentesis	
pyothorax	thoracostomy	
respiratory distress	thorax	
syndrome		

Introduction

The function of the respiratory system is to move air in and out of the lungs. This process is called ventilation, respiration, or breathing. This system functions to deliver oxygen (O_2) via the bloodstream. It also removes a waste product—carbon dioxide (CO_2)—from the blood. This exchange of oxygen and carbon dioxide in the lungs is called external respiration. This same exchange within the hemoglobin of the red blood cells (RBCs) is known as internal respiration.

CASE STUDY

A 5-year-old boy is brought to the pediatrician's office. He has been coughing at night for the past week. Today he presents with shortness of breath, tightness in his chest, and wheezing. The doctor recognizes the child's symptoms as those of asthma and orders a bronchodilator—a drug that relaxes the muscles around the airway—to be delivered using a nebulizer. He also refers the child for allergy testing.

As you read this chapter, consider the following questions:

1. Why is the patient wheezing?
2. Is asthma a life-threatening condition?
3. What is the advantage of using a nebulizer to deliver the bronchodilator?
4. Why did the doctor refer the patient for allergy testing?

Organs of the Respiratory System

The organs of the respiratory system are the nose, pharynx, larynx, trachea, bronchial tree (including the bronchi and bronchioles), and the lungs (Figure 6-1). The nose is made of bones and cartilage and the skin covering them. The openings of the nose are the nostrils, which in medicine are referred to as the **nares.** The hairs of the nostrils prevent large particles from entering the nose through air.

The Nasal Cavity and Paranasal Sinuses

The nasal cavity is simply the hollow space behind the nose. The nasal cavity is divided into a left and right portion by the **nasal septum.** Structures called **nasal conchae** extend from the lateral walls of the nasal cavity. Most of the nasal cavity is lined with a mucous membrane that acts to warm and moisten air as it passes through the nasal cavity. The nasal conchae support this mucus membrane and increase the surface area of the nasal cavity.

The nasal cavity is also lined with cells that possess cilia, which are microscopic, hair-like projections from the mucus membrane. As mucus traps dust and other particles in the nasal cavity, the cilia push the mucus toward the pharynx, where it is swallowed. The enzymes of the stomach then destroy these foreign particles and pathogens, thus assisting in the protection of the respiratory system from disease.

The **paranasal sinuses** are air-filled spaces within the skull bones that open into the nasal cavity. The paranasal sinuses reduce the weight of the skull and equalize pressure between the inside of the skull and the outside environment. The sinuses also give your voice its tone. When your paranasal sinuses are "stopped up" with mucus, they cause the tone of your voice to change. The bones of the skull that contain the sinuses include the frontal, sphenoid, ethmoid, and maxillae bones. When sinus membranes become inflamed due to allergies or infection (sinusitis), they swell, which results in a sinus headache.

The Pharynx

The **pharynx** is an organ of the respiratory system as well as the digestive system. During inspiration, air flows from the nasal or oral cavity into the pharynx. From the pharynx, air flows into the larynx.

The Larynx and Vocal Cords

The **larynx** is more commonly called the voice box. It sits superior to and is continuous with the trachea or windpipe. It functions to move air in and out of the trachea and to produce the sounds of a person's voice. The larynx is mostly made of cartilage and muscle tissue. There are three cartilages in the larynx (Figure 6-2). The largest cartilage is called the **thyroid cartilage,** and it forms the anterior wall of the larynx. During the puberty of a male, testosterone causes the thyroid cartilage to enlarge to produce the "Adam's apple." A smaller cartilage called the **epiglottic cartilage** forms the framework of the epiglottis. The **epiglottis** is the flap-like structure that closes off the larynx during swallowing so that food and liquids do not enter the respiratory system when swallowing occurs. The

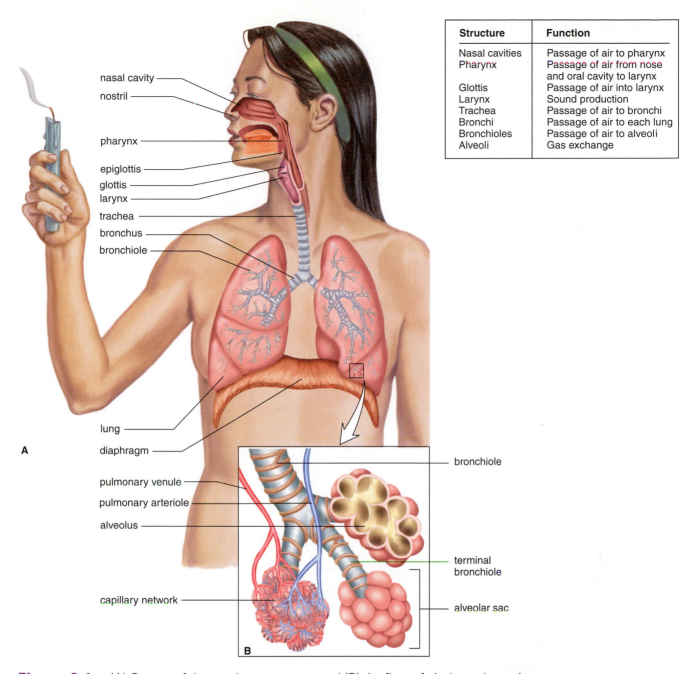

Structure	Function
Nasal cavities	Passage of air to pharynx
Pharynx	Passage of air from nose and oral cavity to larynx
Glottis	Passage of air into larynx
Larynx	Sound production
Trachea	Passage of air to bronchi
Bronchi	Passage of air to each lung
Bronchioles	Passage of air to alveoli
Alveoli	Gas exchange

Figure 6-1. (A) Organs of the respiratory system and (B) the flow of air through respiratory organs.

third cartilage of the larynx is called the **cricoid cartilage.** It forms most of the posterior wall of the larynx and a small part of the anterior wall.

The vocal cords stretch between the thyroid cartilage and the cricoid cartilage. The opening between the vocal cords is called the **glottis** (see Figure 6-2, part C). The upper vocal cords are referred to as *false vocal cords* because they do not produce sound. The lower vocal cords are called *true vocal cords* because muscles stretch and relax them to produce different types of sounds. If the true vocal cords are stretched, the voice becomes higher in pitch. When the true vocal cords are relaxed, the voice becomes lower in pitch. Men have thicker vocal cords, which is why their voices are deeper than female voices.

The Trachea, Bronchi, and Bronchioles

The **trachea** (windpipe) is a tubular organ made of rings of cartilage and smooth muscle. It extends from the larynx to the bronchi. The trachea is lined with cells that possess cilia that constantly move mucus up to the pharynx, where it is swallowed. Mucus traps bacteria, viruses, and any other harmful substances a person inhales—in the same process that occurs in the nasal cavity. The digestive juices of the stomach then destroy the harmful substances. Smoking destroys cilia so the only way a smoker can get mucus out of his trachea is to cough. Smokers often feel the urgency to cough more

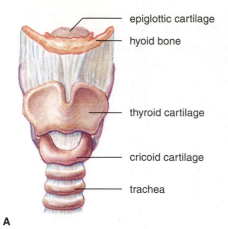

epiglottic cartilage
hyoid bone
thyroid cartilage
cricoid cartilage
trachea

A

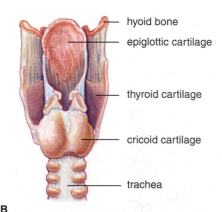

hyoid bone
epiglottic cartilage
thyroid cartilage
cricoid cartilage
trachea

B

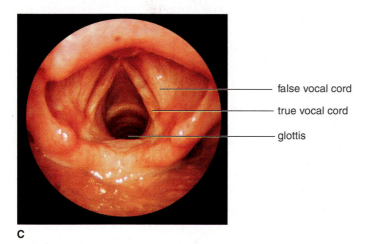

false vocal cord
true vocal cord
glottis

C

Figure 6-2. (A) Anterior view of larynx, (B) posterior view of larynx, and (C) photograph of the vocal cords and glottis.

frequently than nonsmokers in an effort to move mucus to the pharynx.

The distal end of the trachea branches and starts a series of tubes called the **bronchial tree.** The first branches off the trachea are called primary, or main stem, **bronchi.** The branches of the primary bronchi are called secondary bronchi. The secondary bronchi branch into tertiary bronchi. Tertiary bronchi then branch into **bronchioles.** At the ends of the bronchioles are air sacs called alveoli.

Alveoli are very thin sacs made of only one layer of simple squamous epithelial cells and are surrounded by capillaries. They are considered the "working tissue" of the lung because it is in the alveoli where the gaseous exchange of oxygen and carbon dioxide takes place. Many physicians refer to the alveoli as the *pulmonary parenchyma* (parenchymal means "working tissue" of any organ or organ system). Through the process of diffusion, red blood cells in the capillaries release carbon dioxide (refer to carboxyhemoglobin from Chapter 5) into the alveoli. Conversely, the alveoli release oxygen into the blood (refer to oxyhemoglobin in Chapter 5) through the thin walls of the capillaries. This exchange is known as internal or *cellular respiration.*

The Lungs

The lungs are cone-shaped organs that contain connective tissue, the bronchial tree, nerves, lymphatic vessels, and many blood vessels. The right lung is larger than the left (the heart is also in the left **thorax**). The right lung is divided into three lobes, known as the right upper, middle, and lower lobes. The left lung is divided into the left upper and lower lobes. The double-walled membrane that surrounds the lungs is called the **pleura.** The outer membrane is known as the parietal pleura and the innermost membrane is the visceral pleura. The pleura produces a slippery, serous fluid called pleural fluid that helps decrease friction as the membranes move against each other during breathing.

The lungs themselves contain the bronchial tree and alveoli. Some alveolar cells secrete a fatty substance called **surfactant,** which helps maintain the inflation of the alveoli so that they do not collapse in on themselves between inspirations. Premature infants often suffer from respiratory distress syndrome (RDS) or hyaline membrane disease (see the Pathophysiology section at the end of this chapter) because their lungs do not yet create enough surfactant. This causes them to often have great difficulty maintaining adequate lung inflation.

The Mechanisms of Breathing

Breathing, or pulmonary **ventilation,** consists of two events—**inspiration** and **expiration.** During inspiration, or inhalation, air, which is 21% oxygen, flows from the nasal or oropharynx through the sinuses into the larynx, trachea, and bronchial tree, eventually reaching the alveoli of the lungs. Air flows into the airways during inspiration because the thoracic cavity enlarges. When the thoracic cavity enlarges, pressure decreases in the cavity. The atmospheric pressure outside the body is greater than the pressure inside the cavity, and air passively flows from an area of high pressure to an area of low pressure. The events that enlarge the thoracic cavity and therefore lead to inspiration are as follows (Figure 6-3A):

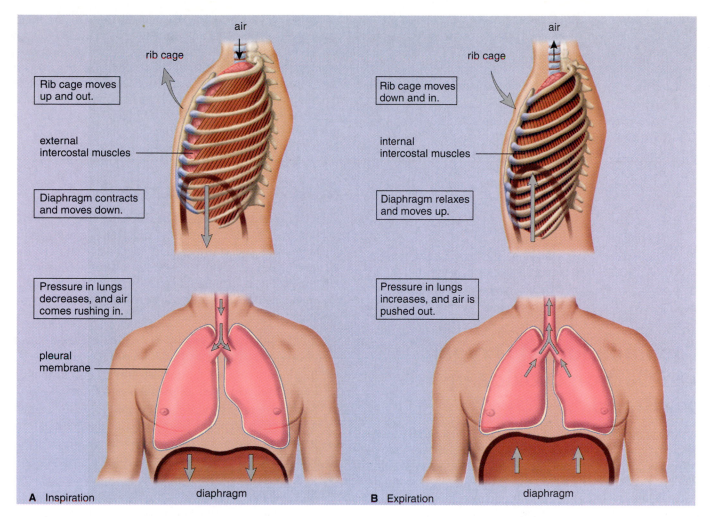

Figure 6-3. (A) Events of inspiration and (B) events of expiration.

- The diaphragm contracts. When the diaphragm contracts, it flattens, which increases the amount of space in the thoracic cavity.
- The intercostal muscles raise the ribs, further enlarging the thoracic cavity.

During expiration, or exhalation, air rich with carbon dioxide flows out of the airways.

Air flows out because the thoracic cavity becomes smaller, which increases the pressure inside the cavity. When the pressure inside the cavity becomes greater than the atmospheric pressure, air flows out. The events that lead to expiration are as follows (Figure 6-3B):

- The diaphragm relaxes. When the diaphragm relaxes, it domes up into the thoracic cavity, which decreases the space in the cavity.
- The intercostal muscles lower the ribs; this further decreases the size of the thoracic cavity.

Breathing is controlled by the respiratory center of the brain, which is located in the pons and medulla oblongata. The medulla oblongata controls both the rhythm and the depth of breathing. The pons controls the rate of breathing.

Other factors that affect breathing are the carbon dioxide levels in the blood and the pH of the blood. When carbon dioxide levels rise in the blood, the rate and depth of breathing increase. The rate and depth of breathing also increase when the blood pH drops. Fear and pain also increase the breathing rate. Breathing rapidly and deeply is called **hyperventilation.** Hyperventilation decreases the amount of carbon dioxide in the blood. However, it should be noted that in patients with chronic obstructive pulmonary disease (COPD), their respiratory rates are stimulated by decreased oxygen levels. Therefore, giving a patient with COPD a high level of oxygen may actually decrease his or her breathing reflex.

The inflation reflex also helps to regulate the depth of breathing. Stretch receptors in pleural membranes are activated when the lungs are stretched past a certain point. This triggers the depth of breathing to decrease to prevent overinflation of the lungs.

There are also normal everyday situations that alter our breathing patterns. Consider these common occurrences:

- Coughing. A deep inspiration occurs and the glottis is closed. As the force of air forces the glottis open, a rush of air is forced up to clear the lower respiratory passages.

- Sneezing. The same process occurs as in coughing except that air is moved to the nasal passages by lowering the uvula. This causes a clearing of the upper respiratory passages.
- Laughing. A deep breath is expelled in short bursts, expressing happiness.
- Crying. The same process occurs as in laughing, but the expression is one of sadness.
- Hiccups. Also spelled hiccoughs; these are spasmodic contractions of the diaphragm against a closed glottis. Interestingly, the purpose for this is not known.
- Yawning. A deep inspiration that increases the amount of air brought to the alveoli, which aids in blood oxygenation.
- Speaking. Air is forced through the larynx, vibrating the vocal cords, whereas words are formed by the tongue, lips, and teeth, allowing for verbal communication.

The Transport of Oxygen and Carbon Dioxide in the Blood

Once oxygen gets into the bloodstream, most of it binds to the hemoglobin in red blood cells. Hemoglobin bound to oxygen is called oxyhemoglobin and is bright red in color. Some oxygen stays dissolved in plasma and does not bind to hemoglobin. Carbon dioxide binds to hemoglobin at the same site that oxygen binds to it. When this occurs, the result is carboxyhemoglobin.

Poisonous to humans, carbon dioxide is particularly dangerous because it is an odorless and clear gas. To allow our blood (hemoglobin) to carry carbon dioxide harmlessly, when carbon dioxide gets into the bloodstream and cerebral spinal fluid, most of it reacts with water to form carbonic acid. As the carbonic acid ionizes, it releases hydrogen and **bicarbonate ions.** These bicarbonate ions attach to hemoglobin, making their way back to the lungs to be exhaled as a waste product by the lungs.

Respiratory Volumes

During different intensities of breathing, different volumes of air move in and out of the lungs. These volumes are called **respiratory volumes** and can be measured to assess the healthiness of the respiratory system. Respiratory capacities can be calculated by adding certain respiratory volumes together. The following are the different types of volumes and capacities (see also Table 6-1):

- Tidal volume: the amount of air that moves in or out of the lungs during a normal breath.
- Inspiratory reserve volume: the amount of air that can be forcefully inhaled following a normal inhalation.
- Expiratory reserve volume: the amount of air that can be forcefully exhaled following a normal exhalation.
- Residual volume: the volume of air that always remains in the lungs, even after a forceful expiration.
- Vital capacity: the total amount of air that can be forcefully exhaled after the deepest inhalation possible.
- Total lung capacity: the total amount of air the lungs can hold.

TABLE 6-1	**Respiratory Air Volumes and Capacities**	
Name	**Volume***	**Description**
Tidal volume (TV)	500 mL	Volume moved in or out of the lungs during a respiratory cycle
Inspiratory reserve volume (IRV)	3,000 mL	Volume that can be inhaled during forced breathing in addition to resting tidal volume
Expiratory reserve volume (ERV)	1,100 mL	Volume that can be exhaled during forced breathing in addition to resting tidal volume
Residual volume (RV)	1,200 mL	Volume that remains in the lungs at all times
Inspiratory capacity (IC)	3,500 mL	Maximum volume of air that can be inhaled following exhalation of resting tidal volume: IC = TV + IRV
Functional residual capacity (FRC)	2,300 mL	Volume of air that remains in the lungs following exhalation of resting tidal volume: FRC = ERV + RV
Vital capacity (VC)	4,600 mL	Maximum volume of air that can be exhaled after taking the deepest breath possible: VC = TV + IRV + ERV
Total lung capacity (TLC)	5,800 mL	Total volume of air that the lungs can hold: TLC = VC + RV

*Values are typical for a tall, young adult.

Educating the Patient

Snoring

Snoring occurs when the muscles of the palate, tongue, and throat relax. Airflow then causes these soft tissues to vibrate. These vibrating tissues produce the harsh sounds characteristic of snoring.

Snoring causes daytime sleepiness and is sometimes associated with a condition known as obstructive sleep apnea (OSA). In OSA, the relaxed throat tissues cause airways to collapse, which prevent a person from breathing. Snoring affects approximately 50% of men and 25% of women older than the age of 40 years. The common causes of snoring include:

- Enlargement of the tonsils or adenoids
- Being overweight
- Alcohol consumption
- Nasal congestion
- A deviated (crooked) nasal septum

The severity of snoring varies among people. The Mayo Clinic's Sleep Disorders Center uses the following scale to determine the severity of snoring:

- Grade 1: Snoring can be heard from close proximity to the face of the snoring person.
- Grade 2: Snoring can be heard from anywhere in the bedroom.
- Grade 3: Snoring can be heard just outside the bedroom with the door open.
- Grade 4: Snoring can be heard outside the bedroom with the door closed.

You can educate patients about making lifestyle modifications and using aids to help reduce their snoring:

- Lose weight
- Change the sleeping position from the back to the side
- Avoid the use of alcohol and medications that cause sleepiness
- Use nasal strips to widen the nasal passageways
- Use dental devices to keep airways open

In addition, patients may benefit from a CPAP (continuous positive airway pressure) machine, which uses a mask attached to a pump that forces air into their passageways while they sleep. If these therapies are not effective, patients may need surgery to trim excess tissues in the throat, such as an **uvulotomy,** or laser surgery to remove a portion of the soft palate.

Pathophysiology

Common Diseases and Disorders of the Respiratory System

Allergic rhinitis is a hypersensitivity reaction to various airborne allergens.

- **Causes.** There are many causes, which may be seasonal such as with hay fever or continual as those caused by dust, molds, colognes, cigarette smoke, animal dander, and mites.
- **Signs and symptoms.** There are numerous signs and symptoms, which may include sneezing; itchy, watery eyes; red, swollen eyelids; congested nasal mucus membranes; and nasal discharge.
- **Treatments.** These commonly include the use of over-the-counter antihistamines and decongestants. Severe cases may be treated with prescription medications such as Allegra® and Zyrtec®. Patients should also avoid known allergens. Air filters and air conditioners will assist in keeping allergen counts down. Seeking the assistance of an allergist for desensitization injections may be an option for long-term management.

Asthma is a condition in which the tubes of the bronchial tree become obstructed as a result of inflammation.

- **Causes.** The causes can include allergens (pollen, pets, dust mites, etc.), cigarette smoke, pollutants, perfumes, cleaning agents, cold temperatures, and exercise (in susceptible individuals).
- **Signs and symptoms.** Symptoms include difficulty breathing, a tight feeling in the chest, wheezing, and coughing, all of which can cause a feeling of suffocation and increased anxiety.
- **Treatment.** Treatment includes avoiding allergens, the use of steroidal and nonsteroidal inhalers such as Advair® and Flovent®, as well as oral medications such as Singulair® and other bronchodilators to

continued ⟶

reduce inflammation. Patients should avoid smoky environments and those who smoke should stop smoking. Strongly scented items such as perfumes, hair products, and cleaning agents should also be avoided.

Atelectasis is more commonly called collapsed lung. It may occur after abdominal or thoracic surgery or because of pleural effusion, which may consist of blood, fluid, air, or pus in the pleural cavity. In order, the medical names for these conditions are **hemothorax, hydrothorax, pneumothorax,** and **pyothorax.**

- **Causes.** These include underlying cystic fibrosis and COPD in which patients may have a chronic form of atelectasis. Cancer patients and those with inflammatory conditions such as pleurisy (pleuritis) may also be subject to chronic atelectasis. Acute atelectasis may occur after any injury to the ribs or trauma to the thorax. Post-surgical patients are also susceptible.

- **Signs and symptoms.** These include **dyspnea** (difficulty breathing), cyanosis (a blue coloration of skin and mucus membranes), diaphoresis (excessive perspiration), anxiety, tachycardia, and intercostal muscle retraction. Depending on the cause of the atelectasis, there may also be chest pain.

- **Treatment.** In acute cases, thoracocentesis may be needed to drain the pleural cavity. For chronic atelectasis, treatment may include chest percussion, postural drainage, coughing, deep breathing exercises, and intermittent positive-pressure breathing (IPPB).

Bronchitis is inflammation of the bronchi and often follows a cold. Bronchitis that occurs frequently often indicates more serious underlying conditions, such as asthma or emphysema. Smokers are much more likely to develop bronchitis than are nonsmokers. Repeated episodes of bronchitis increase a person's chance of eventually developing lung cancer.

- **Causes.** This condition can be caused by viruses and gastroesophageal reflux disease (GERD), a condition in which acids move from the stomach into the esophagus. Exposure to cigarette smoke, pollutants, and the fumes of household cleaners can also contribute to the development of bronchitis.

- **Signs and symptoms.** The signs and symptoms include chills, fever, coughing up yellow-gray or green mucus, tightness in the chest, wheezing, and dyspnea.

- **Treatment.** This condition can be treated with rest, fluids, nonprescription and prescription cough medicines, and the use of a humidifier. Antibiotics are usually prescribed only for smokers. Patients who also have asthma may need to use inhalers. They should also wear masks if they feel they may be exposed to lung irritants.

Chronic obstructive pulmonary disease (COPD) is a group of lung disorders that limit airflow to lungs and usually cause enlargement of the alveoli in the lungs. Emphysema and chronic bronchitis are the most common types of COPD.

- **Causes.** The primary causes are smoking and air pollution.

- **Signs and symptoms.** Common signs and symptoms include dyspnea, **hypoxia** (inadequate oxygenation of the cells), fatigue, and frequent coughing.

- **Treatment.** Treatment should first be focused on lifestyle changes, especially smoking cessation. Other treatment options include respiratory therapy and the use of inhalers. In more serious cases, a lung transplant may be necessary.

Emphysema is a chronic condition that damages the alveoli of the lungs. It is heavily associated with smoking, which causes stretching of the spaces between the alveoli and paralyzes the cilia of the respiratory system.

- **Causes.** The most common causes are cigarette smoking and exposure to cigarette smoke, pollutants, and the dust from grains, cotton, wood, or coal.

- **Signs and symptoms.** Symptoms include shortness of breath that progresses over time, chronic cough, unintended weight loss, and fatigue. Pulmonary function tests and arterial blood gases become progressively more abnormal as the disease progresses. In advanced cases, patients develop characteristic barrel chest caused by the muscular changes in the chest as the patient struggles to breathe.

- **Treatment.** Stopping smoking and preventing exposure to cold environments and pollutants should be the first treatment measures. Vaccinations to prevent the flu and pneumonia as well as antibiotics to control the respiratory infections associated with emphysema may also be administered. In addition, patients can be treated with bronchodilators, supplemental oxygen, inhaled steroids, and respiratory therapy. The most serious cases may require either surgery to remove damaged lung tissue or a lung transplant, without which patients will develop respiratory and/or heart failure, resulting in death.

Influenza is more commonly called the flu. Babies, the elderly, and people with suppressed immune systems and those with chronic respiratory illnesses, such as COPD, are at the highest risk of developing influenza. The flu normally lasts between 5 and 10 days.

- **Causes.** This disease is caused by a number of different viruses that attack the respiratory system. It can be prevented through a yearly flu vaccination. It should be noted that, each year, there are multiple strains of influenza. Therefore, every year, the vaccine available is for the known strains for that year. This should be

continued ⟶

explained to patients so that they understand that a flu shot is needed each year for that year's specific strains of the virus.

- **Signs and symptoms.** Common symptoms include a runny nose (rhinorrhea), sore throat (pharyngitis), sneezing, fever or chills, a dry cough, muscle pain, fatigue, anorexia (loss of appetite), and diarrhea.
- **Treatment.** Over-the-counter analgesics and antipyretics can alleviate the aches and pains as well as the fever associated with the flu. Other treatment options include bed rest, fluids, and antiviral medications.

Laryngitis is an acute inflammation of the larynx. Chronic laryngitis is associated with lung cancer.

- **Causes.** The causes of this condition are varied and include the following: viruses; bacteria; polyp formation in the larynx; excessive talking, shouting, or singing; allergies; smoking; frequent heartburn; the frequent use of alcohol; damage to nerves that supply the larynx; and a stroke (CVA or cerebrovascular accident) that paralyzes vocal cord muscles.
- **Signs and symptoms.** Signs and symptoms include a hoarse voice (dysphonia), sore throat (pharyngitis), a dry cough and throat, and tickling sensations in the throat.
- **Treatment.** The most common treatment options are antibiotics, the management of heartburn, and the avoidance of cigarettes and alcohol, as well as voice rest. The treatment of more serious cases includes removing laryngeal polyps and surgery to tighten the vocal cords.

Legionnaire's disease is an acute type of bacterial pneumonia. As with many respiratory diseases, smokers are much more susceptible to pneumonias than are nonsmokers.

- **Causes.** This disease is caused by Legionnaire bacilli that usually grow in the standing water of air conditioning systems.
- **Signs and symptoms.** The symptoms include fever, which may spike as high as 105°F, fatigue, anorexia, dyspnea, frequent coughing, chest pain, muscle aches, and headache. Complications may include hypotension, arrhythmia, respiratory and renal failure, as well as shock, which is often fatal.
- **Treatment.** Antibiotics, antipyretics, and respiratory therapy, including oxygen and ventilator support if needed. Supportive therapy, such as IV fluids, is also used.

Lung cancer is closely associated with smoking and exposure to secondhand smoke, and kills more people in the United States than any other type of cancer. Smoking accounts for approximately 85% of all lung cancer cases.

- **Causes.** The primary causes are smoking and exposure to radon, asbestos, and industrial carcinogens.
- **Signs and symptoms.** The respiratory symptoms include a cough that worsens over time, **hemoptysis**

(coughing up blood), dyspnea, wheezing, shortness of breath, and recurrent bronchitis. Other symptoms are chest pain, dysphonia, unintended weight loss, and bone pain if the cancer has spread.

- **Classification.** Lung cancer is classified by the following types:
  - *Small cell lung cancer.* This type occurs almost exclusively in smokers. It is the most aggressive type and spreads readily to other organs. Small cell lung cancer that spreads to other organs is termed *extensive*.
  - *Squamous cell lung cancer.* This type of lung cancer arises from the epithelial cells that line the tubes of the lungs. It occurs most commonly in men.
  - *Adenocarcinoma.* This type arises from the mucous-producing cells of the lungs. It develops most commonly in women and nonsmokers.
  - *Large cell carcinoma.* This type of lung cancer arises from the peripheral parts of the lungs.
- **Stages.** Squamous cell lung cancer, adenocarcinoma, and large cell carcinoma are staged as follows:
  - Stage 0: Cancer is found only in the lining of the tubes of the lungs.
  - Stage 1: Cancer has spread from the lining of the tubes to lung tissues.
  - Stage 2: Cancer has spread to the lymph nodes or the chest wall.
  - Stage 3: Cancer has spread to the lymph nodes and to other organs within the chest.
  - Stage 4: Cancer has spread to organs outside the chest.
- **Treatment.** Treatment will vary depending on the type of cancer and the stage. Stopping smoking and avoiding exposure to secondhand smoke should be the first treatment considerations. Common treatment options include chemotherapy and radiation therapy. More serious cases may require the surgical removal of tumors (if they are confined), a lobectomy (the removal of a lung lobe or lobes), or a pneumonectomy (the removal of an entire lung).

Pleural effusion is a buildup of fluid in the pleural cavity.

- **Causes.** Effusions are caused by either an overproduction of pleural fluid or an inadequate absorption of the fluid. These often result from an underlying disease, such as CHF, cirrhosis, tuberculosis, cancer, lupus, or rheumatoid arthritis.
- **Signs and symptoms.** As the fluid builds in the pleural space, the lungs begin to compress, reducing the gaseous exchange of oxygen and carbon dioxide. Infective processes may result in a pus buildup, which is known as **empyema.**
- **Treatment. Thoracocentesis** is done to remove the fluid and/or pus. **Thoracostomy,** which requires insertion of a tube to continually drain the fluid, may

continued ⟶

be required to maintain drainage of the acute phase of the illness. Oxygen may be administered to increase oxygen concentration in the lung. Antibiotics may also be required for any infective process.

Pleuritis or **pleurisy** is a condition in which the pleura becomes inflamed. This often causes the membranes to stick together or can cause an excess amount of fluid to form between the membranes.

- **Causes.** Causes include viruses, pneumonia, autoimmune diseases such as lupus or rheumatoid arthritis, tuberculosis, a pulmonary embolism, inflammation of the pancreas, and trauma to the chest.
- **Signs and symptoms.** Symptoms include fever or chills; a dry cough; shortness of breath; and a sharp, stabbing type of chest pain during respiration.
- **Treatment.** Analgesics may be prescribed to relieve chest pain. Anti-inflammatory drugs, antibiotics, and the removal of fluid around the lungs by thoracocentesis are the primary treatment options.

Pneumoconiosis is the name given to lung diseases that result from years of exposure to different environmental or occupational types of dust. There are three basic types: **anthracosis, asbestosis,** and **silicosis.**

- **Causes.** Anthracosis (black lung disease) results from exposure to coal dusts. Asbestosis results from lung exposure to asbestos. Silicosis arises from exposure to silica sand from sand blasting and ceramic manufacture.
- **Signs and symptoms.** Tachypnea, nonproductive cough, progressive dyspnea on exertion, pulmonary hypertension, recurrent respiratory infections, and eventual right ventricular hypertrophy. In all cases, fibrous tissue takes over healthy lung tissue, which destroys the alveoli and takes over the air passageways.
- **Treatment.** Treatment for all types includes avoiding respiratory infections, using bronchodilators, and using supplemental oxygen as needed. Respiratory therapy can also be useful in assisting patients to rid themselves of respiratory secretions.

Pneumonia, also known as pneumonitis, is characterized by an inflammation of the lungs caused by a bacterial, viral, or fungal infection of the lungs. There are at least 50 different types of pneumonia, and they range from mild to very serious. Double pneumonia refers to inflammation of both lungs.

- **Causes.** Pneumonia can be caused by bacteria, viruses, fungi, and parasites. It can also be caused by foreign matter that enters the lungs (for example, stomach contents that enter the lungs after vomiting), known as *aspiration pneumonia.* This disorder may be prevented by not smoking and, for some types of pneumonia, by pneumococcal vaccinations.
- **Signs and symptoms.** Common signs and symptoms include fever or chills, headache, chest or muscle pain, fatigue, dyspnea, and sputum consisting of rust-colored, green, or yellowish mucus.
- **Treatment.** Rest, fluids, over-the-counter pain medications, and antibiotics are the most common treatments. In severe cases, oxygen and ventilator support may be required.

Pneumothorax is a collection of air in the chest around the lungs, which may cause atelectasis.

- **Causes.** Some causes of this disorder are unknown. Various respiratory diseases and trauma to the chest, such as a stabbing wound, can also contribute to the development of pneumothorax.
- **Signs and symptoms.** The primary symptoms include tightness in the chest or a sharp chest pain, shortness of breath, and a rapid heart rate.
- **Treatment.** The insertion of a chest tube (thoracostomy) to remove air from the chest and surgery to repair chest wounds are the primary treatments.

Pulmonary edema is a condition in which fluids fill spaces within the lungs. This disorder makes it very difficult for the lungs to oxygenate the blood. It most commonly occurs when the heart cannot pump all the blood it receives from the lungs. Left heart failure occurs when blood then backs up in the lungs, causing fluids to seep into lung spaces.

- **Causes.** The causes of this condition are many and include the following: congestive heart failure, myocardial infarction (heart attack), cardiomyopathy, heart valve disorders, lung infections, allergic reactions, smoke inhalation, drowning, various drugs such as narcotics and heroin, chest injuries, and high altitudes. This disorder may be prevented by avoiding high altitudes and smoking. Preventing heart disease may also reduce the chance of developing this disorder.
- **Signs and symptoms.** The symptoms of pulmonary edema are shortness of breath; difficulty breathing, especially when lying down (a condition known as **orthopnea**); a feeling of suffocating; wheezing; a productive cough that produces pink mucus; rapid weight gain; pallor; and profuse sweating, which is known as **diaphoresis.**
- **Treatment.** Treatment includes oxygen therapy, diuretics to eliminate excess fluids, and morphine to reduce anxiety and shortness of breath.

A *pulmonary embolism* is a blocked artery in the lungs. Usually the artery is blocked by a blood clot that has traveled from a vein in the legs. If an artery in the lungs is completely blocked, death can occur quickly from resultant respiratory failure.

- **Causes.** People at the highest risk of developing this condition are those who have had previous heart attacks, cancer, a fractured hip, or chronic lung diseases. Women who use birth control pills and individuals

continued ⟶

who have a pacemaker may be at risk for developing a pulmonary embolism. In addition, long periods of inactivity, increased levels of clotting factors in the blood (usually caused by certain cancers), injury to veins, and a stroke that causes paralysis of the arms or legs may also cause this condition. A sedentary lifestyle as well as auto or airplane travel—or any activity that requires prolonged sitting or standing—are also major risk factors for developing a pulmonary embolism. A half-dose aspirin (formerly known as a baby aspirin) taken daily, as well as plenty of fluids and frequent movement of the arms and legs, may help prevent the development of a pulmonary embolism.

- **Signs and symptoms.** Symptoms include fainting, a sudden shortness of breath, hemoptysis (coughing up blood), wheezing, tachycardia (a rapid heartbeat), diaphoresis (profuse sweating), and chest pain that may spread to a shoulder, arm, or the face.
- **Treatment.** Support stockings can be used to promote circulation. The patient should rest until the blood clot has dissolved and may be prescribed thrombolytic (clot-dissolving) medications, such as TPA. Anticoagulants, typically warfarin (Coumadin), may be used to prevent new blood clots from forming in the deep veins of the body. Finally, surgery may be used to place a filter in the vena cava to prevent blood clots from reaching the lungs.

Respiratory distress syndrome, or RDS, which is formerly known as hyaline membrane disease, kills apparently healthy infants. At highest risk are newborns to infants eight months of age, especially "preemies."

- **Causes.** The etiology is unknown. The underlying problem is known to be a lack of surfactant in the lungs, which helps prevent the alveoli from totally collapsing on expiration. Without surfactant, the alveoli collapse, resulting in poor oxygenation due to difficulty with re-inflation of alveoli.
- **Signs and symptoms.** RDS is usually diagnosed directly after birth, when the infant's breathing becomes rapid and shallow. The infant's nares flare and the accessory muscles are used to aid in respiration. The infant will also exhibit "grunting" noises in an attempt to breathe.
- **Treatment.** Treatment must be immediate, and preferably in a neonatal intensive care unit (NICU). Oxygen therapy, the insertion of an endotracheal tube, ventilator support, and the use of artificial surfactant are all used in an attempt to keep the alveoli inflated. Infants who survive RDS may be at higher risk for respiratory infections later, but as their lungs continue to mature, this threat lessens.

Severe acute respiratory syndrome (SARS) is a relatively new respiratory disease that is very contagious and sometimes fatal.

- **Causes.** SARS is caused by viruses associated with the common cold as well as by unknown viruses. It can be prevented by thoroughly washing the hands, wearing a mask, and avoiding exposure to individuals with this disease.
- **Signs and symptoms.** Signs and symptoms include fever or chills, headache, a dry cough, and muscle aches.
- **Treatment.** Rest and antiviral drugs are the primary treatments.

Sinusitis is an inflammation of the membranes lining the sinuses of the skull.

- **Causes.** Bacteria, excess mucus production in the sinuses (often from the "common cold"), the blockage of sinus openings, and the destruction of cilia that move mucus out of sinuses can cause this disorder.
- **Signs and symptoms.** Fever, cough, headache, pharyngitis, facial pain, and nasal congestion are the common signs and symptoms.
- **Treatment.** Treatment options include the use of nasal decongestants, nasal steroid sprays, a humidifier, applications of heat to the face, and antibiotics. Surgery to clear the sinuses or unblock sinus openings may be required.

Sudden infant death syndrome (SIDS) claims the life of more than 7,000 babies a year in the United States. There are no characteristic signs or symptoms. Usually a baby with this disorder simply goes to sleep and never wakes up.

- **Causes.** The causes of SIDS are unknown but certain risk factors have been identified:
  - Male babies are more likely to die of SIDS.
  - Babies are most susceptible between the ages of 2 weeks and 6 months.
  - Premature or low birth weight babies are more likely to have SIDS.
  - A baby with a sibling who died of SIDS is more likely to also die of this disorder.
  - Babies who are African American or Native American are more likely to die of SIDS.
  - Babies who were prenatally exposed to alcohol, cocaine, heroine, or nicotine are at a higher risk of developing SIDS.
  - Babies who sleep on their stomachs are approximately three times more likely to die of SIDS.
- **Treatment.** Proper sleep positioning on the baby's back is best for all infants, especially those known to be at risk, those with previous apneic episodes, or those who have lost a sibling to SIDS. At-risk infants may also be sent home with an apnea monitor that will sound an alarm if breathing ceases. Research into this disease is ongoing. Support groups are available and are suggested for families who have experienced the tragedy of losing a child to SIDS.

continued ⟶

Common Diseases and Disorders of the Respiratory System *(concluded)*

Tuberculosis (TB) is a disease that kills more than 2 million people worldwide each year. Although it primarily affects the lungs, it can spread to other parts of the body.

- **Causes.** This disease is caused by various strains of the bacterium *Mycobacterium tuberculosis*. Widespread tuberculosis may be complicated by the following factors:
  - HIV infection. HIV infection makes a person more vulnerable to TB.
  - Crowded living conditions. This factor allows TB to spread easily; this disease, therefore, is found in some prisons and homeless shelters.
  - Poverty. Poverty prevents some patients with TB from seeking or completing therapy.
  - Drug-resistant bacterium. Drug-resistant strains of the bacterium that causes TB have increased.
  - Long-term therapy. Current treatments require antibiotic therapy for many months, which some patients with TB do not complete.
- **Signs and symptoms.** The symptoms include a cough that lasts more than 3 weeks, unintended weight loss, fever or chills, fatigue, night sweats, pain when breathing or difficulty breathing, and pain in other affected areas.
- **Treatment.** The first step should be TB testing to detect carriers of this disease, who should then be treated. Drug-resistant cases of TB may require years of drug therapy to treat; this therapy normally lasts 6 months to a year. Isolating the patient during the contagious phase of the disease (usually 2 to 4 weeks after treatment begins) is required. Also, during the initial stages of treatment, the patient should be encouraged to receive adequate bed rest and maintain an adequate, nutritious diet.

Upper respiratory (tract) infection (URI) is the term often used for **coryza,** or the common cold.

- **Causes.** URIs are caused by a family of viruses known as *rhinovirus*. The viruses are airborne and also transmitted by contact with contaminated surfaces and on the hands. Children are frequent sources of transmission.
- **Signs and symptoms.** This is a generally self-limiting condition of approximately one week's duration, which follows an initial incubation period of 2 to 5 days. Symptoms include pharyngitis, nasal congestion, rhinitis, headache, fever, and general malaise. There may be a nonproductive cough, especially at night.
- **Treatment.** Care for this process is usually symptomatic and includes antipyretics, analgesics, decongestants, and cough suppressants. Adequate rest and plenty of fluids to flush the system are also helpful. Antibiotics are ordinarily only prescribed for patients with an underlying illness or complication.

Summary

The major function of the respiratory system is the exchange of oxygen and carbon dioxide between the blood and the atmosphere. In addition to this gas exchange, the respiratory system also regulates blood pH.

The organs of this system include the nose, pharynx, larynx, trachea, bronchial tree, and the lungs. Each of these structures has a role in ventilation (bringing air in and out of the body) and external respiration (the gas exchange of oxygen and carbon dioxide). Understanding this system is important to help patients understand normal lung functioning and what they can do to maintain optimal respiratory function. It is especially important when instructing patients in the use of an inhaler so that proper technique allows for adequate absorption of medication.

CASE STUDY QUESTIONS

Now that you have completed this chapter, review the case study at the beginning of the chapter and answer the following questions:

1. Why is the patient wheezing?
2. Is asthma a life-threatening condition?
3. What is the advantage of using a nebulizer to deliver the bronchodilator?
4. Why did the doctor refer the patient for allergy testing?

Discussion Questions

1. Explain the importance of mucus, cilia, and stomach acid in protecting the respiratory system.
2. List the various respiratory volumes that are commonly measured in the clinical setting. What does each volume represent?
3. Explain the importance of surfactant in respiration. Why is it that premature infants and low-birth weight infants are at higher risk of RDS?

Critical Thinking Questions

1. Smoking destroys cilia in the respiratory tract. Describe how smoking damages the lungs. What causes the "barrel chest" that is characteristic of many patients with emphysema?
2. What effect would breathing in a paper bag have on oxygen concentrations in the blood? Would this be helpful for a person who is hyperventilating? Why or why not?

Application Activities

1. Give the name of the structure for each of the descriptions noted below.
   a. Contains the esophagus, trachea, and larynx
   b. Moves air in and out of trachea; produces sound
   c. The small branches within the lungs
   d. The protective, double-walled sac around the lungs
   e. The pulmonary parenchyma
   f. Keeps us from aspirating while eating or drinking

2. Explain how the cardiovascular system is interrelated with the respiratory system.
3. How many lobes does the left lung have? The right lung? Why are they different in size?

Virtual Fieldtrip

Visit the McGraw-Hill Higher Education Medical Assisting website at www.mhhe.com/medicalassisting3 to complete the following activity:

Cigarette smoking affects all of us, children most of all, and often the tobacco industries target young people to develop new consumers. The site for this exercise has been developed so that parents and others can keep young people safe from the dangers of cigarettes. Once you enter the site's home page, find the icon on the left side labeled "The Tobacco Toll." Choose your state from the list and get the current statistics for your state regarding the following:

- Number of high school students who smoke
- Number of male high school students who use smokeless or spit tobacco
- Number of children (younger than age age 18) who become new daily smokers each year
- Number of children (younger than age 18) exposed to secondhand smoke at home
- Number of cigarette packs bought or smoked by children (younger than age 18) each year
- Number of adults in your state who smoke

1. What are the death statistics in your state from smoking?
2. What are the monetary costs to your state related to smoking?

Open the CD and complete this chapter's practice activities, play the games, listen to the key terms, and test yourself with the interactive review. E-mail, print, and/or save your results to document your proficiency.

CHAPTER 7

The Nervous System

KEY TERMS

action potential
afferent nerves
areflexia
ascending tracts
astrocytes
autonomic
autonomic nervous system (ANS)
axon
blood-brain barrier
brain stem
cell body
central nervous system (CNS)
cerebellum
cerebrospinal fluid (CSF)
cerebrum
cervical enlargement
convolutions
corpus callosum
cortex
cranial nerves
dendrite
depolarized
dermatome
descending tracts
diencephalon
dorsal root
effectors
efferent nerves
epilepsy
ganglia
gray matter
gyri
hyperreflexia

CHAPTER OUTLINE

- General Functions of the Nervous System
- Neuron Structure
- Nerve Impulse and Synapse
- Central Nervous System
- Peripheral Nervous System
- Neurologic Testing

LEARNING OUTCOMES

After completing Chapter 7, you will be able to:

7.1 Explain the difference between the central nervous system and the peripheral nervous system.

7.2 Describe the functions of the nervous system.

7.3 Describe the structure of a neuron.

7.4 Describe the function of a nerve impulse and how a nerve impulse is created.

7.5 Describe the structure and function of a synapse.

7.6 Describe the function of the blood-brain barrier.

7.7 Describe the structure and functions of meninges.

7.8 Describe the structure and functions of the spinal cord.

7.9 Describe the location and function of cerebrospinal fluid.

KEY TERMS (Concluded)

hyporeflexia
hypothalamus
interneuron
lobe
lumbar enlargement
membrane potential
meninges
meningitis
microglia
myelin
nerve fiber
nerve impulse
neuralgia
neuroglia

neuroglial cell
neurons
neurotransmitter
oligodendrocytes
parasympathetic
paresthesias
peripheral nervous system (PNS)
plexus
polarized
reflex
repolarization
Schwann cell
sciatica
seizure

sensory nerves
somatic
somatic nervous system (SNS)
spinal nerves
subarachnoid space
sulci
sympathetic
synaptic knob
thalamus
ventral root
ventricle
vesicles
white matter

7.10 Define reflex and list the parts of a reflex arc.

7.11 List the major divisions of the brain and give the general functions of each.

7.12 Explain the functions of the cranial and spinal nerves.

7.13 Describe the differences between the somatic nervous system and autonomic nervous system.

7.14 Explain the two divisions of the autonomic nervous system.

7.15 Describe the causes, signs and symptoms, and treatments of various diseases and disorders of the nervous system.

Introduction

The nervous system is a highly complex system. It controls all other organ systems and is important for maintaining balance within those systems. Disorders of the nervous system are numerous and often very difficult to diagnose and treat because of the complexity of this system.

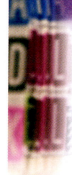

CASE STUDY

A 70-year-old man comes to the family practice office where you are the MA. He complains that he is having trouble with his sense of balance and that it is interfering with his tennis game. He also states his right hand seems to "have a mind of its own" and he can't seem to keep it totally still. His wife observes that his posture is becoming stooped and his reactions seem slowed.

As you read this chapter, consider the following questions:

1. What is the likely diagnosis for this patient?
2. What is the likely cause of this disease?
3. Is there a definitive cure for this disease? What are the treatment options?

General Functions of the Nervous System

The nervous system is divided into two major parts—the **central nervous system (CNS)** and the **peripheral nervous system (PNS).** The CNS consists of the brain and the spinal cord, and the peripheral nervous system consists of peripheral nerves, which are located throughout the rest of the body.

The peripheral nervous system is split into two separate sections: the **somatic nervous system (SNS),** which governs your body's skeletal or voluntary muscles, and the **autonomic nervous system (ANS),** which is charge of your body's automatic functions, such as the respiratory and gastrointestinal systems.

Additionally, there are three separate types of nerve cells or neurons that carry out the actual functions of the nervous system: (1) The **sensory** or **afferent nerves** are responsible for detecting sensory information from the environment or even from inside the body and bringing it to the CNS for interpretation. (2) The **motor** or **efferent nerves** bring information or impulses from the central nervous system to the PNS to allow for movement or action of a muscle or gland. (3) Within the CNS (brain or spinal cord) are the interpretive neurons between the sensory and motor nerves known as **interneurons.** These neurons act as go-betweens or interpreters between the afferent and efferent nerves. An example of this process would be noting a red light while driving. The sensory neurons within your eyes note the color and send the information to the cerebral cortex of your brain where the interpretation takes place. The interneurons pick up the signal and send the information to the motor neurons that you are supposed to stop your vehicle, which in turn sends the instructions to your right foot to step on the brake pedal of your vehicle. This entire transaction, of course, takes place in milliseconds, allowing you to stop in time.

Neuron Structure

Neurons are the functional cells of the nervous system. They transmit electrochemical messages called **nerve impulses** to other neurons and **effectors** (muscles or glands). An important characteristic about neurons is that they lose their ability to divide. Therefore, when neurons are destroyed by disease, they cannot be replaced. However, the **neuroglial cells** or **neuroglia,** which do not transmit impulses, function as support cells for other neurons and never lose their ability to divide. The three types of neuroglia are:

- **Astrocytes**—star-shaped cells within the nervous system that anchor blood vessels to the nerve cells

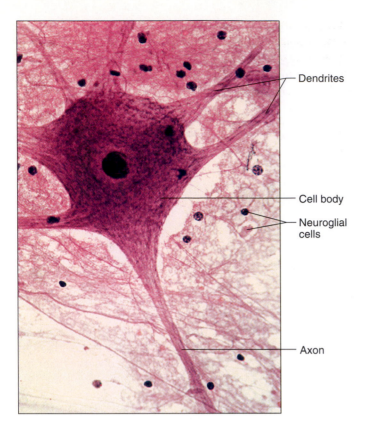

Figure 7-1. A typical neuron surrounded by neuroglial cells.

- **Microglia**—small cells within the nervous system that act as phagocytes watching for and engulfing invaders
- **Oligodendrocytes**—specialized neuroglial cells that assist in the production of the myelin sheath, which will be discussed in further detail later.

All neurons have a **cell body** and processes called **nerve fibers** that extend from the cell body (Figure 7-1).

The cell body is the portion of the neuron that contains the nucleus and the typical organelles of any cell (Chapter 1). It is responsible for generating the large amount of proteins and energy that the neuron needs to carry out its important functions.

Extending from the cell body are nerve fibers. The two types of nerve fibers are **axons** and **dendrites.** A neuron may have one or more dendrites but typically has only one axon. Dendrites are usually short and branch profusely near the cell body. Their function is to receive information for the neuron. Axons are typically long and branch profusely after they have extended far away from the cell body. Their function is to send information (nerve impulses) away from the cell body.

In the peripheral nervous system, neuroglial cells, called **Schwann cells,** wrap themselves around some axons; the axons are coated by the cell membranes of the Schwann cells. The cell membranes contain large amounts of **myelin,** which is a fatty substance. Myelin insulates the axons and allows them to send nerve impulses quickly. The axons thus coated are referred to as **white matter.**

Those not insulated by the myelin sheath are known as **gray matter.**

Nerve Impulse and Synapse

Neuron cell membranes have a cell **membrane potential.** This means the membrane is polarized. Just like a battery is polar—one end is negative and the other end is positive—neuron cell membranes are polar because the inside is negatively charged and the outside is positively charged. In most of the cells in the body, the outside of cell membranes is positively charged because more positive ions are on the outside. The inside of cell membranes is negatively charged because more negative ions are on the inside. This membrane potential is very important for the function of neurons (Figure 7-2).

Potassium and sodium ions are both positively charged and play important roles in generating nerve impulses.

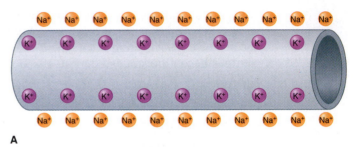

A

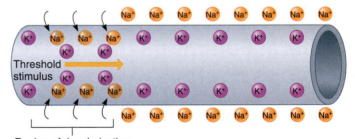

Figure 7-2. Nerve impulse: (A) At rest, or in its polar state, more Na is on the outside of the membrane, which makes the outside positive and the inside negative (less positive). (B) When Na moves into the cell, the membrane depolarizes, meaning that the inside becomes more positive. (C) The membrane repolarizes when K and later Na move to the outside of the cell membrane.

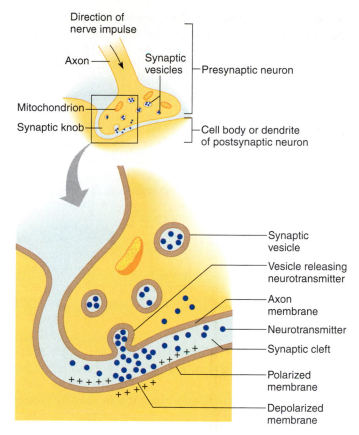

Figure 7-3. Synapse. When a nerve impulse reaches a synaptic knob, it releases a neurotransmitter onto the postsynaptic structure.

When a neuron is at rest or without stimulation, the outside of its membrane is positively charged and the inside is negatively charged because the total of sodium and potassium ions is greater outside the membrane. As long as the neuron is at rest, it remains in this **polarized** state.

However, a neuron will respond to stimuli such as heat, pressure, and chemicals by changing the amount of polarization across its membrane. For example, it can respond to a stimulus by making the outside of its membrane less positive. When this happens, the neuron has **depolarized.** In other words, it has become less polar. To make the outside of the membrane less positive, some of the sodium ions flow to the inside of the cell membrane. If the membrane of an axon becomes depolarized enough, a nerve impulse (**action potential**) is created. A nerve impulse is the flow of electric current along the axon membrane. Eventually, the axon membrane becomes polar again by the return of positively charged ions to the outside of the cell membrane. The return to the original polar (resting) state is called **repolarization.**

An unmyelinated axon does not conduct a nerve impulse as quickly as a myelinated axon does. Also, the speed of the nerve impulse is related to the diameter of the axon. The larger the diameter, the faster the nerve impulse travels to the end of the axon.

When traveling down an axon, a nerve impulse eventually reaches the **synaptic knob** at the end of the axon

branches. These synaptic knobs contain small sacs called **vesicles,** which produce chemicals called **neurotransmitters.** Neurotransmitters are released by the synaptic knob to allow impulse transmission to continue to the postsynaptic structures, which consist of the dendrites, cell bodies, and axons of other neurons (Figure 7-3).

There are about 50 different neurotransmitters. Most neurons release only one type of neurotransmitter, but some will release more than one type. Their functions include causing muscles to contract or relax, causing glands to secrete products, activating neurons to send nerve impulses, or inhibiting neurons from sending nerve impulses.

Central Nervous System

The CNS includes the spinal cord and brain (Figure 7-4). The tissues of the CNS are so delicate that a **blood-brain barrier** and layers of membranes protect them. Tight

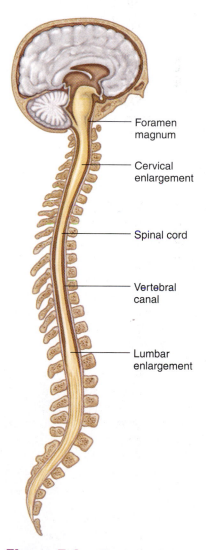

Figure 7-4. The central nervous system (CNS) consists of the brain and spinal cord. The spinal cord ends at the level of the third lumbar vertebra.

The Nervous System **107**

capillaries form the blood-brain barrier. This barrier prevents certain substances from entering the tissues of the CNS. For example, various waste products and drugs do not cross the blood-brain barrier very well. Inflammation, however, can make this barrier more permeable.

Meninges are membranes that protect the brain and spinal cord. The three layers of meninges are dura mater, arachnoid mater, and pia mater. Dura mater is the toughest and outermost layer of the meninges. The space above the dura mater is called the epidural space; below it is the subdural space. The middle layer, named for its spider web-like appearance, is the arachnoid mater. Pia mater is the innermost and most delicate layer. It sits directly on top of the brain and spinal cord and holds blood vessels onto the surface of these structures. Between the arachnoid mater and pia mater is an area called the **subarachnoid space.** It contains **cerebrospinal fluid (CSF),** which cushions the CNS.

Spinal Cord

The spinal cord is a slender structure that is continuous with the brain. The spinal cord descends into the vertebral canal and ends around the level of the first or second lumbar vertebra. The spinal cord is divided into 31 spinal segments: 8 cervical segments, 12 thoracic segments, 5 lumbar segments, 5 sacral segments, and 1 coccygeal segment. The thickening of the spinal cord in the neck

region is called the **cervical enlargement** and contains the motor neurons that control the muscles of the arms. Another thickening of the spinal cord occurs in the lumbar region. This thickening is called the **lumbar enlargement** and contains the motor neurons that control the muscles of the legs (see Figure 7-4).

Gray and White Matter.   When you view a cross-section of the spinal cord, you observe two differently colored areas. The inner tissue is termed gray matter because its color is darker than the outer tissue, which is termed white matter. The gray matter contains neuron cell bodies and their dendrites, whereas the white matter contains myelinated axons. The divisions of the gray matter are called horns, and the divisions of the white matter are called columns (funiculi). The columns contain groups of axons called nerve tracts. A canal runs down the entire length of the spinal cord through the center of the gray matter. This canal is called the central canal and contains CSF (Figure 7-5).

Ascending and Descending Tracts.   One function of the spinal cord is to carry sensory information up to the brain. The tracts that carry sensory information up to the brain are called **ascending tracts.** Another function of the spinal cord is to carry motor information down from the brain to muscles and glands. These tracts are called **descending tracts.**

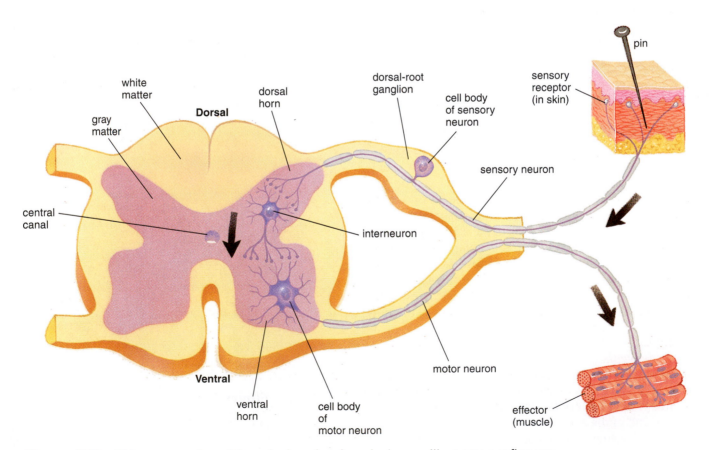

Figure 7-5.   This cross-section of the spinal cord and a spinal nerve illustrates a reflex arc.

Reflexes. Another important function of the spinal cord is to participate in reflexes. A **reflex** is a predictable, automatic response to stimuli. For example, if you touch something very hot, the predictable response is that you will pull your finger away from the hot surface; this type of reflex is called a withdrawal reflex. The information that flows through a typical reflex moves in the following order: from receptors to sensory neurons to interneurons to motor neurons to effectors. In this example of the withdrawal reflex, the receptors are in the skin at the tips of the fingers. These receptors send their information to sensory neurons that relay the information to interneurons in the spinal cord. The interneurons immediately relay the information to motor neurons that activate the muscles (effectors) in the arm. The muscles in the arm coordinate the movement of pulling your finger away from the painful stimulus. A person can consciously inhibit a reflex because the information also goes to the cerebral cortex where a person makes conscious decisions.

Brain

The brain can be divided into four major areas: the cerebrum, the diencephalon, the brain stem, and the cerebellum (Figure 7-6).

Cerebrum. The **cerebrum** is the largest part of the brain. It is divided into two halves called cerebral hemispheres. A thick bundle of nerve fibers called the **corpus callosum** connects the two hemispheres. The grooves on

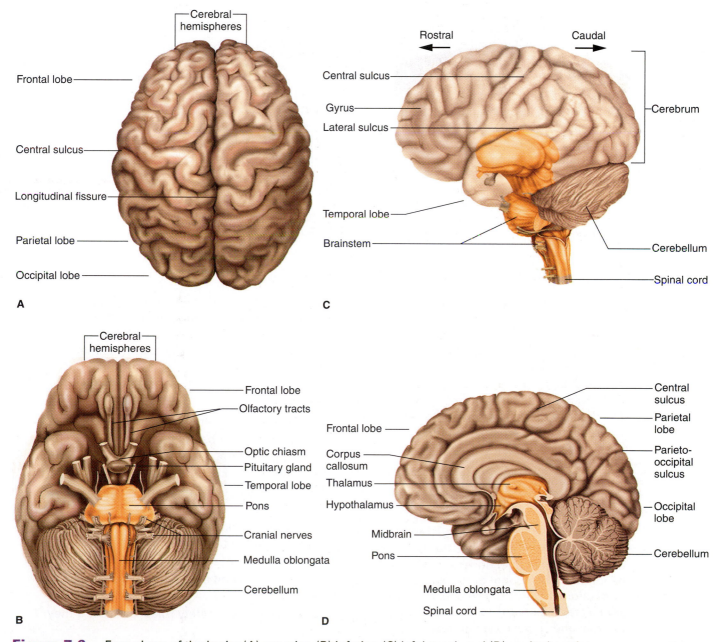

Figure 7-6. Four views of the brain: (A) superior, (B) inferior, (C) left lateral, and (D) sagittal section.

the surface of the cerebrum are called **sulci**. The "bumps" of brain matter between the sulci are called **gyri,** or **convolutions.** A deep groove called the longitudinal fissure runs between the two longitudinal hemispheres.

Lobes. Each cerebral hemisphere is divided into **lobes**—frontal, parietal, temporal, and occipital. The frontal lobes contain motor areas that allow a person to consciously decide to produce a body movement such as walking or tapping a pencil. Somatosensory areas are located in parietal lobes. These areas interpret sensations felt on or within the body. For example, if you feel a light touch on your right hand, the somatosensory area interprets the sensation and where it is occurring. The temporal lobes contain auditory areas that interpret sounds. Visual areas are located in the occipital lobes, and they interpret what a person sees.

Cortex. The outermost layer of the cerebrum is called the cerebral **cortex.** It is composed of gray matter and therefore contains neuron cell bodies and dendrites. This layer contains nearly 75% of all neurons in the entire nervous system. Beneath the cerebral cortex is white matter. Besides interpreting sensory information and initiating body movements, the cortex also stores memories and creates emotions.

Ventricles. **Ventricles** are interconnected cavities within the brain. They are filled with CSF. Recall that this fluid is also found in the subarachnoid space of the meninges and the central canal of the spinal cord. Therefore, CSF is located within the brain and spinal cord and also around the brain and spinal cord. This fluid protects and cushions the central nervous system.

Diencephalon. The **diencephalon** is located between the cerebral hemispheres and is superior to the brain stem. The diencephalon includes the thalamus and hypothalamus. The **thalamus** serves as a relay station for sensory information that heads to the cerebral cortex for interpretation. If sensory information does not pass through the thalamus before it reaches the cerebral cortex, it cannot be interpreted correctly. For example, say you are feeling pain in your left forearm. This information goes up the spinal cord and through the thalamus and then to the cerebral cortex for interpretation. If the information did not go through the thalamus, the cerebral cortex may interpret that you are feeling cold instead of pain in your left forearm. The **hypothalamus** maintains homeostasis by regulating many vital activities such as heart rate, blood pressure, and breathing rate.

Brain Stem. The **brain stem** is a structure that connects the cerebrum to the spinal cord. The three parts of the brain stem are the midbrain, the pons, and the medulla oblongata. The midbrain lies just beneath the diencephalon. It controls both visual and auditory reflexes. An example of a visual reflex is when you see something in your peripheral vision and you automatically turn your head to view it more clearly.

Educating the Patient

Preventing Brain and Spinal Cord Injuries

In the United States alone, almost half a million people a year suffer brain and spinal cord injuries. The most common causes of these injuries are motor vehicle accidents, sports and recreational accidents—especially diving—and violence. People at the highest risk for spinal cord injuries are children and teens. However, most brain and spinal cord injuries can be prevented. You can use the following tips to educate patients on preventing these types of injuries.

Prevention Tips

- Know the depth of water into which you are diving. More than 90% of diving injuries occur in 5 feet of water or less.
- Explore diving areas before diving. For example, know where rocks are located before you dive.
- Do not drive or do any recreational activity while under the influence of alcohol or drugs. Both affect good judgment and control. Alcohol-related traffic crashes are the leading cause of disabling brain and spinal cord injuries.

- Always wear a helmet when riding a bike or motorcycle. Your risk of brain injury is 85% greater during a biking accident if you are not wearing a helmet. Make sure your helmet fits properly.
- Always wear appropriate protective gear while playing any sport.
- Avoid surfing headfirst.
- Always wear your safety belt.
- Make sure children use car seats that are appropriate for their age and weight.
- Be familiar with ways to get help quickly in emergencies.
- Follow traffic rules and signs while walking, biking, or driving.
- Follow safety rules on playgrounds.
- Store firearms and ammunition in separate and locked places.
- Teach children the safety rules to follow if they find a gun.

The pons is a rounded bulge on the underside of the brain stem situated between the midbrain and the medulla oblongata. It contains nerve tracts to connect the cerebrum to the cerebellum. The pons also regulates respiration.

The medulla oblongata is the most inferior portion of the brain stem and is directly connected to the spinal cord. It controls many vital activities such as heart rate, blood pressure, and respiration. It also controls reflexes associated with coughing, sneezing, and vomiting.

Cerebellum. The **cerebellum** is inferior to the occipital lobes of the cerebrum and posterior to the pons and medulla oblongata. It coordinates complex skeletal muscle contractions that are needed for body movements. For example, when you walk, many muscles have to contract and relax at appropriate times. Your cerebellum coordinates these activities. The cerebellum also coordinates fine movements such as threading a needle, playing an instrument, and writing.

Peripheral Nervous System

The peripheral nervous system consists of nerves that branch off the CNS. These nerves are called peripheral nerves and are classified into two types—**cranial nerves** and **spinal nerves.**

Cranial Nerves

Cranial nerves are peripheral nerves that originate from the brain. Roman numerals and names designate the twelve different cranial nerves (Figure 7-7):

I. *Olfactory nerves* carry smell information to the brain for interpretation.

II. *Optic nerves* carry visual information to the brain for interpretation.

III. *Oculomotor nerves* are found within the muscles that move the eyeball, eyelid, and iris.

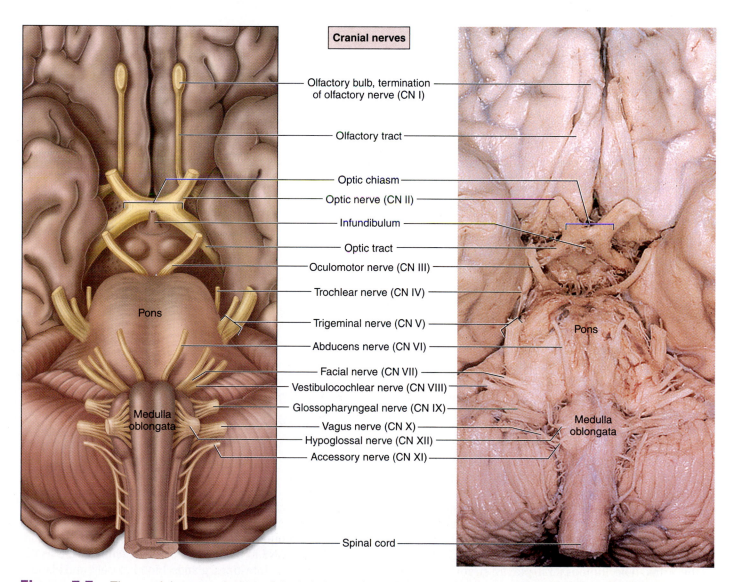

Cranial nerves

- Olfactory bulb, termination of olfactory nerve (CN I)
- Olfactory tract
- Optic chiasm
- Optic nerve (CN II)
- Infundibulum
- Optic tract
- Oculomotor nerve (CN III)
- Trochlear nerve (CN IV)
- Trigeminal nerve (CN V)
- Abducens nerve (CN VI)
- Facial nerve (CN VII)
- Vestibulocochlear nerve (CN VIII)
- Glossopharyngeal nerve (CN IX)
- Vagus nerve (CN X)
- Hypoglossal nerve (CN XII)
- Accessory nerve (CN XI)
- Spinal cord

Pons

Medulla oblongata

Figure 7-7. The cranial nerves. A view of the inferior surface of the brain shows the 12 pairs of cranial nerves.

IV. *Trochlear nerves* act in the muscles that move the eyeball.

V. *Trigeminal nerves* carry sensory information from the surface of the eye, the scalp, facial skin, the lining of the gums, and the palate to the brain for interpretation. They also are found within the muscles needed for chewing.

VI. *Abducens nerves* act in the muscles that move the eyeball.

VII. *Facial nerves* are found in the muscles of facial expression as well as in the salivary and tear glands. These nerves also carry sensory information from the tongue.

VIII. *Vestibulocochlear nerves* carry hearing and equilibrium information from the inner ear to the brain for interpretation.

IX. *Glossopharyngeal nerves* carry sensory information from the throat and tongue to the brain for interpretation. They also act in the muscles of the throat.

X. *Vagus nerves* carry sensory information from the thoracic and abdominal organs to the brain for interpretation. These nerves are also found within the muscles in the throat, stomach, intestines, and heart.

XI. *Accessory nerves* are found within the muscles of the throat, neck, back, and voice box.

XII. *Hypoglossal nerves* are found within the muscles of the tongue.

Spinal Nerves

Spinal nerves are peripheral nerves that originate from the spinal cord (Figure 7-8). There are 31 pairs of spinal nerves: 8 pairs of cervical nerves (numbered C1 through C8), 12 pairs of thoracic nerves (numbered T1 through T12), 5 pairs of lumbar nerves (numbered L1 through L5), 5 pairs of sacral nerves (numbered S1 through S5), and one pair of coccygeal nerves (Co). Except for C1, each spinal nerve innervates a skin segment known as a **dermatome.** A map of the dermatomes with the spinal nerve responsible for the skin area is shown in Figure 7-9.

Two roots, a ventral root and a dorsal root, form each spinal nerve (see Figure 7-5). The **ventral root** contains axons of motor neurons only, and the dorsal root contains axons of sensory neurons only. The **dorsal root** also contains a dorsal root ganglion, which contains the cell bodies of sensory neurons.

Except in the thoracic region, the main portions of spinal nerves fuse together to form nerve **plexuses.** The major nerve plexuses are the cervical, brachial, and lumbosacral. Nerves coming off the cervical plexus supply the skin and the muscles of the neck. The phrenic nerve also originates from the plexus. This nerve controls the diaphragm, which is a muscle that is needed for breathing.

The brachial plexus forms nerves that control muscles in the arms. The lumbosacral plexus supplies the lower abdominal wall, external genitalia, buttocks, thighs, legs,

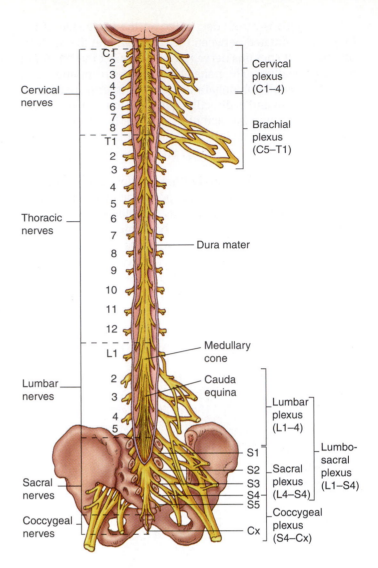

Figure 7-8. Spinal cord, spinal nerves, and plexuses.

and feet. The largest nerve of the body, the sciatic nerve, originates from this plexus. This nerve controls the muscles of the legs.

Somatic and Autonomic Nervous Systems

The peripheral nervous system is divided into a somatic nervous system and an autonomic nervous system. The **somatic** nervous system consists of nerves that connect the CNS to skin and skeletal muscle. The somatic nervous system is often called the "voluntary" nervous system because it controls skeletal muscles, which are under voluntary control. The **autonomic** nervous system consists of nerves that connect the CNS to organs and other structures such as the heart, stomach, intestines, glands, blood vessels, and bladder (among others). The autonomic nervous system controls

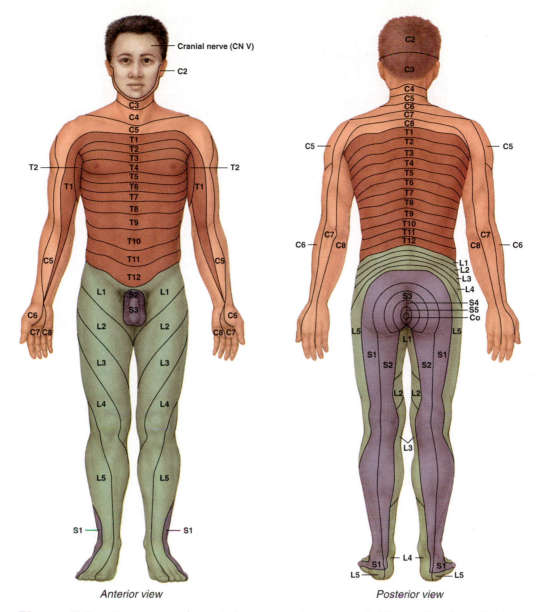

Anterior view   *Posterior view*

Figure 7-9. Dermatome maps. A dermatome is an area of skin supplied by a single spinal nerve. These diagrams only approximate the dermatomal distribution.

organs not under voluntary control, so it is often referred to as the "involuntary" nervous system.

In the autonomic nervous system, motor neurons from the brain and spinal cord communicate to other motor neurons that are located in ganglia. **Ganglia** are collections of neuron cell bodies outside the CNS. The motor neurons of ganglia then communicate to various organs and blood vessels.

The two divisions of the autonomic nervous system are the sympathetic and the parasympathetic (Figures 7-10 and 7-11). The **sympathetic** division prepares organs for "fight-or-flight" situations. In other words, it prepares them for stressful or emergency situations. For example, the sympathetic division prepares the heart for a stressful or frightening situation by increasing the heart rate. The **parasympathetic** division prepares the body for resting and digesting. For example, the parasympathetic division

prepares the heart for resting by keeping the heart rate relatively low. Notice that sympathetic and parasympathetic actions are antagonistic, meaning that they function in opposite ways. Most of the body's organs are under parasympathetic control.

Many neurons of the sympathetic division are located in the thoracic and lumbar regions of the spinal cord. For this reason, this division is also called the thoracolumbar division. The sympathetic neurons usually release the neurotransmitter norepinephrine into organs and glands. Norepinephrine increases the heart and breathing rates, slows down the activity of the digestive glands, slows down the muscles of the stomach and the intestines, and dilates the pupils. Sympathetic nerves also control the constriction of blood vessels. When blood vessels constrict, blood pressure increases, which is a needed response during an emergency situation.

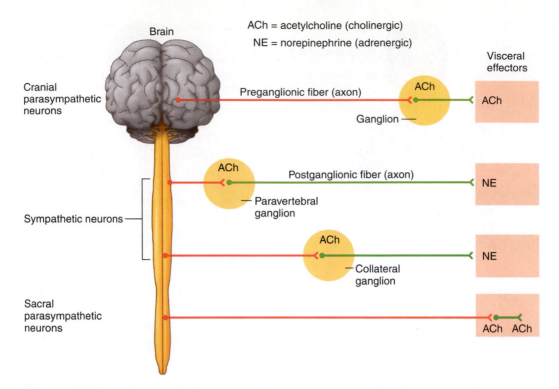

Figure 7-10. Divisions of the autonomic nervous system. Most parasympathetic fibers release acetylcholine onto visceral effectors. Most sympathetic fibers release norepinephrine onto visceral effectors.

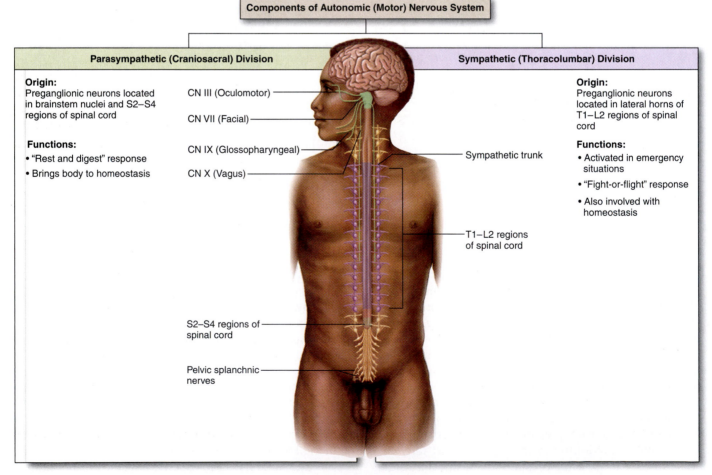

Figure 7-11. Comparison of parasympathetic and sympathetic divisions. The parasympathetic and sympathetic divisions of the ANS have the same basic components, but there are differences in origin and the locations of the preganglionic cell bodies, axon lengths, and the amount of branching.

Many neurons of the parasympathetic division are located in the brain stem and the sacral regions of the spinal cord. For this reason, this division is also referred to as the craniosacral division. All parasympathetic neurons release acetylcholine onto organs and glands. Acetylcholine is a neurotransmitter that slows the heart and breathing rates, constricts the pupils, activates digestive glands, and activates the muscles of the stomach and intestines. Most blood vessels in the body do not receive communication from parasympathetic nerves.

Neurologic Testing

Patients with nervous system disorders may have a wide variety of signs and symptoms, but the most common are headache, muscle weakness, and **paresthesias** (loss of feeling). A typical neurologic examination can determine the following:

- State of consciousness. This state can vary from normal to a state of coma. A patient in a coma cannot respond to stimuli and cannot be awakened. Other terms used to describe states of consciousness include *stupor* (difficulty being awakened), *delirium* (being confused or having hallucinations), *vegetative* (having no cortical function), and *asleep* (can be aroused with normal stimulation).
- Reflex activity. Reflex tests primarily determine the health of the peripheral nervous system.
- Speech patterns. Abnormal speech patterns include a loss of the ability to form words correctly or to form sentences that make sense.
- Motor patterns. Abnormal motor patterns include the loss of balance, abnormal posture, or inappropriate movements of the body. For example, chorea is an exaggerated and sudden jerking of a body part.

Diagnostic Procedures

Common diagnostic procedures to determine neurologic disorders include the following specialized tests:

- Lumbar puncture. Whenever a physician needs to examine CSF, a lumbar puncture is performed. A needle is used to remove CSF from the subarachnoid space usually below the third lumbar vertebra of the spinal column. Analysis of this fluid provides a great deal about the health of a patient. For example, cancer cells in CSF often indicate a brain or spinal cord tumor. White blood cells in this fluid indicate infections such as meningitis. Red blood cells indicate abnormal bleeding.
- Magnetic resonance imaging (MRI). This procedure allows for the brain and spinal cord to be visualized from many angles. It uses powerful magnets to generate images and is useful at detecting tumors, bleeding, or other abnormalities.
- Positron emission tomography (PET) scan. This procedure uses radioactive chemicals that collect in specific areas of the brain. These chemicals allow images of those specific areas to be generated. This test is useful in detecting blood flow to areas of the brain, brain tumors, and the diagnosis of such diseases as Parkinson's and Alzheimer's.
- Cerebral angiography. This procedure uses contrast material that can be visualized in the blood vessels of the brain. It is useful in detecting aneurysms (abnormally dilated blood vessels).
- Computerized tomography (CT) scan. This very common procedure produces images that provide more information than a standard x-ray. It is useful in detecting tumors and other abnormal structures.
- Electroencephalogram (EEG). This test detects electrical activity in the brain. It is useful in diagnosing various states of consciousness.
- X-ray. This procedure is useful in detecting skull or vertebral fractures.

Cranial Nerve Tests

Disorders of the cranial nerves can be determined using the following tests:

- The olfactory nerves (I) are tested by asking a patient to smell various substances.
- Cranial nerves III, IV, and VI are tested by asking a patient to track the movement of the physician's finger. If a patient cannot move her eyeballs properly, there may be damage to one of these nerves. Recall that these nerves control the muscles that move the eyeballs.
- Cranial nerve V controls the muscles needed for chewing. To assess this nerve, a patient is asked to clench his teeth. The physician then feels the jaw muscles. If they feel limp or weak, this nerve may be damaged.
- If a person can no longer make facial expressions, then cranial nerve VII may be damaged. This nerve controls the muscles needed to make facial expressions.
- If a patient cannot extend his tongue and move it from side to side, cranial nerve XII may be damaged. This nerve controls tongue movement.

Reflex Testing

Testing a patient's reflexes allows a physician to evaluate the components of a reflex as well as the overall health of the individual's nervous system. The absence of a reflex is called **areflexia. Hyporeflexia** is a decreased reflex, and **hyperreflexia** is a stronger than normal reflex. The following are common reflex tests:

- Biceps reflex. The absence of this reflex may indicate spinal cord damage in the cervical region.
- Knee reflex. The absence of this reflex may indicate damage to lumbar or femoral nerves.
- Abdominal reflexes. These reflexes are used to evaluate damage to thoracic spinal nerves.

Pathophysiology

Common Diseases and Disorders of the Nervous System

Alzheimer's disease is a progressive, degenerative disease that occurs in the brain.

- **Causes.** Fiber tangles within neurons, degenerating nerve fibers, and a decreased production of neurotransmitters cause the symptoms of this disorder. This disease is associated with advanced age, family history, certain genes, and possibly some environmental factors. Many causes have not yet been determined.
- **Signs and symptoms.** Common symptoms include a loss of memory, confusion, personality changes, language deterioration, impaired judgment, and restlessness.
- **Treatment.** There is no cure, but with medications such as Aricept, Cognex, Razadyne, and Namenda, as well as proper nutrition, physical exercise, social activity, and calm environments, the disease progress may be slowed and managed.

Amyotrophic lateral sclerosis (ALS), commonly known as Lou Gehrig's disease, is a fatal disorder characterized by the degeneration of neurons in the spinal cord and brain.

- **Causes.** Most causes are unknown but they are likely to involve hereditary and environmental factors.
- **Signs and symptoms.** Early symptoms include cramping of hand and feet muscles, persistent tripping and falling, chronic fatigue, and slurred speech. Signs and symptoms that appear in later stages include breathing difficulty and muscle paralysis.
- **Treatment.** There is no cure for this disorder; however, physical, speech, and respiratory therapies help to manage the symptoms. Some medications relieve muscle cramping, but currently only the drug Riluzole is approved by the U.S. Food and Drug Administration (FDA) specifically for ALS.

Bell's palsy is a disorder in which facial muscles are very weak or totally paralyzed.

- **Causes.** This condition can result from damage to cranial nerve VII (the facial nerve), but many times the cause is unknown. It is more common in people with diabetes, the flu, or a cold.
- **Signs and symptoms.** The most common signs and symptoms are a loss of feeling in the face, the inability to produce facial expressions, headache, and excessive tearing or drooling.
- **Treatment.** Treatments include the use of eyedrops, anti-inflammatory medications, and pain relievers. Symptoms usually diminish or go away within 5 to 10 days.

Brain tumors and cancers are abnormal growths in the brain. A brain tumor with cancer cells is termed malignant. Malignant tumors that start in any tissue of the brain are called primary brain cancers. Those that start in body parts and spread to the brain are classified as secondary brain cancers. The most common primary brain tumors are gliomas that arise from neuroglial cells.

- **Causes.** Like most cancers, the causes are gene mutations. Factors associated with gene mutations include exposure to toxins, an impaired immune system, and hereditary factors.
- **Signs and symptoms.** The signs and symptoms depend on size and location of the tumor. Common symptoms include headache, seizures, nausea, weakness in the arms or legs, fatigue, changes in speech patterns, and a loss of memory.
- **Treatment.** Treatment often includes surgery, radiation therapy, chemotherapy, and gene therapy. The success of the treatment depends on the type of tumor, the extent of the diseases, the location of the tumor, the tumor's response to treatment, and the overall health of the patient.

Epilepsy and **seizures** occur when parts of the brain receive a burst of electrical signals that disrupt normal brain functioning. Seizures may be either *petit mal* (partial) or *grand mal* (generalized). Petit mal seizures may appear as loss of awareness of the present, whereas grand mal seizures result in the classic tonic-clonic seizure. Epilepsy is the condition of having repeated, long-term seizures.

- **Causes.** Causes vary but may include birth trauma, high fevers, alcohol and drug withdrawal, head trauma, infections, brain tumors, and certain medications. Many causes are unknown.
- **Signs and symptoms.** The signs and symptoms may include visual disturbances, nausea, generalized abnormal feelings, a loss of consciousness, and uncontrolled muscle contractions and tremors.
- **Treatment.** The primary treatment is medication to prevent seizures. Surgery is sometimes an option in patients with partial seizures.

Guillain-Barré syndrome is a disorder in which the body's immune system attacks part of the peripheral nervous system. It usually has a sudden and unexpected onset.

- **Causes.** The destruction of myelin by the body's immune system produces the signs and symptoms. Viral infections, immunizations, and pregnancy sometimes trigger the disease.
- **Signs and symptoms.** Symptoms may include weakness or tingling sensations in the legs or arms that can progress to paralysis. Difficulty breathing and an abnormal heart rate are more dangerous signs and symptoms. The disease normally runs its course, and with proper medical treatment, it is not fatal.

continued ⟶

Common Diseases and Disorders of the Nervous System *(continued)*

- **Treatment.** Various supportive therapies, such as the use of respirators and heart machines, are necessary until the disease subsides. Physical therapy is used to keep muscles strong.

Headaches affect almost everyone at some point in life. A wide variety of factors produce headaches. Most headaches do not require medical attention, but a physician should evaluate repetitive and severe headaches. Headache types commonly include tension headaches, migraines, and cluster headaches.

Tension headaches are classified as either episodic (random) or chronic (frequent):

Episodic tension headaches are the most common type of tension headache.

- **Causes.** This type of headache is often the result of temporary stress or anger.
- **Signs and symptoms.** Symptoms include pain or soreness in the temples and the contraction of head and neck muscles.
- **Treatment.** Most of these headaches can be managed by taking an over-the-counter (OTC) medicine, and relief usually occurs in 1 or 2 hours.

Chronic tension headaches occur almost daily and persist for weeks or months.

- **Causes.** This type of headache may be the result of stress or fatigue, but it may also be associated with physical problems, psychological issues, or depression.
- **Signs and symptoms.** As with episodic tension headaches, the symptoms include pain or soreness in the temples and the contraction of head and neck muscles.
- **Treatment.** People who suffer from chronic headaches should seek medical treatment.

Migraines are the most severe type of headache. They are responsible for more "sick days" than any other headache type. Almost 30 million people in the United States suffer from migraines.

- **Causes.** Hormones may influence migraines, which may explain why women experience migraines at least three times more often than men do. Migraine headaches are considered vascular headaches because they are associated with the distension of the arteries of the brain.
- **Signs and symptoms.** Migraines often begin as dull pains that develop into throbbing pains accompanied by nausea and sensitivity to light and noise. There are many types of migraines, but the two most common are *migraine with aura* and *migraine without aura*. Auras may include the appearance of jagged lines or flashing lights, tunnel vision, hallucinations, or the detection of strange odors. The auras may last up to an hour and usually go away as the headache begins. Most migraine headaches last about 4 hours but some can last up to a week.

- **Treatment.** When treating migraines, a physician will prescribe a drug to relieve the pain but will also try to identify the factors that trigger it. There are many medicines, both OTC and prescription, available to treat migraines.

Cluster headaches are so named because the attacks come in groups. They are the most severe type of migraines. More men than women experience these types of headaches.

- **Causes.** Some research indicates that alcohol consumption can bring on attacks of cluster headaches.
- **Signs and symptoms.** Common symptoms include a runny nose, watery eyes, and swelling below the eyes. Cluster headaches normally last about 45 minutes to an hour, although they can last longer. It is common for a patient with this disorder to experience 1 to 4 headaches a day during a cluster time span. Cluster time spans can last weeks or months.
- **Treatment.** Various drugs are available for the treatment of these headaches.

Meningitis is an inflammation of the meninges.

- **Causes.** Causes may include bacterial, viral, and fungal infections. Some types of meningitis can be prevented with vaccines.
- **Signs and symptoms.** Fever, headache, vomiting, stiffness in the neck, sensitivity to light, drowsiness, and joint pain usually accompany this disorder.
- **Treatment.** The treatment varies depending on the type of meningitis. Intravenous antibiotics are used for bacterial meningitis, supportive therapy for viral meningitis, and antifungal drugs for fungal meningitis. Bacterial meningitis can be fatal.

Multiple sclerosis (MS) is a chronic disease of the central nervous system in which myelin is destroyed.

- **Causes.** The causes are mostly unknown, but some known causes are viruses, genetic factors, and immune system abnormalities.
- **Signs and symptoms.** Depending on the type of MS, symptoms can range from mild to severe. In severe cases, a person will lose the ability to walk or speak.
- **Treatment.** There is no cure for MS, but supportive treatments may lessen the symptoms. Some medications including interferon, Copaxone, prednisone, and Solu Medrol are available to treat and slow the progression of symptoms.

Neuralgias are a group of disorders commonly referred to as nerve pain. They most frequently occur in the nerves of the face.

- **Causes.** There are many causes of neuralgia, including trauma, chemical irritation of the nerves, bacterial infections, and diabetes. Many times the causes are unknown.

continued ⟶

Common Diseases and Disorders of the Nervous System *(concluded)*

- **Signs and symptoms.** Sudden and severe skin pain are the most common symptoms. The pain repeatedly occurs in the same body area. Numbness of skin areas is also common.
- **Treatment.** Many times the disorder goes away spontaneously, and treatment, other than pain medication, is not needed. Other treatments include injections of anesthetics or surgery to remove the affected nerves.

Parkinson's disease is a motor system disorder. It is slowly progressive and degenerative.

- **Causes.** Most causes are undetermined, although it is known that patients with this disease lack certain chemicals (neurotransmitters) in the brain. Brain tumors, certain drugs, carbon monoxide, or repeated head trauma may produce Parkinson's disease.
- **Signs and symptoms.** The most common signs and symptoms include tremor and stiffness of the arms and legs as well as a lack of coordination and balance. Masked faces, where the patient shows little or no facial emotion, is also common, as is stooped posture with a shuffling gait.
- **Treatment.** There is no cure, but medications such as dopamine, Selegiline, and Symmetrel alleviate some symptoms and slow the progression of this disease. Surgery is useful in some cases of Parkinson's.

Sciatica occurs when the sciatic nerve is damaged.

- **Causes.** The sciatic nerve is commonly damaged by excessive pressure on the nerve from prolonged sitting or lying down. It is also easily damaged from trauma to the pelvis, buttocks, or thighs.
- **Signs and symptoms.** The most usual symptoms include numbness, pain, or tingling sensations on the back of a leg or foot. Weakness of leg and foot muscles can also develop.
- **Treatment.** This disorder is usually treated with pain and anti-inflammatory medication or steroids. Physical therapy is also needed following trauma to the nerve.

Stroke occurs when brain cells die because of an inadequate blood flow. Stroke is sometimes referred to as a "brain attack." The medical term is *cerebrovascular accident* (CVA). It is not uncommon for a stroke to be preceded by *transient ischemic attacks* (TIAs) or *mini strokes*, which are caused by brief interruptions of blood supply to the brain.

- **Causes.** Most strokes are caused by the blockage of an artery in the neck or brain. They may also be caused by aneurysms that burst.
- **Signs and symptoms.** Signs and symptoms may include paralysis, speech problems, memory and reasoning deficits, coma, and possibly death. Symptoms will vary depending on the location of the stroke within the brain.
- **Treatment.** Because neurons in the brain cannot be replaced, the effects of a stroke can be permanent. However, physical, occupational, and speech therapy are often very useful in lessening the effects of a stroke.

Summary

The functions of the nervous system include detecting and interpreting sensory information, making decisions about that information, and responding to and carrying out motor functions based on those decisions. The cells responsible for these functions are neurons. There are two divisions of the nervous system. The CNS consists of the brain and spinal cord. The PNS is made up of cranial nerves and spinal nerves. All organs are under the control of the nervous system. Knowledge of this system is essential when assisting the physician during a neurologic exam.

CASE STUDY QUESTIONS

Now that you have completed this chapter, review the case study at the beginning of the chapter and answer the following questions:

1. What is the likely diagnosis for this patient?
2. What is the likely cause of this disease?
3. Is there a definitive cure for this disease? What are the treatment options?

Discussion Questions

1. Explain the relationship between the central nervous system and the afferent and efferent nerves, and what role the interneurons play in this relationship.
2. What is the function of neuroglia? Give the names and functions of each of the three types of neuroglial cells.
3. What are the two divisions of the autonomic nervous system? How do these two divisions differ?

Critical Thinking Questions

1. In some diseases, such as multiple sclerosis and Guillain-Barré, myelin is destroyed. What is the function of myelin in the nervous system, and how can the destruction of myelin contribute to the signs and symptoms of both of these diseases?
2. Meningitis is an inflammation of the protective covering of the central nervous system. Why is it important for physicians to know whether the cause of meningitis is viral, bacterial, or fungal when treating a patient with meningitis?

Application Activities

1. Give the Roman numeral designations and functions of the following cranial nerves:
   a. Olfactory nerve
   b. Glossopharyngeal nerve
   c. Trigeminal nerve
   d. Vestibulocochlear nerve
   e. Trochlear nerve
2. What are the uses of the following diagnostic procedures?
   a. Lumbar puncture
   b. MRI
   c. CT scan
   d. Cerebral angiography
3. Name the layers of the meninges, outermost to innermost, including the names of the spaces between the layers when applicable. Include where the CSF is found.
4. What is a dermatome? What skin condition, caused by a virus attacking a nerve root, is associated with this term? (You may want to refer to the Chapter 2, The Integumentary System.)

Virtual Fieldtrip

Visit the McGraw-Hill Higher Education Medical Assisting website at www.mhhe.com/medicalassisting3 to complete the following activity:

Using the National Library of Medicine's reference website, search for the term *seizures* and then choose the topic "Types of Seizures."

- Explain the differences among tonic-clonic seizures, simple partial seizures, and complex partial seizures.
- What is the name for the warning sign that some patients experience prior to a seizure?

Open the CD and complete this chapter's practice activities, play the games, listen to the key terms, and test yourself with the interactive review. E-mail, print, and/or save your results to document your proficiency.

CHAPTER 8

The Urinary System

KEY TERMS

afferent arterioles
Bowman's capsule
calyces
cystitis
detrusor muscle
distal convoluted tubule
efferent arterioles
glomerular filtrate
glomerular filtration
glomerulonephritis
glomerulus
hilum
incontinence
loop of Henle
micturition
nephrons
proximal convoluted
  tubule
pyelonephritis
renal calculi
renal column
renal corpuscle
renal cortex
renal medulla
renal pelvis
renal pyramids
renal sinus
renal tubule
renin
retroperitoneal
trigone

CHAPTER OUTLINE

- The Kidneys
- Urine Formation
- The Ureters, Urinary Bladder, and Urethra

LEARNING OUTCOMES

After completing Chapter 8, you will be able to:

8.1 Describe the structure, location, and functions of the kidney.
8.2 Define the term *nephron* and describe its structure.
8.3 Explain how nephrons filter blood and form urine.
8.4 List substances normally found in urine.
8.5 Describe the locations, structures, and functions of the ureters, bladder, and urethra.
8.6 Explain how urination is controlled.
8.7 Describe the causes, signs and symptoms, and treatments of various diseases and disorders of the urinary system.

KEY TERMS (Concluded)

tubular reabsorption	urea	urethra
tubular secretion	ureters	uric acid

Introduction

The organs of the urinary system are the kidneys, ureters, urinary bladder, and urethra (Figure 8-1). This system functions to remove waste products from the bloodstream. These waste products are excreted from the body in the form of urine. Nephrons are microscopic structures within the kidneys that filter blood, remove waste products, and form urine.

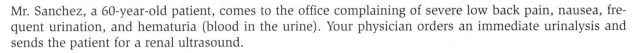

CASE STUDY

Mr. Sanchez, a 60-year-old patient, comes to the office complaining of severe low back pain, nausea, frequent urination, and hematuria (blood in the urine). Your physician orders an immediate urinalysis and sends the patient for a renal ultrasound.

As you read this chapter, consider the following questions:

1. What is the likely diagnosis for Mr. Sanchez?
2. What noninvasive therapies will be tried to help him?
3. Will surgery be needed?
4. What lifestyle changes might be suggested for Mr. Sanchez?

The Kidneys

The kidneys are responsible for removing metabolic waste products from the blood. These metabolic wastes are combined with water and ions to form urine, which is excreted from the body. The kidneys also secrete the hormone erythropoietin, which stimulates the red bone marrow to produce red blood cells, and the hormone **renin,** which helps to regulate blood pressure. All three of these functions are important in maintaining the body's internal environment or homeostasis, which is a balanced, stable state within the body.

The kidneys are bean-shaped organs that are reddish brown in color. Tough, fibrous capsules cover them. The kidneys are **retroperitoneal** in position, which means that they lie behind the peritoneal cavity. They lie on either side of the vertebral column at about the level of the lumbar vertebrae; the left kidney is slightly higher than the right, which is displaced by the liver.

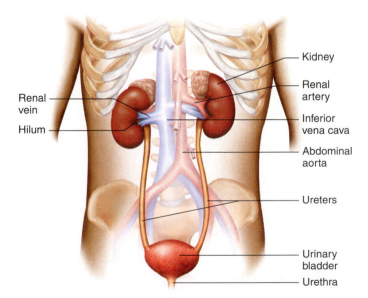

Figure 8-1. Organs of the urinary system.

The surface area of the concave depression of the kidney is called the **renal sinus.** The renal artery, renal vein, and ureter enter the kidney here in the area known as the **hilum.** The ureter is the tube that drains urine from the kidney, carrying it to the bladder. Inside the kidney, this same area is called the **renal pelvis,** formed by the expansion of the ureter inside the kidney. The renal pelvis itself further divides into small tubes known as **calyces** (*calyx* is singular).

The outermost layer of the kidney is the **renal cortex,** and the middle portion is the **renal medulla.** The renal medulla is divided into triangular-shaped areas called **renal pyramids.** The renal cortex covers the pyramids and also dips down between the pyramids. The portion of the cortex between pyramids is called a **renal column** (Figure 8-2).

Blood enters the kidney through the renal artery, goes through the filtration process explained in the next section, and then exits the kidney via the renal vein.

Nephrons

Waste products are removed from the blood by **nephrons.** Each kidney contains about one million nephrons, which are located in the renal medulla. Nephrons are made of a **renal corpuscle** and a **renal tubule** (Figure 8-2). A renal corpuscle is composed of a mass of capillaries called a **glomerulus,** and the capsule that surrounds the glomerulus is called the **Bowman's capsule.** The renal corpuscle is where blood filtration occurs.

Renal tubules extend from the Bowman's capsule of a nephron. The three parts of a renal tubule are the **proximal convoluted tubule,** the **loop of Henle,** and the **distal convoluted tubule.** The proximal convoluted tubule is directly attached to the Bowman's capsule and eventually straightens out to become the loop of Henle. The loop of Henle curves back toward the renal corpuscle and starts to twist again, becoming the distal convoluted tubule. Distal convoluted tubules from several nephrons merge together to form collecting ducts. These ducts collect urine and deliver it to the renal pelvis, which in turn empties urine into the ureters (Figures 8-2 and 8-3).

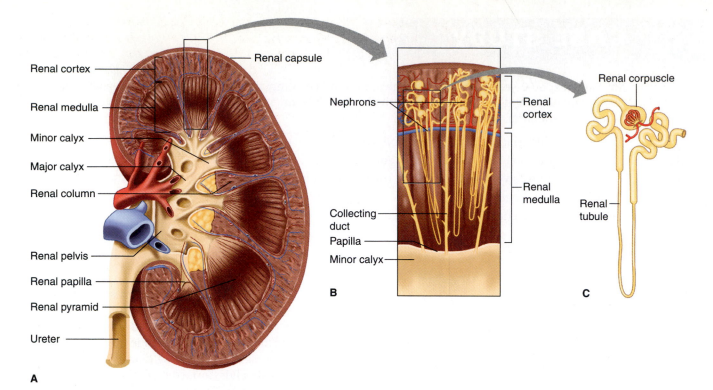

Figure 8-2. (A) Longitudinal section of a kidney, (B) the location of nephrons, and (C) a single nephron.

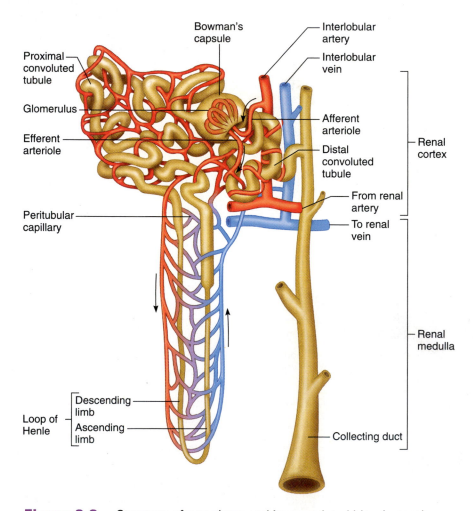

Figure 8-3. Structure of a nephron and its associated blood vessels.

Afferent arterioles bring blood to the tightly packed, increasingly narrow capillaries of the glomeruli. This narrowing is what causes the filtration of the blood by forcing blood through the capillary walls, similar to what occurs when water drips through a coffee filter in a drip coffeemaker. **Efferent arterioles** deliver blood to peritubular capillaries, which are wrapped around the renal tubules of the nephron. Blood leaves the peritubular capillaries through the veins of the kidneys. By the time the blood leaves the peritubular capillaries, it has been cleansed of waste products. Blood flows through a nephron in the following pathway:

afferent arteriole → glomerulus → efferent arteriole → peritubular capillaries → the veins of the kidney

Urine Formation

The three processes of urine formation are **glomerular filtration, tubular reabsorption,** and **tubular secretion.**

Glomerular Filtration

Glomerular filtration takes place in the renal corpuscles of nephrons. In this process, the fluid part of blood is forced from the glomerulus (the capillaries) into Bowman's capsule (Figure 8-4). The fluid in the Bowman's capsule is called the **glomerular filtrate.**

Glomerular filtration depends on filtration pressure, which is the amount of pressure that forces substances (filtrate) out of the glomerulus into the Bowman's capsule.

It is largely determined by blood pressure. If a person's blood pressure is too low, glomerular filtrate will not form. If filtration pressure increases, the rate of filtration and the amount of glomerular filtrate also increase.

The sympathetic nervous system (SNS) largely controls the rate of filtration. If blood pressure or blood volume drops, the SNS causes the afferent arterioles in the kidneys to constrict. When this constriction occurs, glomerular filtration pressure decreases and less glomerular filtrate is formed. When less glomerular filtrate is formed, less urine is ultimately formed. This allows the body to retain fluids that are needed to raise blood pressure and blood volume.

Tubular Reabsorption

Tubular reabsorption is the second process in urine formation. In this process, the glomerular filtrate flows into the proximal convoluted tubule (Figure 8-5A). The body needs to keep many of the substances (nutrients, water, and ions) that are found in glomerular filtrate. In tubular reabsorption, all the necessary substances in the glomerular filtrate pass through the wall of the renal tubule into the blood of the peritubular capillaries.

Water reabsorption varies depending on the presence of two hormones—antidiuretic hormone (ADH) and aldosterone. Both of these hormones increase water reabsorption, which decreases urine production. This retention of fluid and the resultant increase in blood pressure is one of the reasons why diuretics, which rid the body of excess fluid, are successful in treating some forms of hypertension.

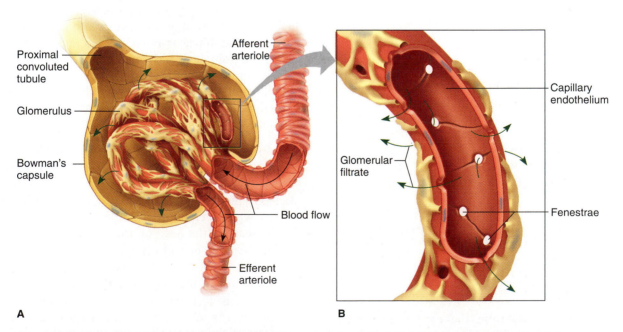

Proximal convoluted tubule

Glomerulus

Bowman's capsule

Afferent arteriole

Blood flow

Efferent arteriole

Capillary endothelium

Glomerular filtrate

Fenestrae

A

B

Figure 8-4. Glomerular filtration. (A) Substances move out of glomerular capillaries and into Bowman's capsule. (B) Glomerular capillaries have large holes called fenestrae that allow substances to move out of them and into Bowman's capsule.

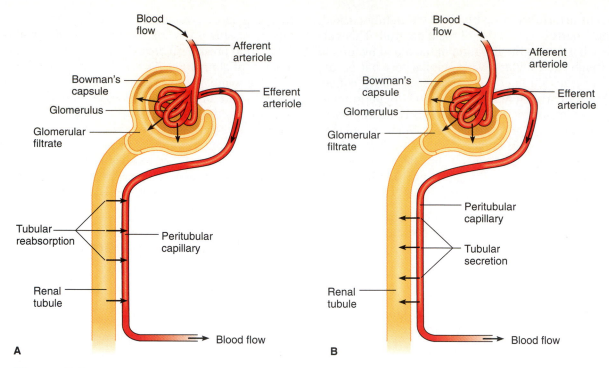

Figure 8-5. (A) Tubular reabsorption. Substances move from the glomerular filtrate into the blood of peritubular capillaries. (B) Tubular secretion. Substances move out of the blood of the peritubular capillaries into the renal tubule.

Tubular Secretion

Tubular secretion is the third process of urine formation. In tubular secretion, substances move out of the blood in the peritubular capillaries and into the renal tubules (Figure 8-5B). Substances that are secreted include drugs, hydrogen ions, and waste products. All of these secreted substances will be excreted in the urine.

Urine Composition

The final solution that reaches the collecting ducts of the kidneys is urine. Urine is mostly made of water but also normally contains **urea, uric acid,** trace amounts of amino acids, and various ions. Urea and uric acid are waste products formed by the breakdown of proteins and nucleic acids. The secretion of these waste materials assists in maintaining the body's acid-base balance.

The Ureters, Urinary Bladder, and Urethra

The Ureters

Ureters are long, muscular tubes that carry urine from the kidneys to the urinary bladder. They propel urine toward the bladder through rhythmic muscular contractions of the ureters called peristalsis.

Urinary Bladder

The urinary bladder is a distensible (expandable) organ that is located in the pelvic cavity. Its function is to store urine (up to 600 mL on average) until it is eliminated from the body. The internal floor of the bladder contains three openings—one for the urethra and two for the ureters. These three openings form a triangle called the **trigone** of the bladder. The wall of the bladder contains smooth muscle, called the **detrusor muscle.** This muscle contracts to push urine from the bladder into the urethra (Figure 8-6).

The process of urination is called **micturition.** The stretching of the bladder triggers this process—usually when the bladder contains approximately 150 mL of urine. The major events of micturition are the following:

1. The urinary bladder distends as it fills with urine.
2. The distension stimulates stretch receptors in the bladder wall, signaling the micturition center in the spinal cord.
3. Parasympathetic nerves stimulate the detrusor muscle, which begins rhythmic contractions that trigger the sense of the need to urinate.
4. The brain stem and cerebral cortex send impulses to voluntarily contract the external urethral sphincter and to inhibit the micturition impulse.
5. Upon the decision to urinate, the external urethral sphincter is relaxed and impulses from the pons and hypothalamus start the micturition reflex.
6. Contraction of the detrusor muscle occurs and urine is expelled through the urethra.

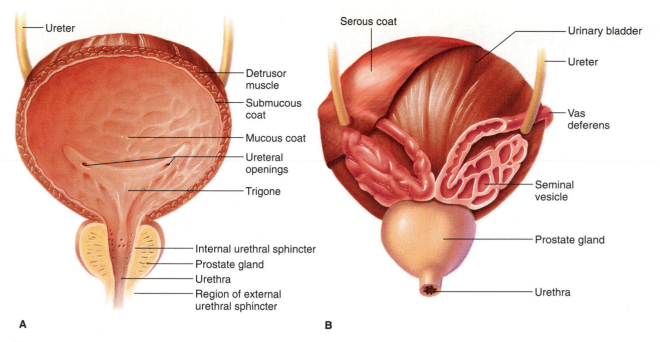

Figure 8-6. Male urinary bladder: (A) anterior view and (B) posterior view.

The Urethra

The **urethra** is a tube that moves urine from the bladder to the outside world. In females, the urethra is much shorter than in males. This anatomic difference, combined with the fact that the anus, vagina, and urethra are in close proximity in females, makes them much more susceptible to urinary tract infections.

Educating the Patient

Preventing Urinary Cystitis in Women

In females, the openings for the digestive, urinary, and reproductive systems are all within close proximity to each other in a highly functional design. However, when you combine this design with the female's shorter urethra (relative to men), women are much more likely than men to suffer from urinary tract infections (UTIs) and cystitis, more commonly known as bladder infections. As a medical assistant, if you understand why this is so, you will not only be able to assist your female patients when they have a UTI, with its pain (dysuria), urgency, and frequency, but you will also be able to give them helpful tips to prevent these painful episodes. Educate your female patients to take these steps:

1. *Urinate when the urge occurs.* By "holding it," urine stays in the bladder and the upper urethra, allowing bacteria to grow and causing infection.

2. *Drink lots of clear fluids.* This is known as "pushing fluids." The more clear liquids you drink, the more urine is created and the system is flushed on a regular basis. Cranberry juice is highly recommended as a preventative fluid, as well as part of the treatment if infection does occur.

3. *Wipe front to back.* Teach your female patients that after a bowel movement, they should wipe "front to back." Doing so prevents contamination of both the vagina and urethra by gastrointestinal (GI) bacteria (*E. coli*). Maintaining excellent hygiene in the perineal area is a very important component of UTI and cystitis prevention.

4. *Urinate after sexual intercourse.* Explain to your sexually active patients that urinating immediately after sexual intercourse will also help prevent episodes of cystitis.

If despite preventative methods cystitis or UTI does strike, reassure your patient that antibiotics and lots of fluids should take care of the problem. If the patient suffers from more than three infections during a year, a urologic workup may be advisable to look for underlying anatomical anomalies.

Pathophysiology

Common Diseases and Disorders of the Urinary System

Acute kidney (renal) failure is a sudden loss of kidney function.

- **Causes.** There are many causes and risk factors of kidney failure, including burns, dehydration, low blood pressure, hemorrhaging, allergic reactions, obstruction of the renal artery, various poisons, alcohol abuse, trauma to the kidneys and skeletal muscles, blood disorders, blood transfusion reactions, kidney stones, urinary tract infections, enlarged prostate, childbirth and immune system disorders, and food poisoning involving the bacteria *E. coli*.

- **Signs and symptoms.** The signs and symptoms include decreased urine production or no urine production, excessive urination, swelling of the extremities, bloating, mental confusion, coma, seizures, hand tremors, nosebleeds, easy bruising, pain in the back or abdomen, hypertension, abnormal heart or lung sounds, abnormal urinalysis, and an increase in potassium levels.

- **Treatment.** The first treatment measure is modifying the diet to decrease the amount of protein consumed. Controlling fluid intake and potassium levels is also recommended. Antibiotics and dialysis may also be needed. If the underlying cause can be treated, acute renal failure may be reversed and kidney function returned to normal.

Chronic kidney (renal) failure is a condition in which the kidneys slowly lose their ability to function. The patient may be asymptomatic until the kidneys have lost about 90% of their function.

- **Causes.** This disorder results from diabetes, hypertension, glomerulonephritis, polycystic kidney disease, kidney stones, obstruction of the ureters, and acute kidney failure.

- **Signs and symptoms.** The list of signs and symptoms is extensive and includes headache, mental confusion, coma, seizures, fatigue, frequent hiccups, itching, easy bruising, abnormal bleeding, anemia, excessive thirst, fluid retention, nausea, hypertension, abnormal heart or lung sounds, weight loss, white spots on the skin or increased pigmentation, high potassium levels, an increased or decreased urine output, urinary tract infections, and abnormal urinalysis results.

- **Treatment.** This disorder can be treated with antibiotics; blood transfusions; medications to control anemia; restriction of fluids, electrolytes, and protein; control of high blood pressure; and dialysis. The most serious cases may require surgery to repair a ureteral obstruction or a kidney (renal) transplant.

Cystitis is a urinary bladder infection. Women are much more likely to develop this disorder than men because of the short length of their urethras. The urethral opening in women is also close to the anal opening, allowing bacteria from this area to be more easily introduced into the urinary tract.

- **Causes.** This infection is caused by different types of bacteria (especially those that are found in the rectum) and may be caused by the placement of a catheter in the bladder. Good hygiene, urinating promptly when the urge occurs, and, for females, wiping from front to back can help to prevent this infection.

- **Signs and symptoms.** Common symptoms include fatigue, chills, fever, and a painful, frequent need to urinate, often with only small amounts of urine produced. Urine is often cloudy and blood may be present in the urine.

- **Treatment.** This infection is treated with antibiotics and pain medication when needed. The patient should also be urged to push (drink) lots of clear liquids.

Glomerulonephritis is an inflammation of the glomeruli of the kidney. Chronic glomerulonephritis is one of the causes of chronic renal disease.

- **Causes.** This disorder is caused by renal diseases, immune disorders, and bacterial infections.

- **Signs and symptoms.** The signs and symptoms are hiccups, drowsiness, coma, seizures, nausea, anemia, high blood pressure, increased skin pigmentation, abnormal heart sounds, abnormal urinalysis results, blood in the urine, and a decreased or increased urine output.

- **Treatment.** Treatment begins with a low-sodium, low-protein diet. Medications to control high blood pressure, corticosteroids to reduce inflammation, and dialysis are other treatment options.

Incontinence is a condition in which a person (other than a child) cannot control urination. This condition can be either temporary or long lasting. Women are more likely to develop incontinence than men are.

- **Causes.** This condition can be caused by various medications, excessive coughing (for example, in smokers), UTIs, nervous system disorders, and bladder cancer. In men, prostate problems can lead to the development of this disorder. The weakness of the urinary sphincters from surgery, trauma, or pregnancy can also cause incontinence. It may be prevented by avoiding urinary bladder irritants such as coffee, cigarettes, diuretics, and various medications.

- **Signs and symptoms.** The primary symptom is the involuntary leakage of urine.

continued ⟶

Common Diseases and Disorders of the Urinary System *(concluded)*

- **Treatment.** Treatment includes various medications, incontinence pads, removal of the prostate, Kegel exercises to increase the control of urinary sphincters, and surgery to repair damaged bladders or urethral sphincters.

Polycystic kidney disease is a disorder in which the kidneys enlarge because of the presence of many cysts within them. The disease develops relatively slowly, with symptoms worsening over time.

- **Causes.** The causes are hereditary (via an inherited dominant gene from a parent).
- **Signs and symptoms.** Fatigue, hypertension, anemia, pain in the back or abdomen, joint pain, heart murmurs, the formation of kidney stones, kidney failure, blood in the urine, and liver disease are the symptoms of this disorder.
- **Treatment.** Treatment includes medications to control anemia and high blood pressure, blood transfusions, draining of the cysts, dialysis, and surgery to remove one or both kidneys.

Pyelonephritis is a type of complicated UTI. It begins as a bladder infection and spreads to one or both kidneys. This condition can develop suddenly, or it may be chronic.

- **Causes.** This disorder is caused by bacteria, a bladder infection, kidney stones, or an obstruction of the urinary system ducts.
- **Signs and symptoms.** Signs and symptoms include fatigue, mental confusion, fever, nausea, pain in the back or abdomen, enlarged kidneys, painful urination, and cloudy or bloody urine.
- **Treatment.** Treatment includes intravenous fluids, pain medication, and antibiotics.

Renal calculi are more commonly called kidney stones. These stones can become lodged in the ducts within the kidneys or ureters.

- **Causes.** This condition is caused by gouty arthritis, defects of the ureters, overly concentrated urine, and urinary tract infections.
- **Signs and symptoms.** The signs and symptoms include fever, nausea, severe back or abdominal pain, a frequent urge to urinate, blood in the urine, and abnormal urinalysis results.
- **Treatment.** Treatment includes pain medication, intravenous fluids, medications to decrease stone formation, surgery to remove kidney stones, and lithotripsy (a procedure that uses shock waves to break up stones).

Summary

The kidneys, ureters, bladder, and urethra work together to remove waste products from the blood. The nephrons of the kidneys are involved in filtering the blood and urine formation. The ureters, bladder, and urethra are responsible for eliminating urine from the body. The kidneys also play an important role in regulating blood cell production by producing the hormone erythropoietin to stimulate the red bone marrow to produce red blood cells. They also help to control blood pressure by producing the hormone renin, which helps regulate blood pressure. Knowledge of the anatomy and physiology of the urinary system is important when collecting urine specimens, performing urinary testing, and assisting with cystoscopy.

REVIEW

CASE STUDY QUESTIONS

Now that you have completed this chapter, review the case study at the beginning of the chapter and answer the following questions:

1. What is the likely diagnosis for Mr. Sanchez?
2. What noninvasive therapies will be tried to help him?
3. Will surgery be needed?
4. What lifestyle changes might be suggested for Mr. Sanchez?

Discussion Questions

1. Describe the three steps in the formation of urine.
2. Normal urine contains only trace amounts of protein. Explain why a urinalysis showing a large amount of protein would be of concern.
3. Why are diuretics successful in treating some forms of hypertension?
4. Explain the functions of the kidneys.

Critical Thinking Questions

1. Why are females more likely than males to develop urinary tract infections?
2. Why would it not be surprising for a patient suffering from kidney failure to also be anemic?
3. The position of the kidneys is retroperitoneal. What would be the easiest way for a surgeon to reach a kidney?
4. Explain why patients with polycystic kidney disease tend to be less successful with kidney transplants than patients who have chronic renal failure related to other diagnoses.

Application Activities

1. Define the following parts of a kidney:
   a. Renal pyramid
   b. Renal cortex
   c. Renal medulla
   d. Renal pelvis
2. Name the three openings of the urinary bladder.
3. What is the name of the tubes that carry urine from the kidneys to the bladder? What is the name of the tube that carries urine from the bladder to outside of the body?
4. Explain the events of urination (micturition).

Virtual Fieldtrip

Visit the McGraw-Hill Higher Education Medical Assisting website at www.mhhe.com/medicalassisting3 to complete the following activity:

Use the National Kidney Foundation website and choose the *Kidney Diseases* tab to complete the following activities:

- What are some of the complications of chronic kidney disease?
- What test is now considered essential for tracking the progression of chronic kidney disease? What is the purpose of this test and how is it performed?
- How many Americans have chronic kidney failure and how many more may be at risk?

Now enter the *Organ Donation* area from the list on the left-hand side of the screen. Access the *Organ Donation* area (presently a PDF file, which you will have to download) and write a short paper based on the information you find on organ donation.

Open the CD and complete this chapter's practice activities, play the games, listen to the key terms, and test yourself with the interactive review. E-mail, print, and/or save your results to document your proficiency.

The Reproductive Systems

CHAPTER OUTLINE

- The Male Reproductive System
- The Female Reproductive System
- Pregnancy
- The Birth Process
- Contraception
- Infertility

KEY TERMS *(Concluded)*

fertilization
fetal period
fibroid
fimbriae
flaccid
follicle-stimulating
   hormone (FSH)
follicular cells
foramen ovale
fulgurated
fundus
glans penis
gonadotropin-releasing
   hormone (GnRH)
human chorionic
   gonadotropin (HCG)
hysterectomy
impotence
infundibulum
inner cell mass
interstitial cell
labia majora
labia minora
lactiferous
lactogen
luteinizing hormone (LH)
mammary glands
menarche
menopause
menses

menstrual cycle
mesoderm
mons pubis
morula
motility
myometrium
neonatal period
neonate
oocyte
oogenesis
ova
oviduct
ovulation
oxytocin (OT)
parathyroid hormone
   (PTH)
parturition
perimetrium
perineum
placenta
polar body
postnatal period
premenstrual syndrome
   (PMS)
prenatal period
prepuce
primary germ layer
primordial follicle
progesterone
prostaglandins

prostate gland
prostatitis
relaxin
rugae
scrotum
semen
seminal vesicles
seminiferous tubules
spermatids
spermatocytes
spermatogenesis
spermatogenic cells
spermatogonia
testes
testosterone
transurethral resection of
   prostate
umbilical cord
uterus
vagina
vaginal introitus
vaginitis
vas deferens
vasectomy
vestibule
vulva
vulvovaginitis
yolk sac
zona pellucida
zygote

KEY TERMS

acrosome
aldosterone
alveolar glands
amnion
areola
Bartholin's glands
benign prostatic
   hypertrophy
blastocyst
bulbourethral glands
cervical orifice
cervicitis
cervix
cesarean section
chlamydia
cleavage
clitoris
corpus luteum
Cowper's glands
cryptorchidism
ductus arteriosus
ductus venosus
dysmenorrhea
ectoderm
effacement
embryonic period
endoderm
endometriosis
endometrium
epididymis
epididymitis
episiotomy
erectile tissue
estrogen
fallopian tubes

LEARNING OUTCOMES

After completing Chapter 9, you will be able to:

9.1 List the organs of the male reproductive system and give the locations, structures, and functions of each.

9.2 Describe how sperm cells are formed.

9.3 Describe the substances found in semen.

9.4 Describe the processes of erection and ejaculation.

9.5 List the actions of testosterone.

9.6 Describe the causes, signs and symptoms, and treatment of various disorders of the male reproductive system.

9.7 List the organs of the female reproductive system and give the locations, structures, and functions of each.

9.8 Explain how ova develop.

9.9 List the actions of estrogen and progesterone.

9.10 Explain how and when ovulation occurs.

9.11 Describe what happens to an ovum after ovulation occurs.

9.12 List the purpose and events of the menstrual cycle.

9.13 Define menopause and explain what causes it.

9.14 Describe the causes, signs and symptoms, and treatment of various disorders of the female reproductive system.

9.15 Explain how and where fertilization occurs.

9.16 Describe the process of implantation.

9.17 Explain the difference between an embryo and a fetus.

9.18 Describe the changes that occur in a woman during pregnancy

9.19 List several birth control methods and explain why they are effective.

9.20 List the causes of and treatments for infertility.

9.21 Describe the causes, signs and symptoms, and treatments of the most common sexually transmitted diseases.

Introduction

The male and female reproductive systems function together to produce offspring. The female reproductive system nurtures a developing offspring. If a female breastfeeds, her breasts, considered accessory organs of both her reproductive and integumentary systems, are also used to nurture the newborn baby. The male and female reproductive systems also produce a number of important hormones before and during the reproductive years.

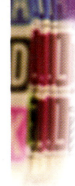

CASE STUDY

Last week, a 27-year-old female came to the doctor's office complaining of abnormal vaginal discharge, pain during urination, and pain in her abdominopelvic area. Her symptoms have been occurring for a couple of weeks but have recently started to get worse. She says that her sexual partner also has an abnormal discharge coming from his penis but is not experiencing any pain. The doctor diagnoses her with a urinary tract infection (UTI) and a sexually transmitted disease (STD) caused by bacteria. The doctor also tells the patient that she has peritonitis, which is inflammation in the abdominopelvic cavity. The patient is treated with antibiotics and pain medication. The doctor tells her that her sexual partner must also be treated with antibiotics.

As you read this chapter, consider the following questions:

1. What STDs are caused by bacteria?
2. How did the infection spread to the patient's abdominopelvic cavity?
3. Why is her sexual partner not experiencing pain in his abdominopelvic cavity?
4. Why is it important for her sexual partner to be treated with antibiotics?
5. Why is it common for women with STDs to also have UTIs?

The Male Reproductive System

Testes

Testes are the primary organs of the male reproductive system because they produce the sex cells (sperm) of the male (Figure 9-1). They also produce the male hormone **testosterone.** Most males have two testes that are held just below the pelvic cavity in the **scrotum.** During the fetal stage, the testes develop in the abdominopelvic cavity of the fetus. Shortly before or soon after birth, the testes descend into the scrotal sac located just below the pelvic cavity. A fibrous capsule encloses each testis and invades the testis to divide it into lobules. Each lobule is filled with **seminiferous tubules,** which are filled with **spermatogenic cells.** These cells give rise to sperm cells. Between the seminiferous tubules are the **interstitial cells,** which produce testosterone.

Sperm Cell Formation. Spermatogenic cells of the seminiferous tubules begin the process of making sperm cells, but the sperm cells do not mature until they travel to the **epididymis. Spermatogenesis** is the process of sperm cell formation. At the beginning of spermatogenesis, the cells are called **spermatogonia.** Spermatogonia contain 46 chromosomes. These cells undergo mitosis (refer to Figure 1-10), and the resulting cells are called primary **spermatocytes.** Primary spermatocytes also contain 46 chromosomes. At about the time of puberty, primary spermatocytes undergo a process called meiosis (Figures 9-2 and 9-3A). In meiosis, each primary spermatocyte divides to make two secondary spermatocytes. Each secondary spermatocyte divides to make two **spermatids.** Therefore, from one primary spermatocyte, four spermatids are formed. Spermatids develop flagella to become mature sperm cells. They contain only 23 chromosomes.

Structure of Sperm Cells. A mature sperm (Figure 9-3B) has the following three parts: the head, the midpiece, and the tail.

The Head. The head is oval in structure and holds a nucleus with 23 chromosomes. The head is covered with an enzyme-filled sac called an **acrosome,** which helps the sperm penetrate an ovum at the time of fertilization.

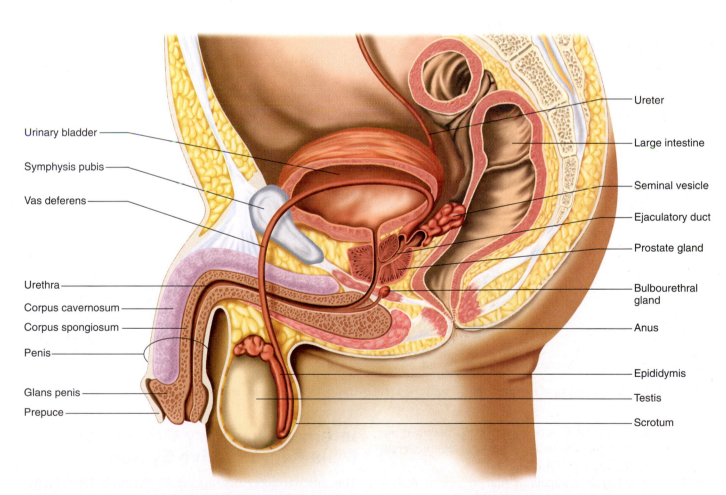

Figure 9-1. Sagittal view of male reproductive organs. The male reproductive system produces sperm and delivers them in a form that keeps them viable long enough to fertilize an ovum.

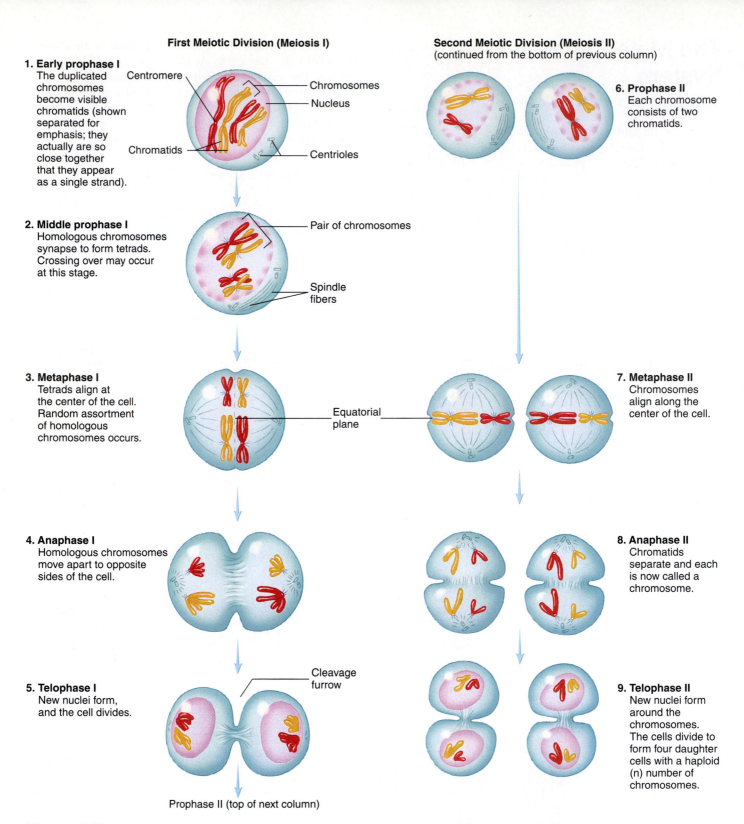

Figure 9-2. The process of meiosis, including prophase, metaphase, anaphase, and telophase.

The Midpiece. This portion of the sperm is between the head and tail. It is filled with mitochondria that generate the energy needed by the cell to move.

The Tail. The tail is a flagellum that moves in such a way as to propel the sperm forward in the female reproductive tract.

Internal Accessory Organs of the Male Reproductive System

The internal accessory organs of the male reproductive system are the epididymis, **vas deferens, seminal vesicles, prostate gland,** and **bulbourethral** or **Cowper's glands.**

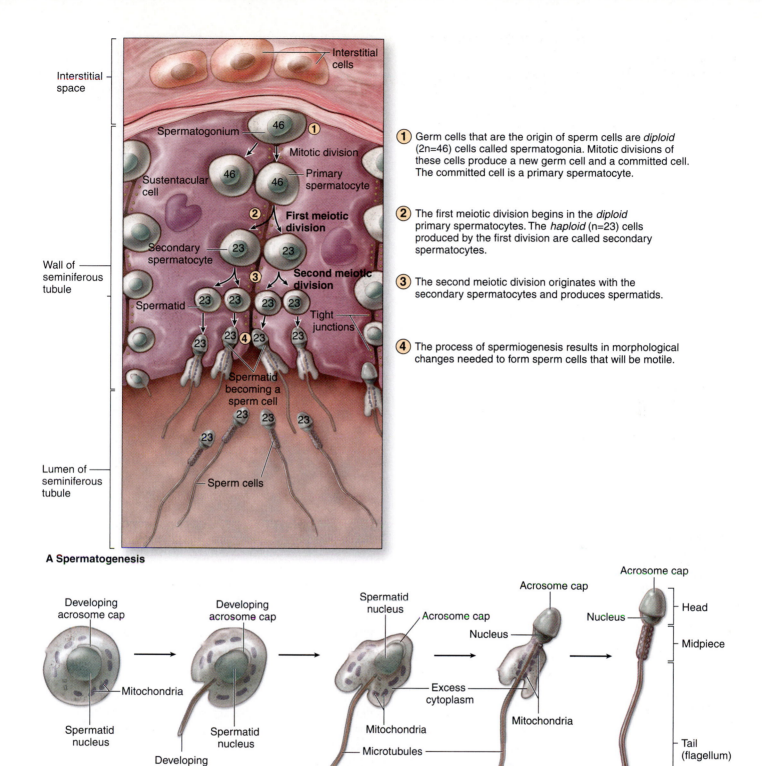

A Spermatogenesis

Interstitial space

Interstitial cells

Spermatogonium — 46 ①

Mitotic division

Sustentacular cell

46 — Primary spermatocyte

② First meiotic division

Secondary spermatocyte — 23 · 23

③ Second meiotic division

Spermatid — 23 23 · 23 23 — Tight junctions

23 · 23 ④ 23 · 23

Spermatid becoming a sperm cell

Wall of seminiferous tubule

Lumen of seminiferous tubule

Sperm cells — 23 · 23 · 23 · 23

① Germ cells that are the origin of sperm cells are *diploid* (2n=46) cells called spermatogonia. Mitotic divisions of these cells produce a new germ cell and a committed cell. The committed cell is a primary spermatocyte.

② The first meiotic division begins in the *diploid* primary spermatocytes. The *haploid* (n=23) cells produced by the first division are called secondary spermatocytes.

③ The second meiotic division originates with the secondary spermatocytes and produces spermatids.

④ The process of spermiogenesis results in morphological changes needed to form sperm cells that will be motile.

B Spermiogenesis

Developing acrosome cap — Mitochondria — Spermatid nucleus

Developing acrosome cap — Spermatid nucleus — Developing flagellum

Spermatid nucleus — Acrosome cap — Excess cytoplasm — Mitochondria — Microtubules — Developing flagellum

Acrosome cap — Nucleus — Excess cytoplasm — Mitochondria

Acrosome cap — Nucleus — Head — Midpiece — Tail (flagellum)

Figure 9-3. Spermatogenesis and Spermiogenesis. (A) The processes of spermatogenesis and spermiogenesis take place in the wall of the seminiferous tubule. (B) Structural changes occur during spermiogenesis as a sperm cell forms from a spermatid.

Epididymis. An epididymis sits on top of each testis. It is a highly coiled tube that receives spermatids from seminiferous tubules as these cells are formed. Inside the epididymis, spermatids mature to become sperm cells.

Vas Deferens. A tube called a vas deferens is connected to each epididymis. These tubes carry sperm cells from an epididymis to the urethra in the pelvic cavity of the male. When a male has a **vasectomy,** these tubes are cut and tied, or **fulgurated,** to prevent sperm from reaching the ovum.

Seminal Vesicle. Seminal vesicles are sac-like organs that secrete an alkaline fluid rich in sugars and **prostaglandins.** The sugars are used by sperm cells to make energy, and the prostaglandins stimulate muscular contractions in the female reproductive system. These muscular contractions, known as peristalsis, help to propel sperm forward in the female reproductive tract. Seminal vesicles release their product into the vas deferens just before ejaculation. Seminal fluid makes up approximately 60% of semen volume.

Prostate Gland. The muscular prostate gland surrounds the proximal portion of the urethra. It produces a milky, alkaline fluid and secretes this fluid into the urethra just before ejaculation. The alkaline nature of this fluid helps to protect the sperm when they enter the acidic environment of the female vagina. Prostatic fluid makes up approximately 40% of semen volume. During ejaculation, the muscular contractions of the prostate assist with the expulsion of semen.

Bulbourethral Glands. Bulbourethral glands, or Cowper's glands, are inferior to the prostate gland. They produce a mucus-like fluid that is secreted before ejaculation into the urethra. This fluid lubricates the end of the penis in preparation for sexual intercourse.

Semen. **Semen** is a mixture of sperm cells and fluids from the seminal vesicles, prostate gland, and bulbourethral glands. This mixture is alkaline and contains nutrients and prostaglandins. Total semen volume is between 1.5 and 5.0 mL per ejaculate, with a sperm count of between 40 and 250 million/mL. A normal sperm count is considered to be more than 80 million.

External Organs of the Male Reproductive System

The two male external reproductive organs are the scrotum and the penis (see Figure 9-1).

Scrotum. The scrotum is a pouch of skin that holds the testes. It is lined with a serous membrane that secretes serous fluid to ensure that the testes move freely within it. The scrotum holds the testes away from the rest of the body, keeping their temperature about one degree lower than the rest of the body, which is necessary for the viability of the sperm.

Penis. The penis is a cylindrical organ that moves urine and semen to outside of the body. The shaft, or body, of the penis contains specialized tissue called **erectile tissue** that surrounds the urethra, which runs the length of the penis. The end of the penis is enlarged into a cone-shaped structure called the **glans penis.** If a male has not been circumcised, a piece of skin, called the **prepuce,** covers the glans penis. The function of the penis is to deliver sperm to the female reproductive tract. The penis also functions in urination because it contains the urethra, which drains urine from the bladder.

Erection, Orgasm, and Ejaculation

During sexual arousal, the parasympathetic nervous system causes erectile tissue of the penis to become engorged with blood, which produces erection of the penis. During orgasm, sperm cells are propelled out of the testes toward the urethra. The secretions of the prostate, seminal vesicles, and bulbourethral glands are also released into the urethra. The movement of the sperm and secretions into the urethra is called emission. The process of ejaculation occurs when semen is forced out of the urethra. After ejaculation, sympathetic nerve fibers cause the erectile tissue to release blood, and the penis gradually returns to a **flaccid** or nonerect state.

Male Reproductive Hormones

The hypothalamus, anterior pituitary gland, and the testes secrete hormones that regulate male reproductive functions. At the onset of puberty and throughout his life, the hypothalamus releases a hormone called **gonadotropin-releasing hormone (GnRH).** GnRH stimulates the anterior pituitary gland to release **follicle-stimulating hormone (FSH)** and **luteinizing hormone (LH).** FSH causes spermatogenesis to begin, and LH stimulates interstitial cells to produce testosterone.

Testosterone is responsible for the development of male secondary sex characteristics, which are the characteristics that are typically unique to males. Examples of these characteristics are chest hair, thick facial hair, a thickening and strengthening of muscles and bones, and the thickening of vocal cords that produces a deeper voice. Testosterone also stimulates the maturation of male reproductive organs.

Testosterone levels are regulated by negative feedback in the following cycle: Blood testosterone levels increase to above normal levels, which cause the hypothalamus to release GnRH. In response, the anterior pituitary ceases the secretion of LH and FSH, in turn causing the testosterone level to fall. When the testosterone level falls below normal, GnRH is again secreted by the hypothalamus, triggering the release of LH and FSH by the anterior pituitary, and the cycle begins again.

Pathophysiology

Common Diseases and Disorders of the Male Reproductive System

Benign prostatic hypertrophy or BPH is the nonmalignant enlargement of the prostate gland. This condition is common in older men.

- **Causes.** BPH is related to the hormonal changes that occur as part of the aging process.
- **Signs and symptoms.** Men with BPH often complain of frequent urination, especially at night, as well as painful urination and difficulty starting or stopping the urinary stream, including "dribbling" at the end of urination.
- **Treatment.** Diagnosis is often confirmed by digital rectal exam (DRE), when the physician inserts a gloved finger into the rectum and palpates the prostate. Blood tests (PSA) and a biopsy may be done to rule out cancer. Once this is ruled out, medications such as Avodart® or Flomax® may manage the problem or **transurethral resection of the prostate** (TURP) may be performed to remove the enlarged tissue.

Epididymitis is inflammation of an epididymis. Most cases start out as an infection of the urinary tract that spreads to an epididymis.

- **Causes.** The causes include the use of certain medications, placement of a catheter in the urethra, and bacteria—especially those that cause gonorrhea and chlamydia.
- **Signs and symptoms.** Signs and symptoms include fever, pain in the testes, a lump in the testes, swelling of the scrotum, painful ejaculation, blood in the semen, pain during urination, discharge from the urethra, and enlarged lymph nodes in the pelvic area.
- **Treatment.** Treatment includes pain medication, antibiotics for both the patient and his sexual partner, elevation of the scrotum, and ice packs applied to the scrotum.

Impotence or *erectile dysfunction* (ED) is a disorder in which a male cannot achieve or maintain an erect penis to complete sexual intercourse. It is estimated that half of all men between the ages of 40 and 70 years have some degree of impotence. Most causes are physical and not psychological.

- **Causes.** Psychological causes include anxiety, stress, and depression. Common physical causes include diabetes, high blood pressure, anemia, coronary artery disease (CAD), peripheral vascular disease (PVD), low testosterone production, various medications, smoking, excessive alcohol consumption, and drugs such as cocaine, marijuana, and heroin.
- **Signs and symptoms.** Signs and symptoms are an inability to achieve an erection or an inability to maintain an erection long enough to complete sexual intercourse.

- **Treatment.** The first treatment step should be lifestyle changes to quit smoking and stop using alcohol or drugs. Counseling to reduce anxiety and depression may also be helpful. Other treatment options include oral medications such as Viagra® or Cialis®, penile injections of medications, and penile implants if oral medications do not work.

Prostate cancer is one of the most common cancers found in men older than age 40 and the risk of developing prostate cancer increases with age. Awareness about this malignancy is growing and access to screenings such as DRE (digital rectal exam) is becoming widely available. Therefore, many cases in the United States are being diagnosed before symptoms even occur.

- **Causes.** The causes are mostly unknown, although decreased testosterone production may contribute to the development of this disease, explaining why risk increases with age.
- **Signs and symptoms.** Common symptoms include anemia, weight loss, incontinence, difficulty starting or stopping urination, painful urination, pain in the lower back or abdomen, pain during bowel movements, high levels of PSA (prostate-specific antigen) in the blood, blood in the urine, and bone pain in advanced cases, when cancer cells, known as metastases, have spread to the bone.
- **Treatment.** Treatments include hormone therapy, chemotherapy, radiation therapy to shrink or destroy the tumor, as well as surgery to remove the prostate, known as *prostatectomy*.

Prostatitis is an inflammation of the prostate gland. If it develops suddenly, it is called *acute prostatitis*. The slow development of this condition is termed *chronic prostatitis*.

- **Causes.** This condition can be caused by excessive alcohol consumption, bacterial infection, a catheterization, trauma to the urethra or urinary bladder, and scarring of the urethra or prostate because of frequent infections. Urinating frequently can help to prevent this infection.
- **Signs and symptoms.** Signs and symptoms include fever; pain in the scrotum, pelvic area, or abdomen; difficult, frequent, and/or painful urination; blood in the urine; painful ejaculation; blood in the semen; discharge from the urethra; a low sperm count; and white blood cells in urine or semen.
- **Treatment.** This condition is treated with antibiotics. Surgery may also be required to repair any damage to the urethra.

Testicular cancer. Testicular cancer is a malignant growth of one or both testicles. Unlike prostate cancer, which

continued ⟶

Common Diseases and Disorders of the Male Reproductive System *(concluded)*

tends to occur in older males, testicular cancer occurs in males ages 15 to 30 and is a much more aggressive type of malignancy.

- **Causes.** Predisposing factors include **cryptorchidism** (undescended testicles during infancy). Family history may also be a factor.

- **Signs and symptoms.** A hard, painless lump in one testicle is a common early symptom. Patients may

complain of groin or abdominal pain as the disease progresses.

- **Treatment.** Orchiectomy or removal of the involved testis is usually performed, followed by radiation therapy and chemotherapy. Caught in the early stages, testicular cancer has up to a 95% success rate, verifying the need for males to perform testicular self-exams on a monthly basis.

The Female Reproductive System

Ovaries and Ovum Formation

The ovaries are the primary sex organs of the female because they produce the sex cells, called **ova,** of the female (Figures 9-4 and 9-5). They also produce **estrogen** and **progesterone,** the female hormones. Most females have two ovaries. They are oval in shape and are located in the pelvic cavity. Each ovary is divided into an inner area called the medulla and an outer area called the cortex. The medulla contains nerves, lymphatic vessels, and many

blood vessels. The cortex contains small masses of cells called ovarian follicles. Epithelial tissue and dense connective tissue cover each ovary.

Before a female child is born, **primordial follicles** develop in her ovarian cortex. Each primordial follicle contains a large cell called a primary **oocyte** (immature ovum) and smaller cells called **follicular cells.** Unlike males, who make sperm cells throughout their entire life, a female is born with the maximum number of primary oocytes she will ever produce.

Oogenesis is the process of ovum formation. At the onset of puberty, some primary oocytes are stimulated to continue meiosis (see Figure 9-2). When a primary oocyte

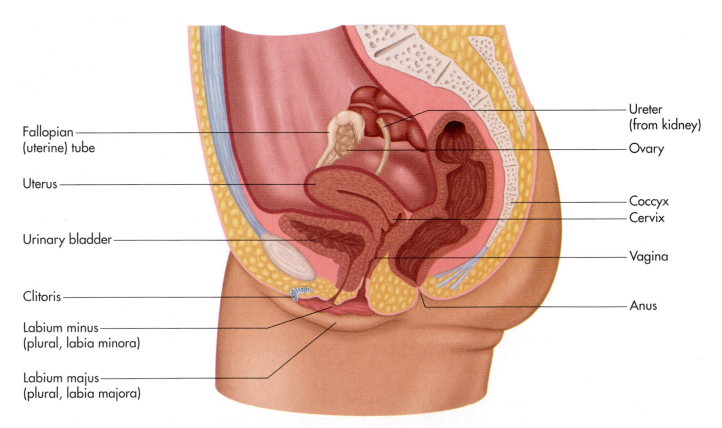

Fallopian (uterine) tube

Uterus

Urinary bladder

Clitoris

Labium minus (plural, labia minora)

Labium majus (plural, labia majora)

Ureter (from kidney)

Ovary

Coccyx

Cervix

Vagina

Anus

Figure 9-4. Sagittal view of female reproductive organs. The female reproductive system produces ova for fertilization and provides the place and means for a fertilized ovum to develop.

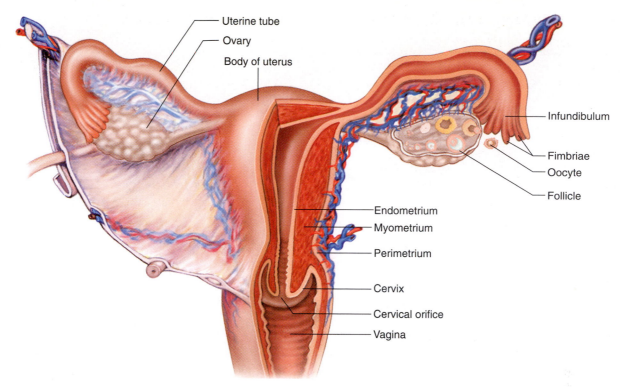

Figure 9-5. Anterior view of internal female reproductive organs. Ovulation of an oocyte is also demonstrated.

Labels in figure:
- Uterine tube
- Ovary
- Body of uterus
- Infundibulum
- Fimbriae
- Oocyte
- Follicle
- Endometrium
- Myometrium
- Perimetrium
- Cervix
- Cervical orifice
- Vagina

divides, it becomes one **polar body** (a nonfunctional cell) and a secondary oocyte. It is the secondary oocyte that is released from an ovary each month during a process called **ovulation.** When the secondary oocyte is fertilized, it divides to form a mature, fertilized ovum. Therefore, the process of meiosis begins before a female is born and is completed only if a secondary oocyte is fertilized. The mature ovum contains 23 chromosomes; when it combines with a sperm cell, the resulting cell contains 46 chromosomes.

Internal Accessory Organs of the Female Reproductive System

The female reproductive internal accessory organs are the **fallopian tubes, uterus,** and **vagina.**

Fallopian Tubes. A fallopian tube or **oviduct** opens near each ovary and the other end connects to the uterus. The fringed, expanded end of a fallopian tube near an ovary is called an **infundibulum** and **fimbriae.** The infundibulum and its fimbriae function to "catch" an ovum as it leaves an ovary. Fallopian tubes are muscular tubes that are lined with mucus membrane and cilia. This construction allows the tube to propel the ovum toward the uterus using peristalsis and the sweeping motions of cilia.

Uterus. The uterus is a hollow, muscular organ that functions to receive a developing embryo and sustain its development. The upper domed portion of the uterus is called the **fundus,** the main portion is called the body, and the narrow,

lower portion that extends into the vagina is called the **cervix.** The opening of the cervix is called the **cervical orifice.**

The wall of the uterus has three layers—the **endometrium, myometrium,** and **perimetrium.** The endometrium is the innermost lining of the uterus. It is vascular with a rich blood supply and also contains numerous tubular glands that secrete mucus. The myometrium is the middle, thick, muscular layer. The perimetrium is a thin layer that covers the myometrium. It secretes serous fluid that coats and protects the uterus.

Vagina. The vagina is a tubular, muscular organ that extends from the uterus to the outside of the body. The muscular folds of the vagina, called **rugae,** allow it to expand to receive an erect penis during sexual intercourse, and provide a passageway for delivery of offspring as well as for uterine secretions. The opening of the vagina is posterior to the urinary opening and anterior to the anal opening. The wall of the vagina has three layers—an innermost mucosal layer that secretes mucus, a middle muscular layer, and an outermost fibrous layer. The opening of the vagina to the outside is known as the *vaginal os,* the vaginal orifice, or the **vaginal introitus.**

External Accessory Organs of the Female Reproductive System

Mammary glands are the accessory organs of the female reproductive and integumentary systems (Figure 9-6). Their reproductive function is the secretion of milk for newborn offspring.

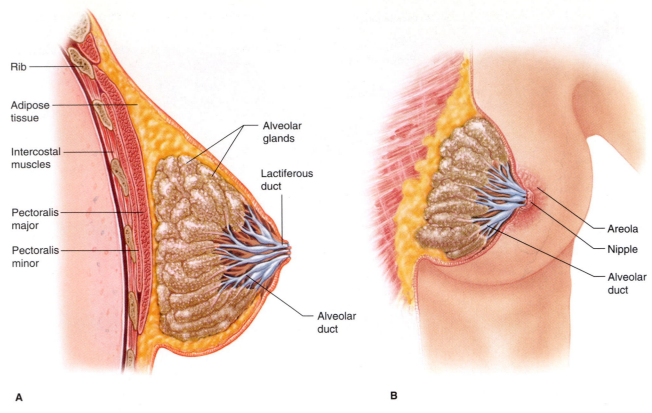

Figure 9-6. Mammary glands: (A) sagittal view and (B) anterior view.

Labels in figure:
Rib
Adipose tissue
Intercostal muscles
Pectoralis major
Pectoralis minor
Alveolar glands
Lactiferous duct
Alveolar duct
Areola
Nipple
Alveolar duct
A
B

Mammary glands are located beneath the skin in the breast area. A nipple is located near the center of each breast. The pigmented area that surrounds the nipple is called the **areola.** Each gland is made of 15 to 20 lobes and contains **alveolar glands** that make milk under the influence of the hormone prolactin. The hormone **oxytocin (OT)** induces **lactiferous** ducts to deliver milk through openings in the nipples. If a woman wants to breast-feed, she must produce adequate amounts of prolactin and oxytocin.

External Genitalia of the Female Reproductive System

The female external genitalia, collectively known as the **vulva,** include the following structures: **mons pubis, labia majora, labia minora, clitoris,** urethral meatus, vaginal orifice, **Bartholin's glands,** and **perineum.**

Labia Majora.   The labia majora are rounded folds of adipose tissue and skin that serve to protect the other external female reproductive organs. At their anterior ends, the labia majora form the mons pubis, which is a fatty area that overlies the pubic symphysis. The labia majora and mons pubis are typically covered in pubic hair in post-pubescent females.

Labia Minora.   The labia minora are folds of skin between the labia majora. They are pinkish in color because of their high degree of vascularity. They merge together anteriorly to form a hood over the clitoris.

The space enclosed by the labia minora is called the **vestibule.** The Bartholin's glands, sometimes referred to as the vestibular glands, secrete mucus into this area during sexual arousal. This mucus eases insertion of the penis into the vagina.

Clitoris.   The clitoris is anterior to the urethral meatus. It contains the female erectile tissue and is rich in sensory nerves.

Perineum.   The perineum is the area between vagina and anus. This is the area that is sometimes "clipped" during the birth process, in a procedure known as an **episiotomy.**

Erection, Lubrication, and Orgasm

During sexual arousal, nervous stimulation causes the clitoris to become erect and the Bartholin's glands to become active. At the same time, the vagina elongates. If the clitoris is sufficiently stimulated, an orgasm occurs. During orgasm, the walls of the uterus and fallopian tubes contract to help propel sperm toward the upper ends of the fallopian tubes.

Female Reproductive Hormones   Beginning at puberty, the hypothalamus secretes increasing amounts of GnRH. This causes the anterior pituitary gland to release FSH and LH, which stimulate the ovary to produce estrogen and progesterone, and also to mature the ovarian follicles. The estrogen and progesterone are responsible for the female secondary sex characteristics: breast development, increased vascularization of the skin, and increased fat deposits in the breasts, thighs, and hips.

Female Reproductive Cycle   The female reproductive cycle is also called the **menstrual cycle.** It consists of regular changes in the uterine lining that leads to a monthly "period," or bleeding. The first menstrual period is known as **menarche. Menopause** is the termination of the menstrual cycle because of normal aging of the ovaries. The following steps are the major hormonal changes that occur during one reproductive cycle:

1. The anterior pituitary gland releases FSH, which stimulates an ovarian follicle to mature.

2. The maturing follicle secretes estrogen. Estrogen causes the uterine lining to thicken.

3. The anterior pituitary gland releases a sudden surge of LH, which triggers ovulation.

4. Following ovulation, follicular cells of the follicle become a **corpus luteum.**

5. The corpus luteum secretes progesterone, which causes the uterine lining to become more vascular and glandular.

6. If the released oocyte is not fertilized, the corpus luteum degenerates, causing estrogen and progesterone levels to fall.

7. The decline in estrogen and progesterone levels causes the uterine lining to break down, and **menses** (bleeding) starts.

8. When the anterior pituitary releases FSH, the reproductive cycle begins again.

Pathophysiology

Common Diseases and Disorders of the Female Reproductive System

Breast cancer. According to the American Cancer Society, breast cancer is the second leading cause of cancer deaths in women after lung cancer. Depending on tumor size and how far cancer cells have spread, breast cancer is classified in stages from 0 to 4, with stage 4 cancer being the most serious. Early diagnosis through regular mammograms and breast self-exams greatly increases the success of treatment.

- **Causes.** The causes are largely unknown, although breast cancer may be related to hormonal changes or the presence of certain genes.
- **Signs and symptoms.** Signs and symptoms include a lump in the breast that is usually painless and firm, a lump in the armpit, discharge from the nipples, dimpled skin on the breast or nipple, and breast pain. Swelling of the breast into the adjacent arm and bone pain may be present in advanced cases. Inflammatory breast cancer may present only as a painless rash of the affected breast with none of the other typical symptoms.
- **Treatment.** Nonsurgical treatment methods include hormone therapy, radiation therapy, and chemotherapy. Surgical options include surgery to remove affected lymph nodes, lumpectomy (surgery to remove a lump), and mastectomy (surgery to remove a breast).

Cervical cancer generally develops slowly. With early detection by a yearly Pap smear (a test looking for abnormal cervical cells), treatment is often successful. It should be noted that the new recommendation for Pap smear screenings is now every other year if a woman's previous screenings have been negative for 5 years and if the woman is in a monogamous relationship and not on birth control pills.

- **Causes.** A weak immune system may be a factor in the development of this cancer. Risk factors also include sexual intercourse early in life, multiple sexual partners, and infection with the human papilloma virus (HPV).
- **Signs and symptoms.** Primary symptoms include frequent vaginal discharge, sporadic vaginal bleeding, vaginal bleeding after sexual intercourse, and abnormal cells in the cervix. Patients who are in later stages of this disease may experience pain in the pelvic area or legs, or bone fractures.
- **Treatment.** Radiation therapy, chemotherapy, the removal or destruction of diseased tissue with cryosurgery or laser surgery, and the removal of the uterus (**hysterectomy**) are the treatments for this disease.

Cervicitis is defined as an inflammation of the cervix, which is usually caused by an infection.

- **Causes.** Causes include bacterial or viral infections and allergic reactions to spermicidal creams and latex condoms.
- **Signs and symptoms.** Frequent vaginal discharge, pain during intercourse, and vaginal bleeding after intercourse are common signs and symptoms.
- **Treatment.** This condition is treated with antibiotics and by changing the method of contraception.

continued ⟶

Common Diseases and Disorders of the Female Reproductive System (continued)

Dysmenorrhea is the condition of experiencing severe menstrual cramps that limit normal daily activities.

- **Causes.** Causes include anxiety, endometriosis, pelvic inflammatory disease, fibroid tumors in the uterus, ovarian cysts, abnormally high levels of prostaglandins, and multiple sexual partners.
- **Signs and symptoms.** Common symptoms are abdominal pain, including sharp or dull pain in the pelvic area just prior to and during the menstrual period.
- **Treatment.** Nonsurgical treatments include pain medication, anti-inflammatory drugs, medications that inhibit prostaglandin formation, oral contraceptives, and antibiotics in the case of pelvic inflammatory disease. Surgical treatments include hysterectomy and surgery to remove cysts or fibroids.

Endometriosis is a condition in which tissues that make up the lining of the uterus grow outside the uterus.

- **Causes.** The cause of this disorder is unknown; it may be inherited.
- **Signs and symptoms.** Signs and symptoms include infertility, heavy bleeding from the uterus, pain in the abdomen or pelvis, painful periods, spotting between periods, and pain during sexual intercourse.
- **Treatment.** Oral contraceptives, pain medications, and various hormone therapies may be prescribed. Surgical treatments include laser surgery to remove endometrial tissue outside the uterus and hysterectomy.

Fibrocystic breast disease is the presence of abnormal cystic tissues in the breasts. The cysts within the breasts vary in size related to the menstrual cycle. It is a common disorder and occurs in more than 60% of women in the United States between the ages of 30 and 50. It is rare in women who have gone through menopause because it is related to hormonal changes occurring during the menstrual cycle.

- **Causes.** This disorder is caused by hormonal changes associated with the menstrual cycle and ingestion of various dietary substances, including caffeine, nicotine, and sugar. Birth control pills may also aggravate this condition.
- **Signs and symptoms.** Common symptoms include breasts that feel "lumpy," breast tenderness or pain, itchy nipples, and dense tissues as seen in a mammogram. The masses are usually firm and vary in size related to the stage of the menstrual cycle.
- **Treatment.** Treatments include changing one's diet, taking vitamin supplements such as vitamin E, B complex, and magnesium. Pain control may be affected by wearing support bras.

Fibroids are benign (noncancerous) tumors that grow in the uterine wall. They are known to affect one out of four women in their 30s and 40s and appear to be more common in women of African descent.

- **Causes.** The causes are mostly unknown, although it has been found that tumors enlarge as estrogen levels increase. Heredity does appear to play a role.
- **Signs and symptoms.** The signs and symptoms are pressure in the abdomen, severe menstrual cramps, abdominal gas, heavy menstrual bleeding, and intermenstrual bleeding. Back and leg pain may also occur.
- **Treatment.** Treatment includes pain medications, hormone treatments to shrink tumors, surgery to remove tumors, hysterectomy, and surgery to decrease the blood supply to the uterus.

Ovarian cancer is considered more deadly than other types of cancer because its signs and symptoms are usually mild or indistinct until the disease has spread to other organs, making early detection difficult. Current statistics suggest that about 1 woman in 67 will develop ovarian cancer.

- **Causes.** The causes are unknown, although the presence of certain genes has been indicated as a risk factor. Some oral contraceptives may lower the risk of developing this disease.
- **Signs and symptoms.** Abdominal and pelvic discomfort, unusual menstrual cycles, indigestion, bloating, nausea, and excessive hair growth are signs and symptoms. Diagnosis is made after ultrasound, a CA 125 blood test, and an ovarian biopsy.
- **Treatment.** Treatment options include radiation therapy, chemotherapy, and surgery to remove the ovaries and reproductive organs.

Premenstrual syndrome (PMS) is a collection of symptoms that occur just before a menstrual period.

- **Causes.** The causes are mostly unknown, although hormone fluctuations during the menstrual cycle are implicated.
- **Signs and symptoms.** The signs and symptoms include anxiety, depression, irritability, acne, fatigue, food cravings, bloating, aches in the head or back, abdominal pain, breast tenderness, muscle spasms, diarrhea, weight gain, and loss of sex drive.
- **Treatment.** PMS is commonly treated with pain medications, diuretics, medications to treat depression or anxiety, and oral contraceptives. Many women have also found changes in diet, including limiting caffeine, sugar, and sodium, helpful. The addition of B complex vitamins may also be helpful.

Vaginitis (inflammation of the vagina) and **vulvovaginitis** (inflammation of the vulva and vagina) are usually associated with an abnormal vaginal discharge. Some vaginal discharge is normal for all women, and it varies

continued ⟶

Common Diseases and Disorders of the Female Reproductive System *(concluded)*

throughout the menstrual cycle. Normal vaginal discharge is clear, whitish, or yellowish in color.

- **Causes.** This condition can be caused by yeast infections, tampon use, poor hygiene, bacteria, antibiotics, and STDs. Vaginitis may be prevented through good hygiene and safer sex practices.
- **Signs and symptoms.** Common symptoms include fever, vulvar and vaginal itching and swelling, an abnormal increase or decrease in the amount of vaginal discharge, an abnormal color of vaginal discharge (brown, green, or pinkish), a change in the consistency of vaginal discharge (frothy or cheeselike), and vaginal discharge that has an abnormal odor.
- **Treatment.** The patient may be given medications for fungal or bacterial infections, or the patient and her sexual partner may be treated for sexually transmitted diseases.

Uterine (endometrial) cancer is most common in postmenopausal women. In the United States, it accounts for approximately 6% of cancer deaths in women.

- **Causes.** The causes are mostly unknown, although it may be related to increased levels of estrogen.
- **Signs and symptoms.** Signs and symptoms include abdominal pain, abnormal bleeding from the uterus, pelvic pain, and a thin, white vaginal discharge in postmenopausal women.
- **Treatment.** Treatment includes radiation therapy, chemotherapy, and surgery to remove the uterus, fallopian tubes, and ovaries.

Pregnancy

Fertilization

Pregnancy is defined as the condition of having a developing offspring in the uterus. Pregnancy results when a sperm cell unites with an ovum in a process called **fertilization** (Figure 9-7).

Prior to fertilization, an ovum is released from an ovary and it travels through a fallopian tube. During sexual intercourse, the male deposits semen into the vagina. Sperm cells must travel up through the uterus to the fallopian tubes to fertilize the ovum.

Prostaglandins in semen stimulate the flagella of sperm cells to undulate, causing the swimming action of sperm. Prostaglandins also stimulate muscles in the uterus

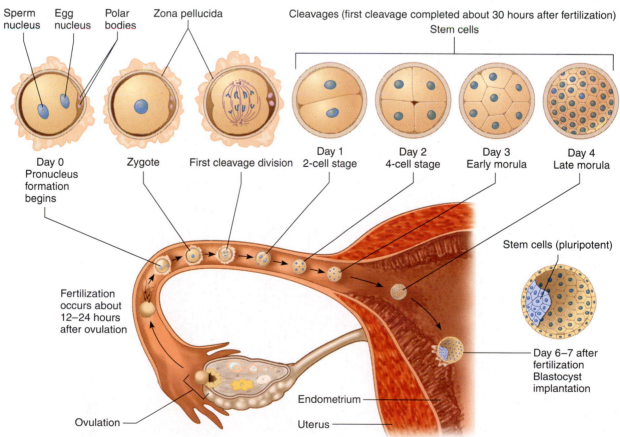

Figure 9-7. Stages of early embryo development.

and fallopian tubes to contract. These contractions (peristalsis) help the sperm reach the ovum. Normally about 10 to 14 days after ovulation, high estrogen levels stimulate the uterus and cervix to secrete a thin watery fluid that also promotes the movement of sperm toward the ovum.

Although many sperm cells normally reach an ovum, only one sperm cell unites with the ovum, penetrating the follicular cells and a layer called the **zona pellucida,** which surround the cell membrane of the ovum. The acrosome of this sperm releases enzymes to help the sperm penetrate the membrane of the ovum. Once a sperm unites with an ovum, enzymes are released by the ovum preventing other sperm from invading it by causing the zona pellucida to become hard and therefore impenetrable to other sperm.

The nucleus of the ovum (with 23 chromosomes) and the nucleus of the sperm (with 23 chromosomes) eventually fuse together to make one nucleus that contains 46 chromosomes. The cell that is formed by this union is called a **zygote.**

The Prenatal Period

The **prenatal period** is the time before the offspring is born. The prenatal period is divided into an **embryonic period** (weeks 2 through 8 of pregnancy) and a **fetal period** (week 9 to the delivery of the offspring). It is further divided into three periods known as *trimesters,* which consist of three calendar months each.

About one day after the zygote forms, it begins to undergo mitosis at a relatively rapid rate. This rapid cell division is called **cleavage** and the resulting ball of cells is called a **morula.** The morula travels down the fallopian tube to the uterus. Fluid then invades the morula, and this

organism is called a **blastocyst.** The blastocyst implants in the endometrial wall of the uterus. The process of moving from zygote formation to implantation of the blastocyst takes about one week. Once the blastocyst implants, a group of cells in the blastocyst, called the **inner cell mass,** gives rise to an embryo. Other cells in the blastocyst, along with cells of the uterus, eventually form the **placenta.**

The Embryonic Period. The embryonic period extends from the second week of pregnancy to the end of the eighth week of development. During this stage, the placenta, **amnion, umbilical cord,** and **yolk sac** form along with most of the internal organs and external structures of the embryo (Figure 9-8). The cells of the inner cell mass organize into layers called **primary germ layers.** All organs are formed from the primary germ layers, which include the ectoderm, mesoderm, and endoderm.

- The **ectoderm** gives rise to nervous tissue and some epithelial tissue.
- The **mesoderm,** the middle layer, gives rise to connective tissues and some epithelial tissue.
- The **endoderm** gives rise to epithelial tissues only.

The placenta allows nutrients and oxygen from maternal blood to pass to embryonic blood. It also allows waste products from the fetal blood to pass into maternal blood. The amnion is a protective, fluid-filled sac that surrounds the embryo. The umbilical cord contains three blood vessels—one umbilical vein that carries oxygenated blood from the placenta to the embryo and two umbilical arteries that carry deoxygenated blood from the embryo back to the placenta.

The yolk sac makes new blood cells for the fetus as well as cells that eventually become sex cells of the baby.

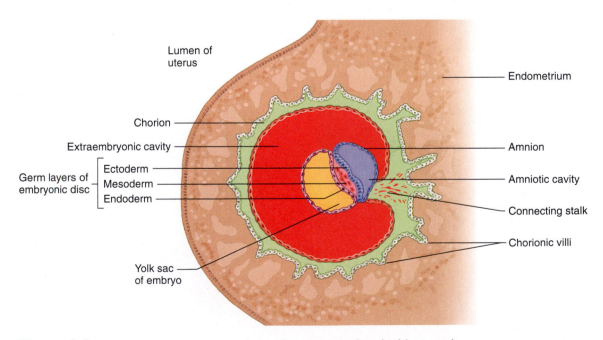

Figure 9-8. Primary germ layers and membranes associated with an embryo.

By the end of the embryonic stage, the baby closely resembles a human because all external structures (arms, hands, legs, feet, etc.) have formed.

The Fetal Period. The fetal period begins at the end of the eighth week of development and ends at birth. During this period, the growth of the offspring, which is now called a fetus, is rapid. By the twelfth week bones have begun to harden and the external reproductive organs are distinguishable as male or female.

The growth rate of the fetus slows down in the fifth month but skeletal muscles become active. In the sixth month, the fetus starts to gain substantial weight. In the seventh month, the eyelids open. In the last three months of pregnancy, fetal brain cells divide rapidly and organs continue to grow. The testes of the male descend into the scrotum. The last organ systems to completely develop are the digestive and respiratory systems. By the end of the ninth month, the fetus is usually positioned upside down in the uterus in preparation for delivery.

Fetal Circulation

Throughout prenatal development, the placenta and umbilical blood vessels carry out the exchange of nutrients, oxygen, and waste products between maternal and fetal blood. Therefore, the fetus does not need to send blood to the lungs to pick up oxygen nor does it need to send blood to the liver to process nutrients.

Fetal circulation has some important differences from normal circulation, which are illustrated in Figure 9-9. In the fetal heart, a hole called the **foramen ovale** is located between the right and left atria. Therefore, in the fetal heart, most blood flows from the right atrium into the left atrium. In the adult heart, blood flows from the right

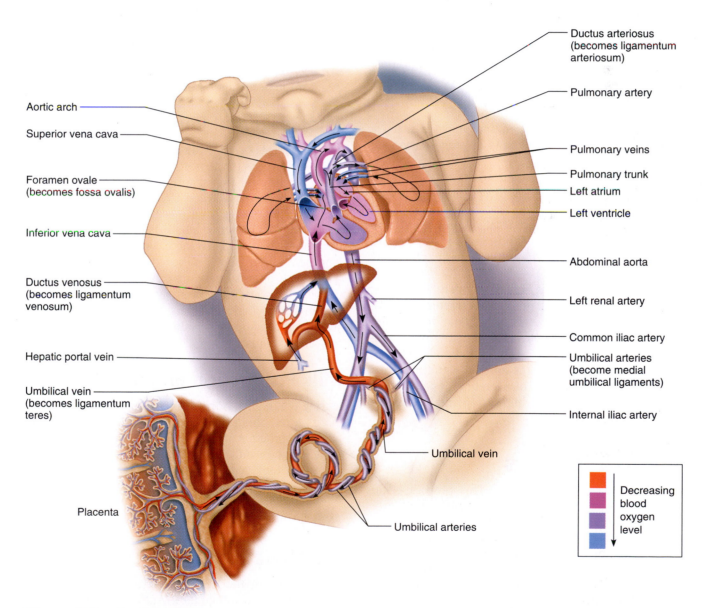

Figure 9-9. Fetal circulation.

atrium into the right ventricle so it can be pumped to the lungs. However, some fetal blood does flow from the right atrium into the right ventricle, and the right ventricle then delivers the blood to the pulmonary trunk.

In the fetus, there is also a connection between the pulmonary trunk and the aorta called the **ductus arteriosus.** This connection allows blood to flow from the pulmonary trunk into the aorta. In the adult, this connection does not exist and blood flows from the pulmonary trunk to the lungs.

The fetus also contains a blood vessel that allows most of the blood to bypass the liver. This vessel is called the **ductus venosus.** After a baby is born, the foramen ovale, ductus arteriosus, and ductus venosus normally close.

Hemoglobin within the fetus has a much higher affinity for oxygen than does the normal hemoglobin that is found after birth and growth. Therefore, the fetus's blood is adapted to carry more oxygen.

Hormonal Changes During Pregnancy

Many hormonal changes take place when a woman is pregnant. Following implantation of the embryo, the cells of the embryo begin to secrete **human chorionic gonadotropin (HCG).** HCG maintains the corpus luteum in the ovary so it will continue to secrete estrogen and progesterone. The placenta also secretes large amounts of progesterone and estrogen.

Progesterone and estrogen stimulate the uterine lining to thicken and inhibit the anterior pituitary gland from secreting FSH and LH to prevent ovulation during pregnancy. Estrogen and progesterone also stimulate the development of the mammary glands, inhibit uterine contractions, and stimulate the enlargement of female reproductive organs.

Another hormone called **relaxin,** which comes from the corpus luteum, inhibits uterine contractions and relaxes the ligaments of the pelvis in preparation for childbirth. The placenta also secretes **lactogen,** a hormone that stimulates the enlargement of mammary glands. **Aldosterone,** which is secreted from the adrenal gland, increases sodium and water retention. The secretion of **parathyroid hormone (PTH)** increases, helping to maintain high calcium levels in the blood.

The Birth Process

The birth process ends pregnancy. This process begins when progesterone levels fall. When progesterone levels fall, uterine contractions are no longer inhibited and the uterus secretes prostaglandins. Prostaglandins stimulate uterine contractions, which cause the posterior pituitary gland to release oxytocin. Oxytocin stimulates strong uterine contractions until the birth process ends. The birth process itself occurs in three stages after the fetus settles into position in the mother's pelvis (Figure 9-10A)

1. *Dilation* (Figure 9-10B). The cervix thins and softens known as **effacement,** dilating to approximately 10 cm. Regular contractions occur at this stage and the amniotic sac ruptures. If rupture does not occur, the sac may be surgically punctured. This stage normally last 8 to 24 hours.

2. *Expulsion* (Figure 9-10C). Also known as **parturition,** this is the actual childbirth stage. Forceful contractions and abdominal compressions force the fetus from the uterus into the vagina. This stage may take 30 minutes or only a few minutes.

3. *Placental stage* (Figure 9-10D). This stage is also referred to as the *afterbirth.* Approximately 10 to 15 minutes after the birth, the placenta separates from the uterine wall and is expelled. Uterine contractions continue during this stage and the blood vessels constrict to prevent hemorrhage. Normal blood loss is less than 350 mL (12 oz).

If the fetus is not in the usual head-down position, the child is said to be breech, in which the buttocks or feet present first. If the fetus cannot be turned manually, forceps may be used to assist in the birth. Alternately, a **cesarean section** (C-section) may be performed to deliver the infant through the abdominal wall.

The Postnatal Period

The **postnatal period** is the 6-week period following birth. The first 4 weeks of the postnatal period is called the **neonatal period** and the offspring is called a **neonate.** The neonatal period is marked by adjustment to life outside the uterus. The lungs of the neonate must expand, which is why the first breath of a baby is forceful. The liver of the newborn is immature, so the baby must obtain most of its glucose from fat stores in the skin. The newborn urinates a lot because the kidneys are too immature to concentrate urine well. In addition, body temperature tends to be unstable. The umbilical vessels of the newborn must constrict, and the foramen ovale, ductus arteriosus, and ductus venosus must close.

Milk Production and Secretion

During pregnancy, hormones stimulate the breasts to enlarge. After childbirth, prolactin causes the mammary glands to produce milk. The hormone oxytocin stimulates the ejection of milk from mammary gland ducts. As long as milk is removed from the mammary glands, milk production will continue. Once a female stops breast-feeding, the hypothalamus will inhibit the release of prolactin and oxytocin so that milk production will stop.

Contraception

Birth control methods, also referred to as contraception, reduce the risk of pregnancy. Although many methods of birth control are available, some are more reliable than

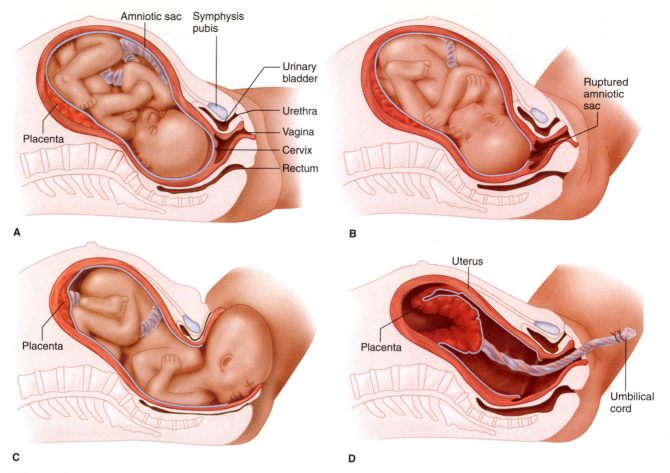

Figure 9-10. Stages of the birth process: (A) the fetal position before birth, (B) dilation of the cervix, (C) delivery of the fetus, and (D) delivery of the placenta.

others. The following are the most commonly used birth control methods:

- Coitus interruptus. The penis is withdrawn from the vagina before ejaculation. This method is not very reliable because small amounts of semen may enter the vagina before ejaculation.
- Rhythm method. The rhythm method requires abstinence from sexual intercourse around the time a female is ovulating. However, predicting ovulation can be difficult; therefore, this type of contraception can be unreliable.
- Mechanical barriers. Mechanical barriers prevent sperm from entering the female reproductive tract. They include condoms, diaphragms, and cervical caps. Sperimicides are often used in conjunction with barrier methods, particularly condoms and diaphragms.
- Chemical barriers. Chemical barriers destroy sperm in the female reproductive tract. They primarily include spermicides.
- Oral contraceptives. Birth control pills are oral contraceptives. These pills normally include low doses of estrogen or progesterone that prevent the LH surge necessary for ovulation. These pills therefore prevent ovulation. Newer oral contraceptives are being devel-

oped in which the woman takes the pill daily for three months and then is off for a week, so that a period only occurs four times a year.

- Injectable contraceptives. Depo-Provera is one brand of injectable contraceptive. It prevents ovulation and alters the lining of the uterus so that implantation of a blastocyst is not likely.
- Insertable contraceptives. NuvaRing® is one of the newest forms of contraception. The ring is inserted vaginally by the patient and is left in for 3 weeks. It is removed at the beginning of the fourth week to allow for menstruation, in the same schedule as most oral contraceptives.
- Contraceptive implants. Contraceptive implants are small rods of progesterone that are implanted beneath the skin. They also prevent ovulation.
- Transdermal contraceptives. Commonly called "the Patch," transdermal contraceptives are applied to the skin once a week and removed on the seventh day for a three-week cycle. No patch is applied during the fourth week to allow for the menstrual period.
- Intrauterine devices. An intrauterine device (IUD) is a small, solid device that a physician places in the uterus. It prevents the implantation of a blastocyst.

The Reproductive Systems **145**

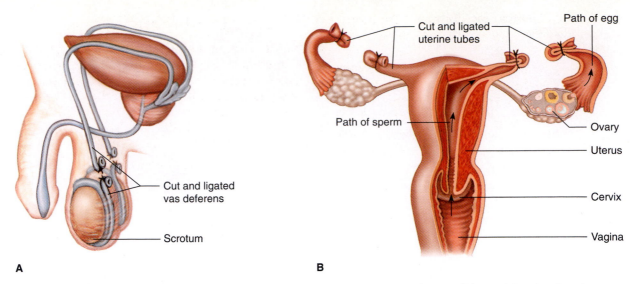

Figure 9-11. (A) Vasectomy involves cutting and ligating the vas deferens. (B) Tubal ligation involves cutting and ligating each fallopian tube.

- Surgical methods. *Tubal ligation* is a surgical method used in females to prevent pregnancy. In this process, each fallopian tube is cut and tied or fulgurated to prevent sperm from reaching the oocyte. *Vasectomy* is a surgical method used in males to prevent pregnancy. In this process, each vas deferens is cut and tied or fulgurated to prevent sperm from being ejaculated. Figure 9-11 illustrates these methods.

Infertility

Infertility is the inability to conceive a child. If a couple has never been pregnant and has tried for 12 months to achieve pregnancy, they are said to have primary infertility. If a couple has had at least one pregnancy but has not been able to get pregnant after 1 year, they are said to have secondary infertility.

In the United States, about 15% of infertility causes are unknown, about 35% are the result of problems in the male, and about 50% are because of problems in the female. Common causes of infertility as a result of male factors include the following:

- Impotence
- Retrograde ejaculation
- Low or absent sperm count
- Use of various medications or drugs
- Decreased testosterone production
- Scarring of the male reproductive tract from sexually transmitted diseases
- Previous mumps infection that infected the testes
- Inflammation of the epididymis or testes

Infertility because of female factors includes these common causes:

- Scarring of fallopian tubes from STDs
- Pelvic inflammatory disease
- Inadequate diet
- Lack of ovulation
- Lack of menstrual cycles
- Endometriosis
- Abnormal shape of the uterus or cervix
- Hormone imbalances
- Cysts in ovaries
- Being older than age 40

Women are most likely to get pregnant in their early 20s. By the time a woman reaches the age of 40, her chance of conceiving a child is less than 10% each month. In general, infertility in men is not age-related.

Infertility Tests

A number of tests are used to diagnose infertility. They include the following:

- Semen analysis. This test determines the thickness of semen and the number and **motility** of sperm cells in a sample.
- Monitoring of morning body temperature. If a woman's body temperature does not rise slightly once a month, which is best determined by taking her temperature first thing in the morning, a woman may not be ovulating.
- Blood hormone measurements. In females, various hormone levels can be monitored to predict ovulation and the general health of ovaries. In males, testosterone levels are primarily measured.
- Endometrial biopsy. This test determines the health of the uterine lining.

- Urinary analysis for luteinizing hormone. The absence of this hormone in urine may indicate a lack of ovulation.
- Hysterosalpingogram. This type of x-ray uses contrast media to visualize the shape of the uterus and the fallopian tubes. If a woman has excess scar tissue in her fallopian tubes, the contrast cannot run through them.
- Laparoscopy. Laparoscopy is a procedure that is used to visualize pelvic organs.

Treatment of Infertility

Many treatments are available for infertility, but often there is no cure for this condition. Common treatments include surgery to repair abnormal or scarred fallopian tubes, fertility drugs to increase ovulation, and hormone therapies. In cases where infertility cannot be cured, procedures such as artificial insemination, in vitro fertilization, or the use of a surrogate may help a couple to have a child.

Pathophysiology

Sexually Transmitted Diseases

AIDS or acquired immunodeficiency syndrome develops from advanced stages of the HIV virus. The incubation period in adults is between 8 and 15 years, and the majority of adults with the disease are between the ages of 25 and 45. The greatest risk factor for contracting the virus is unprotected sexual activity. Homosexual men constitute a large percentage of AIDS in the United States, but virtually no one is immune.

- **Causes.** The human immunodeficiency virus (HIV) causes AIDS.
- **Signs and symptoms.** These are numerous and include decreased T-cell count, flu-like symptoms, and a host of opportunistic infections, including *pneumocystis carinii pneumonia* (PCP), Kaposi's sarcoma (KS), and cytomegalovirus (CMV).
- **Treatment.** Antiviral medications have been successful in decreasing the viral load and maintaining T-cell counts in some patients, but there are many side effects to these drugs and a strict medicine regime. Other medications include drugs to support the immune system and to treat opportunistic infections as they arise.

Chlamydia is the most commonly reported STD in the United States. Chlamydia may be grossly underreported because, for women, there are often no symptoms until the disease has spread.

- **Causes.** Chlamydia is caused by the bacterium *Chlamydia trachomata.*
- **Signs and symptoms.** For females, there may be no symptoms. If they do occur, it will be 2 to 3 weeks after exposure. Symptoms may include abnormal vaginal discharge and burning on urination. As the disease progresses to other reproductive organs (pelvic inflammatory disease), there may be abdominal pain, pain during intercourse, and intermenstrual bleeding. Men may have a penile discharge and pain on urination. In women, pelvic inflammatory disease (commonly referred to as PID) is a common cause of infertility; men seldom have serious complications related to chlamydia.
- **Treatment.** It is important for both partners to be treated to avoid reinfection. Effective antibiotics against chlamydia include azithromycin and doxycycline. Patients must complete the medication cycle and avoid sexual contact until both partners are cured. Because of the high rate of reinfection, women should be retested 3 to 4 months after treatment.

Genital warts, also known as *Condyloma acuminata,* are one of the most common STDs in the world. It is important to note that not everyone infected with human papillomavirus (HPV) has symptoms. HPV has been implicated in an increased risk of cervical cancer in women.

- **Causes.** Human papillomavirus or HPV.
- **Signs and symptoms.** Genital warts appear weeks or months after infection in the vulva, vagina, and cervix in women. In men, warts appear on the scrotum and penis. They have also been known to appear around the anus and on the thighs and groin. It is important to note that HPV can be spread even if the patient has no outward signs of the disease.
- **Treatment.** Imiquimod cream, 20% podophyllin antimiotic solutions, and TCA (trichloroacetic acid) may be used to remove warts. Cryosurgery, cautery, and laser surgery may also be used; however, the virus remains in the patient's body. Currently, there is no treatment to rid the body of the virus. Vaccines to prevent infection with HPV are being developed and tested.

Gonorrhea is a bacterial STD that is very common in the United States. The Centers for Disease Control and Prevention (CDC) estimates 700,000 new infections per year.

- **Causes.** Gonorrhea is caused by *Neisseria gonorrhoea,* a bacteria that thrives in the warm, moist areas of the reproductive tract, urethral tract, mouth, throat, eyes, and anus.
- **Signs and symptoms.** Men often have no symptoms. If they do appear, it will be 2 to 3 days after exposure,

continued ⟶

Sexually Transmitted Diseases *(concluded)*

when the patient will experience burning on urination and/or white, yellow, or greenish penile discharge. Women may also be asymptomatic, but common symptoms include dysuria, increased vaginal discharge, and intermenstrual bleeding. Gonorrheal infections, like chlamydia, may lead to PID in women. In men, it may lead to epididymitis.

- **Treatment.** Antibiotics are effective against gonorrhea and both partners must be treated. There are, however, drug-resistant strains of gonorrhea developing, making successful treatment more difficult. It is not unusual for a patient with gonorrhea to also be diagnosed with chlamydia or other STDs, which will also need to be tested for and treated if found to be present. In addition, gonorrhea lives well and actively in the throat, even if there is not an active genitourinary infection, which can lead to additional co-infection.

Herpes simplex infections include those caused by both herpes simplex 1 and herpes simplex 2.

- **Causes.** Herpes viruses cause both infections. In most cases, herpes simplex 1 causes oral blisters known as *cold sores,* and herpes simplex 2 causes what is commonly known as *genital herpes,* although herpes simplex 1 has also been known to cause the genital type of infection. The herpes infection may also be passed from an infected mother to her child during pregnancy and birth with potentially fatal outcomes.
- **Signs and symptoms.** Many infected persons have minimal or no symptoms. Typical symptoms of genital herpes include blisters on or around the genitals or rectum. These blisters break, leaving tender ulcers in their wake for 2 to 4 weeks. The number and severity of outbreaks tend to decrease over a period of years.
- **Treatment.** There is no treatment to rid the patient of the herpes virus; however, antiviral medications such as Acyclovir® may shorten outbreaks when they occur. Daily suppressive therapies with medications like Valtrex® may reduce the risk of transmission. Pregnant women with active outbreaks should deliver the child via a C-section.

Pubic lice are known commonly as *crabs* and medically as *Pediculosis pubis.*

- **Causes.** These can be caused by a parasitic infestation in the genital area, most commonly spread through sexual contact.
- **Signs and symptoms.** Symptoms include itching in the genital area with visible evidence of eggs known as *nits,* as well as crawling lice. Lice only live while on a human body. If they fall off the body, they will die in 24 to 48 hours.

- **Treatment.** Patient should use a lice-killing shampoo of 1% permethrin or pyrethin. All laundry and clothing must be washed in hot water with the use of a hot dryer cycle for at least 30 minutes. Nits remaining in hair may be removed by hand. All partners should be treated and sexual contact should be avoided until treatment is completed.

Syphilis is the one bacterial STD whose incidence in women is decreasing, according to the CDC. However, it is increasing in males, especially in those who have sex with other males (MSM).

- **Causes.** Syphilis is caused by the bacterium *Treponema pallidum.*
- **Signs and symptoms.** Primary-stage syphilis usually involves the appearance of a painless sore known as a chancre, which appears 10 to 90 days after exposure. It will remain for 3 to 6 weeks, disappearing even without treatment. If untreated, the disease lies dormant, progressing to the second stage, which is characterized by a nonpruritic rash and lesions in the mucus membranes. The rash may be associated with flu-like symptoms. Again, all symptoms disappear without treatment. After a long latent period without symptoms, often years later, the third stage becomes apparent with damage to the brain, eyes, heart, blood vessels, liver, and bones. This damage may lead to muscular incoordination, paralysis, numbness, blindness, dementia, and, finally, death.
- **Treatment.** The cure for syphilis in its early stage is a single dose of intramuscular (IM) penicillin. Additional doses are needed for disease present longer than a year. Other antibiotics are also effective for patients allergic to penicillin. Sexual contact must be avoided until treatment is completed to avoid further spread of the disease.

Trichomoniasis (also known as trichomonas infection or the abbreviation "trich") is a common, curable STD.

- **Causes.** Trichomonas infection is caused by the protozoan parasite *Trichomonas vaginalis.*
- **Signs and symptoms.** The vagina is the most common site of infection for females; the urethra for males. Male patients may have penile irritation, dysuria, or a mild penile discharge, but more often than not, men have no symptoms. Females often have a frothy yellow-green vaginal discharge with a strong "fishy" odor to it. Itching and irritation of the vulva is also common.
- **Treatment.** Oral *metronidazole* (Flagyl®) is the treatment of choice. Both partners, even those who are asymptomatic, must be treated to avoid reinfection. Sexual contact should be avoided until after treatment is completed.

Summary

The ability to reproduce is one of the basic characteristics of life. The male and female reproductive systems work together to produce offspring. The male produces sperm and delivers them to the female. The female produces ova and, once fertilization occurs, her body nurtures the fetus until birth. The medical assistant must understand the anatomy and physiology of the reproductive systems in order to assist with exams and procedures such as colposcopy and vasectomy. Knowledge of the system is also important when teaching patients about breast and testicular self-examination and prevention and treatment of STDs.

REVIEW

CHAPTER 9

CASE STUDY QUESTIONS

Now that you have completed this chapter, review the case study at the beginning of the chapter and answer the following questions:

1. What STDs are caused by bacteria?
2. How did the infection spread to the patient's abdomino-pelvic cavity?
3. Why is her sexual partner not experiencing pain in his abdominopelvic cavity?
4. Why is it important for her sexual partner to be treated with antibiotics?
5. Why is it common for women with STDs to also have UTIs?

Discussion Questions

1. Describe the components of semen. What is the function of each component?
2. Explain the functions of GnRH, FSH, and LH in the male and female reproductive systems.
3. Outline the basic events of the prenatal period from conception to the fetal period.

Critical Thinking Questions

1. Discuss the pros and cons of the following birth control methods.
   a. Coitus interruptus and rhythm method
   b. Mechanical methods, such as the diaphragm and cervical cap
   c. Oral contraceptives
   d. Insertable and implantable contraceptives
2. Why do condoms prevent the spread of STDs, whereas most other methods of birth control do not?
3. What changes occur as a result of a tubal ligation? As a result of a vasectomy?

Application Activities

1. Describe the functions of the following parts of a sperm:
   a. Head
   b. Midpiece
   c. Tail
2. List the primary sex organs of the male and the hormones produced by them. List the primary sex organs of the female and the hormones produced by them.
3. List the structures that are derived from the following embryonic germ layers:
   a. Endoderm
   b. Mesoderm
   c. Ectoderm

Virtual Fieldtrip

Visit the McGraw-Hill Higher Education Medical Assisting website at www.mhhe.com/medicalassisting3 to complete the following activity:

Use the Medline website from the NIH (National Institutes of Health), moving to the area on Health and Wellness. Locate the areas on Sexual Health and, from there, on STDs. Halfway down the page in the left-hand column is a list of common STDs. Choose one and obtain more information regarding this STD, answering the following questions:

1. What is the causative agent?
2. Can the condition be caused by exposure other than sex? Is so, how?
3. What are some symptoms of this condition for both males and females?
4. What are some treatment options? Is there a cure? Are there sequelae (long-term effects) to this infection or condition and, if so, what are they?
5. How can this condition be prevented?

At your instructor's discretion, create a poster or other presentation based on your research to educate others about your findings.

Open the CD and complete this chapter's practice activities, play the games, listen to the key terms, and test yourself with the interactive review. E-mail, print, and/or save your results to document your proficiency.

The Lymphatic and Immune Systems

CHAPTER OUTLINE

- The Lymphatic System
- Defenses Against Disease
- Antibodies
- Immune Responses and Acquired Immunities
- Major Immune System Disorders

LEARNING OUTCOMES

After completing Chapter 10, you will be able to:

10.1 List the pathways and organs of the lymphatic system and give their locations.

10.2 Define lymph and tell how it is circulated in the body.

10.3 Define the terms *infection, pathogen,* and *antigen.*

10.4 List and describe the nonspecific body defense mechanisms.

10.5 Explain the signs and causes of inflammation.

10.6 Explain what is meant by specific body defenses.

10.7 Define B cells and T cells and describe their locations and functions.

10.8 Explain the importance of MHC proteins.

10.9 List the different types of T cells and describe their functions.

10.10 Explain how antibodies fight infection.

10.11 List the different types of antibodies and tell how they differ.

10.12 Define complement proteins and give their function.

10.13 Explain the difference between the primary immune response and secondary immune response.

10.14 Explain the four different types of acquired immunities.

10.15 Describe the function of a vaccine.

10.16 Define the terms *cancer* and *carcinogen.*

10.17 Describe how cancers are diagnosed and treated.

10.18 Explain how cancers are classified.

10.19 Describe how allergies develop.

10.20 Describe the causes, signs and symptoms, and treatments of other common immune disorders.

KEY TERMS

allergens
anaphylaxis
antihistamines
autoimmune disease
benign
biopsy
carcinogen
complement
cytokines
epinephrine
febrile
hapten
humors
immunoglobulins
infection
inflammation
innate immunity
interferon
interstitial fluid
lymph
lymphedema
lymphokines
lysozyme
major histocompatibility complex (MHC)
malignant
monokines
mononucleosis
natural killer (NK) cells
phagocytosis
splenectomy
systemic lupus erythematosus (SLE)

Introduction

The immune system is responsible for protecting the body against bacteria, viruses, fungi, toxins, parasites, and cancer. It works with the organs of the lymphatic system, the thymus, spleen, and lymph nodes, to clear the body of these disease-causing agents.

A few days ago a 17-year-old female came to the doctor's office very concerned that she had a "serious, possibly fatal, illness." She had been running a slight fever for the past week, had been very tired, had tender lymph nodes in her neck, and had been losing weight without dieting. Her chart indicated that she had never been sexually active and had never used intravenous drugs.

As you read this chapter, consider the following questions:

1. Is it likely that this patient has a life-threatening illness?
2. What tests should be done to diagnose this patient?
3. Based on her symptoms, what disease or disorder is this patient more likely to have?
4. Is the patient contagious? What precautions should she take to avoid spreading her illness?

The Lymphatic System

The lymphatic system is a network of connecting vessels that collects fluids between cells. These lymphatic vessels then return this fluid, called **lymph,** to the bloodstream. The lymphatic system also picks up lipids from the digestive organs and transports them to the bloodstream. Finally, the lymphatic system functions to defend the body against disease-causing agents called pathogens.

Lymphatic Pathways

Lymphatic pathways start with tiny vessels called lymphatic capillaries. The lymphatic capillaries merge together to make lymphatic vessels. Lymphatic vessels eventually merge together to make lymphatic trunks, and the trunks merge into lymphatic collecting ducts.

Lymphatic capillaries extend into the spaces between cells called interstitial spaces. Lymphatic capillaries have very permeable, thin walls that are designed to pick up fluids in interstitial spaces. Once fluid enters the lymphatic capillaries, it is called lymph. Lymphatic capillaries deliver lymph to lymphatic vessels, and lymphatic vessels deliver the fluid to lymph nodes. The cells inside lymph nodes can remove pathogens from lymph or start an immune response against the pathogen.

Lymph leaves lymph nodes through efferent lymphatic vessels. Efferent lymphatic vessels eventually deliver lymph to lymphatic trunks, and the trunks deliver the lymph to lymphatic collecting ducts. There are two major lymphatic collecting ducts in the body—the thoracic duct and the right lymphatic duct. Both of these ducts empty lymph into the bloodstream, usually near the right and left subclavian veins in the thoracic cavity (see Figures 10-1, 10-2, and 10-3).

The right lymphatic duct is much smaller than the thoracic duct. The right lymphatic duct collects all the lymph from the right side of the head and neck, the right arm, and the right side of the chest. The thoracic duct collects lymph from the left side of the head and neck, the left arm, the left side of the thorax, the entire abdominopelvic area, and both legs (Figure 10-3).

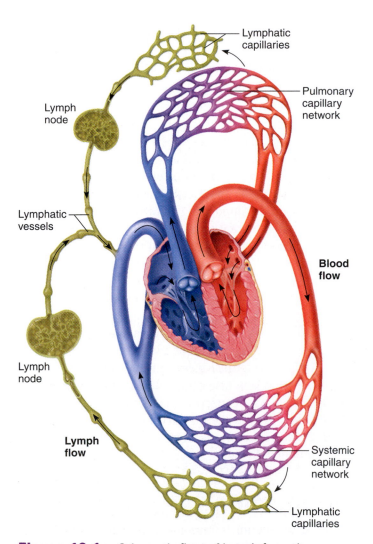

Figure 10-1. Schematic flow of lymph from the lymphatic capillaries to the bloodstream.

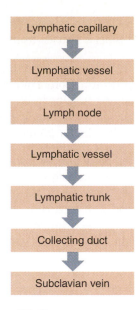

Figure 10-2. Lymphatic pathway.

Tissue Fluid and Lymph

Fluid constantly leaks out of blood capillaries into the spaces between cells. This fluid is high in nutrients, oxygen, and small proteins. Most of this fluid is picked up by body cells. However, some of the fluid persists between cells. This fluid is called **interstitial** (tissue) **fluid** and is destined to become lymph.

Once lymph enters lymphatic vessels, it is pushed through the vessels by the squeezing action of neighboring skeletal muscles. Lymphatic vessels contain valves that prevent the backflow of lymph. Breathing movements also squeeze lymphatic vessels and therefore promote lymph movement. If lymph is not pushed through a lymphatic vessel, it will leak back out of the lymphatic capillaries. When this happens, swelling of the surrounding tissue occurs. This condition is called edema.

Lymph Nodes

Lymph nodes are very small, glandular structures that usually cannot be felt very easily. They are located along the paths of larger lymphatic vessels and are spread throughout the body, but they do not occur in the nervous system. One side of a lymph node, called the hilum, is indented. Nerves and blood vessels enter the node through the hilum.

Some lymphatic vessels carry lymph to a lymph node on the side away from the hilum. These vessels are called afferent lymphatic vessels (afferent, meaning "to"). About four or five afferent vessels are associated with each node. Lymphatic vessels that carry lymph out of a node are called efferent vessels (efferent, meaning "away from"). A lymph node usually has only one or two efferent vessels. Because more lymph enters the node than can exit at one time, lymph tends to pool, or stay, in the node for some period of time.

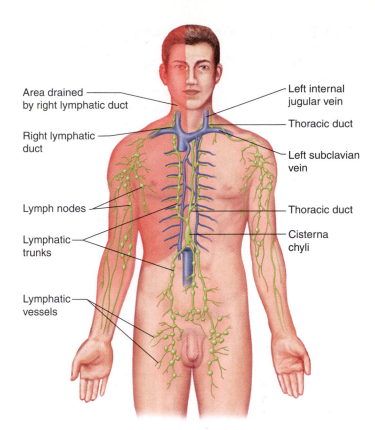

Figure 10-3. Areas drained by the right lymphatic duct (shaded) and thoracic duct (not shaded).

Two important cell types are found inside the node—macrophages and lymphocytes. Macrophages digest unwanted pathogens in the lymph as it sits in the node, and the lymphocytes start an immune response against the pathogen. Lymph nodes are also responsible for the generation of some lymphocytes (see Figure 10-4).

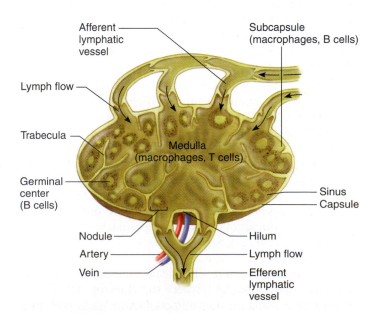

Figure 10-4. Section of a lymph node.

The Thymus and Spleen

The thymus is a soft, bilobed organ located just above the heart in the mediastinum. The thymus in an infant is quite large because it assists with the production of lymphocytes for the child's immature immune system. As a person ages, the thymus shrinks, becoming almost nonexistent as the immune system is fully functional. The thymus carries out the same functions as a lymph node but is also responsible for the production of lymphocytes and the hormone called thymosin. Thymosin stimulates the production of mature lymphocytes.

The spleen is the largest lymphatic organ. It is located in the upper-left quadrant of the abdominal cavity. The spleen is filled with blood, macrophages, and lymphocytes. It filters blood in much the same way that lymph nodes filter lymph. The spleen also removes worn-out red blood cells from the bloodstream. If the spleen is injured or diseased, a **splenectomy** may be done, and then the patient's liver takes over most of its functions.

Defenses Against Disease

An **infection** is the presence of a pathogen in or on the body. A pathogen is a disease-causing agent such as a bacterium, virus, toxin, fungus, or protozoan. The body has mechanisms to protect itself against pathogens in general; these mechanisms are called nonspecific defenses or **innate immunity.** The body also has mechanisms to protect itself against very specific pathogens; these mechanisms are called immunities and are considered specific defenses.

Nonspecific Defenses

The nonspecific mechanisms that protect bodies against pathogens include species resistance, mechanical and chemical barriers, and **phagocytosis.** Fever and **inflammation** are also effective in protecting the body from invading organisms.

Species Resistance. Species resistance simply means that a species typically gets only diseases that are unique to that species. For example, humans do not get diseases that affect plants. Humans also do not get most diseases that affect animals.

Mechanical Barriers. The covering of the body (skin) and the linings of the tubes of the body (mucous membranes) provide mechanical barriers against pathogens. Intact skin is impermeable to most pathogens. Intact mucous membranes, although generally impermeable, do permit the entry of a few pathogens.

Chemical Barriers. Chemicals and enzymes in body fluids provide chemical barriers that destroy pathogens. For example, acids in the stomach destroy pathogens that are swallowed. **Lysozymes** in tears destroy pathogens on the surface of the eye. Salt in sweat also kills bacteria, and **interferon** in blood blocks viruses from infecting cells.

Phagocytosis. Neutrophils and monocytes are the most active phagocytes in blood. They can also leave the bloodstream to attack pathogens in other tissues. When a monocyte leaves the bloodstream, it becomes a macrophage, which is simply a larger phagocytic cell.

Fever. An elevated body temperature is a fever. Patients experiencing a fever are said to be **febrile.** Fever causes the liver and spleen to take iron out of the bloodstream. Many pathogens need iron to survive in a body, so when their iron sources are gone, they die. Fever also activates phagocytic cells in the body to attack pathogens.

Inflammation. When an area of the body becomes injured or infected with a pathogen, inflammation can result. In inflammation, blood vessels in the injured area dilate and become leaky. Because blood vessels dilate, more blood enters the area, bringing phagocytic white blood cells (WBC) to the area to attack the pathogen. The blood also brings proteins to replace injured tissues and clotting factors to stop any bleeding. The clotting factors also "wall off" the area so that pathogens cannot spread. Because blood vessels become leaky, more fluid accumulates in the injured area, which leads to edema. The excess fluid often irritates pain receptors. The four cardinal signs of inflammation are redness, heat, swelling, and pain.

Specific Defenses

Specific defenses are called immunities. They protect the body against very specific pathogens. For example, a person who has chickenpox develops a specific defense that prevents that person from getting chickenpox again. However, this specific defense does not protect the person from any other disease. For example, a person may contract herpes zoster (shingles), which is caused by the same varicella virus as chickenpox. A person may not get chickenpox again, but the virus may resurface as herpes zoster.

Antigens are very simply defined as foreign substances in the body. Pathogens have many antigens on their surfaces. The immune system is programmed to recognize antigens in the body. Foreign substances in the body too small to start an immune response by themselves are called **haptens.** Many times, haptens join to proteins in the blood where they are then able to trigger an immune response. Penicillin is an example of a hapten.

Antibodies and **complements** are the major proteins involved in specific defenses. Lymphocytes and macrophages are the major WBCs involved in specific defenses. The cells of the lymphatic system produce proteins known as **cytokines,** which assist in immune response regulation. Lymphocytes and macrophages produce cytokines known as **monokines.** Monokines assist in regulation of the immune response by increasing B cell production and stimulating red bone marrow to produce more WBCs.

B Cells and T Cells. Two major types of lympho-cytes are B cells and T cells. Although both B cells and T cells circulate in the blood, most of the lymphocytes in blood are T cells. B cells and T cells are also found in lymph nodes, the spleen, the thymus, the lining of diges-tive organs, and bone marrow.

Both T cells and B cells recognize antigens in the body; however, they respond to antigens in different ways. T cells bind to antigens on cells and attack them directly. This type of response is called a cell-mediated response. T cells also respond to antigens by secreting cytokines called **lymphokines,** which increase T-cell production and directly kill cells that have antigens. B cells do not attack antigens directly. B cells respond to antigens by becoming plasma cells. The plasma cells then make anti-bodies against the specific antigen. The antibodies end up attaching to antigens in the **humors** (fluids) of the body;

this response is called a humoral or antibody-mediated response.

B cells become activated when a specific antigen binds to receptors on their surfaces. Each group of B cells only recognizes one type of antigen. Once activated, B cells di-vide to make plasma cells and memory B cells. Plasma cells make antibodies. Antibodies go out into the fluids of the body and bind to the antigens that activated the B cells. Memory B cells trigger a stronger immune response the next time the person is exposed to the same antigen (Figures 10-5 and 10-6).

Before a T cell can respond to an antigen, it must be activated. T-cell activation begins when a macrophage ingests and digests a pathogen that has antigens on it. The macrophage then takes some of the antigens from the pathogen and puts them on its cell membrane next to a large protein complex called a **major histocompatibility**

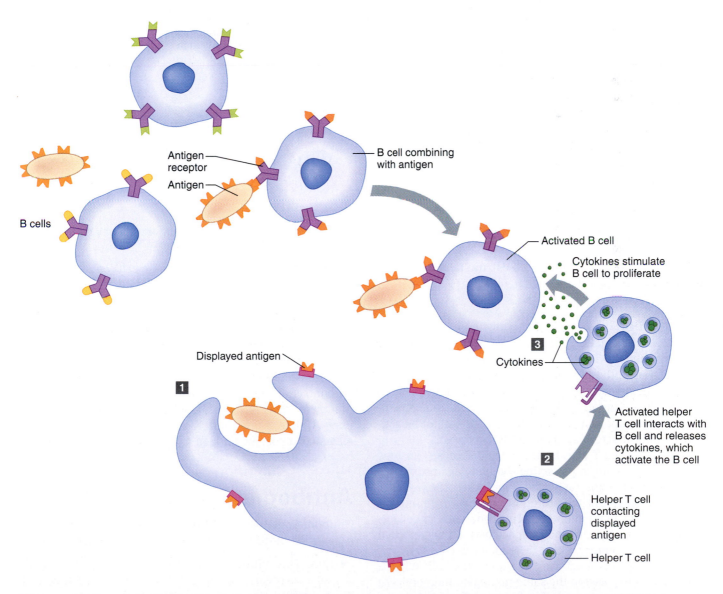

Figure 10-5. T cell and B cell activation. (1) A macrophage displays an antigen on its cell membrane. (2) A helper T cell binds to the antigen on the macrophage and becomes activated. (3) An activated helper T cell releases cytokines to help an activated B cell proliferate. Notice that the B cell must also bind to an antigen to become activated.

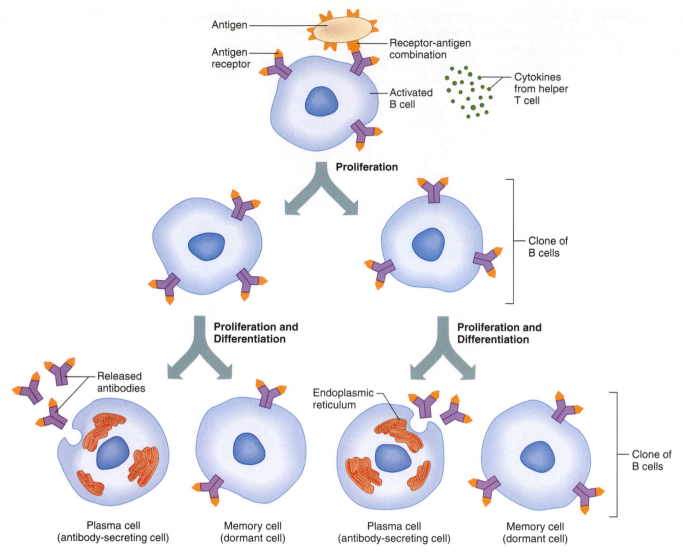

Labels in figure:

Antigen

Antigen receptor

Receptor-antigen combination

Cytokines from helper T cell

Activated B cell

Proliferation

Clone of B cells

Proliferation and Differentiation

Proliferation and Differentiation

Released antibodies

Endoplasmic reticulum

Clone of B cells

Plasma cell (antibody-secreting cell)

Memory cell (dormant cell)

Plasma cell (antibody-secreting cell)

Memory cell (dormant cell)

Figure 10-6. An activated B cell multiplies to become memory cells and plasma cells. Plasma cells secrete antibodies.

complex **(MHC).** Every human being has unique MHC (similar to an internal fingerprint) and it is present on every cell in their body. A T cell that has a receptor for the antigen recognizes and binds to the antigen and the MHC on the surface of the macrophage. The T cell is now activated and begins to divide to form other types of T cells and T memory cells. It is important to note that T cells cannot be activated without macrophages and MHC proteins.

Some activated T cells form cytotoxic T cells. This type of T cell is important in protecting the body against viruses and cancer cells. Other activated T cells become helper T cells, which carry out many important roles in immunity. Helper T cells increase antibody formation, memory cell formation, B cell formation, and phagocytosis. Some activated T cells become memory T cells. The memory cells "remember" the pathogen that activated the original T cell. When a person is later exposed to the same pathogen, memory cells trigger an immune response that is more effective than the first immune response. The production of memory cells prevents a person from suffering from the same disease twice.

Natural Killer (NK) Cells. Natural killer (NK) cells are another type of lymphocyte. They primarily target cancer cells but also protect the body against many types of pathogens. Like cytotoxic T cells, NK cells kill harmful cells on contact. They secrete chemicals that produce holes in the membranes of harmful cells, which cause the cells to burst. Unlike B cells and T cells, NK cells do not have to recognize a specific antigen to start destroying pathogens.

Antibodies

Antibodies are also called **immunoglobulins.** The following is a list of different types of immunoglobulins (Ig):

- IgA. This antibody is found in secretions of the body such as breast milk, sweat, tears, saliva, and mucus. It prevents pathogens from entering the body.

- IgD. This antibody is found on the cell membranes of B cells. It is thought to control the activity of the B cells

- IgE. This antibody is found wherever IgA is located. It is involved in triggering allergic reactions.
- IgG. This antibody primarily recognizes bacteria, viruses, and toxins. It can also activate complements, which are proteins in serum that attack pathogens.
- IgM. This antibody is very large and primarily binds to antigens on food, bacteria, or incompatible blood cells. It also activates complements.

When antibodies bind to antigens, they take one of the following actions:

- They allow phagocytes to recognize and destroy antigens.
- They make antigens clump together, causing them to be destroyed by macrophages. This is how incompatible blood cells are destroyed.
- They cover the toxic portions of antigens to make them harmless.
- They activate complements. Complements are proteins in serum that attack pathogens by forming holes in them. Complement proteins also attract macrophages to pathogens and can stimulate inflammation.

Immune Responses and Acquired Immunities

A primary immune response occurs the first time a person is exposed to an antigen. This response is slow and takes several weeks to occur. In this response, memory cells are made. A secondary immune response occurs the next time a person is exposed to the same antigen. This response is very quick and usually prevents a person from developing a disease from the antigen. Memory cells carry out the secondary immune response.

A person is born with very few immunities but normally develops them as long as the person's immune system is healthy. The four types of immunities a person can acquire are: (1) natural acquired active immunity, (2) artificially acquired active immunity, (3) naturally acquired passive immunity, and (4) artificially acquired passive immunity.

Naturally Acquired Active Immunity

A person develops this immunity by being naturally exposed to an antigen and subsequently making antibodies and memory cells against the antigen. Having an infectious disease caused by pathogens leads to the development of this type of immunity. This immunity is usually long lasting.

Artificially Acquired Active Immunity

A person develops this immunity by being injected with a pathogen and then subsequently making antibodies and memory cells against the pathogen. Immunizations or vaccines cause this type of immunity. This type is usually long lasting.

Naturally Acquired Passive Immunity

A person is given this immunity through his mother. When a mother breast-feeds, she passes antibodies to her baby through breast milk. A mother also passes antibodies to her baby across the placenta. This type of immunity is short-lived.

Artificially Acquired Passive Immunity

A person is given this immunity when she is injected with antibodies. If a snake bites a person, a physician will inject the patient with antibodies (antivenom) to neutralize the venom. This type of immunity is short lived.

Major Immune System Disorders

A number of diseases and disorders can challenge the immune system. Among them, HIV infection, AIDS, cancer, and allergies are the most significant.

Cancer

Cancer is defined as the uncontrolled growth of abnormal cells. Healthy cells normally know when to stop reproducing, but cancer cells have lost this ability. Occasionally, normal cells create growths, but these are **benign,** meaning they are not cancerous. Cancer cells, however, often form growths called **malignant** tumors, which may become fatal. In many cases, these cancerous cells or tumors damage normal cells of tissues and organs, which cause organ systems to fail.

At least 200 different types of cancers are known. In the United States, the three most common cancer types in men are prostate, lung, and colon cancer. The three most common types in women are breast, lung, and colon cancer. Lung cancer is the leading killer of all types of cancer for all people.

Causes. The causes of cancer are mostly unknown but certain risk factors have been identified. These factors include a suppressed immune system, radiation, tobacco, and some viruses. Many other factors are suspected. One of the best ways to prevent cancer is to not smoke and to avoid other known risk factors. A factor that is known to cause the formation of cancer is called a **carcinogen.**

Diagnosis. Most cancers are diagnosed with a **biopsy,** which is a removal of tissues for examination. CT scans are also used to help diagnose most cancer types. Other

TABLE 10-1 Cancer Staging

Stage	Description
Stage 0	Very early cancer. Cancer cells are localized in a few cell layers.
Stage I	Cancer cells have spread to deeper cell layers, or some may have spread to surrounding tissues.
Stage II	Cancer cells have spread to surrounding tissues but are considered contained in the primary cancer site.
Stage III	Cancer cells have spread beyond the primary cancer site to nearby areas.
Stage IV	Cancer cells have spread to other organs of the body.
Recurrent	Cancer cells have reappeared after treatment.

diagnostic tests include blood counts, an analysis of blood chemistry, and x-rays.

Signs and Symptoms. The symptoms of different types of cancer vary but the following are usually observed in most types: fever, chills, unintended weight loss, fatigue, and a general sense of not feeling well.

Treatment. The treatment of cancer differs depending on the type and stage of cancer. The stage of cancer refers to how large a tumor is and how far cancer cells have spread throughout the body. Table 10-1 provides a summary of cancer staging.

If tumors are localized and have not spread, the cancer can often be successfully treated by surgically removing the tumor. Other treatment options are chemotherapy and radiation therapy. Even if a cancer cannot be cured, its progression can sometimes be slowed, allowing patients to live additional years.

Allergies

An allergic reaction is an immune response to a substance, such as pollen, that is not normally harmful to the body. An allergy can also be an excessive immune response. Substances that trigger allergic responses are called **allergens.**

Allergic reactions involve IgE antibodies and mast cells. When IgE antibodies bind to allergens, they cause mast cells to release histamine and heparin. These chemicals trigger allergic reactions. A patient receiving allergy shots is being injected with tiny amounts of the allergen. This causes the body to produce IgG antibodies that will prevent IgE antibodies from binding to the allergen. IgG antibodies do not trigger immune responses because they do not activate mast cells.

Most allergies do not cause life-threatening conditions, but some do. One life-threatening condition that can result is **anaphylaxis.** In this condition, blood vessels dilate so quickly that blood pressure drops too quickly for organs to adjust. Without treatment, patients may go into anaphylactic shock and die.

Signs and Symptoms. The signs and symptoms of allergies vary depending on what part of the body is exposed to allergens. Allergens that are inhaled often cause a runny nose, sneezing, coughing, or wheezing. An allergen that is ingested causes nausea, diarrhea, or vomiting. Skin allergens cause rashes. Allergens in the blood, such as penicillin for people who are allergic to it, are often the most life-threatening because they can affect many organ systems.

Treatment. Many allergies are effectively treated with over-the-counter medications called **antihistamines.** Prescription-strength antihistamines are also available. Various types of nasal sprays and decongestants can also reduce the symptoms of allergies. When a person experiences anaphylaxis, an injection of **epinephrine** is usually an effective treatment. Epinephrine causes vasoconstriction, which increases blood pressure.

Pathophysiology

Common Diseases and Disorders of the Immune System

As science and medicine develop a better understanding of the immune system and its relationship to causing disease, multiple diseases and disorders involving many body systems are now thought to have an *autoimmune* component. An **autoimmune disease** is one where the body begins to attack its own antigens. Examples of autoimmune diseases include scleroderma, rheumatoid arthritis (Chapter 3), multiple sclerosis (Chapter 7),

continued ⟶

Common Diseases and Disorders of the Immune System *(continued)*

glomerulonephritis (Chapter 8), Crohn's disease (Chapter 11), and insulin-dependent (Type I) diabetes mellitus (Chapter 12), as well as others.

In this section, we will focus on specific immune system disorders. For other diseases with possible or probable autoimmune components, please refer to the appropriate body system pathophysiology section for further information.

Acquired immunodeficiency syndrome (AIDS) is the development of severe signs and symptoms caused by the human immunodeficiency virus (HIV) as it destroys lymphocytes—particularly T lymphocytes—leaving the immune system weakened and susceptible to many other diseases. Because a person may be infected with HIV for years before developing symptoms, it is important for all high-risk individuals to be tested.

- **Causes.** AIDS is caused by the human immunodeficiency virus (HIV).
- **Signs and symptoms.** Symptoms of AIDS include T-cell counts below 200 (normal is more than 400); fever; diaphoresis; weakness; weight loss; frequent infections, including herpetic ulcers of the mouth, skin, and genitals; TB; yeast infections of the mouth, esophagus, and vagina; meningitis; and encephalitis. Cytomegalovirus (CMV), a specific type of herpetic virus, may also affect the eyes and other internal organs. Kaposi's sarcoma is a skin cancer commonly seen in AIDS patients.
- **Treatment.** There is no cure for AIDS, but in the United States, treatments are available that significantly delay the progression of the disease for many patients. Treatments include the use of various antiviral drugs, but many of these drugs have serious side effects. Antibiotics are also used to treat infections.

Chronic fatigue syndrome (CFS) is a condition in which a person feels severe tiredness that cannot be relieved by rest and is not related to other illness.

- **Causes.** The causes are primarily unknown, although the Epstein-Barr virus (EBV) is suspected as a possible cause. This condition may also be caused by an autoimmune response against the nervous system.
- **Signs and symptoms.** The most common symptom is severe fatigue. Other signs and symptoms include mild fever, sore throat, tender lymph nodes in the neck or armpit, general body aches, joint pain, sleep disturbances, and depression.
- **Treatment.** Treatment includes antiviral drugs, medications to treat the depression associated with this condition, and pain medications.

Lymphedema is the blockage of lymphatic vessels. These vessels typically drain excess fluids from various areas of the body.

- **Causes.** This condition may be caused by parasitic infections, trauma to the vessels, tumors, radiation

therapy, cellulitis (a skin infection), and surgeries such as mastectomies and biopsies in which lymph tissues have been removed.

- **Signs and symptoms.** The common symptom is tissue swelling that lasts longer than a few days or increases over time.
- **Treatment.** Treatment options include compression stockings for swelling in the legs or arms, elevation of the affected limb, or surgery to remove abnormal lymphatic tissue. Physical and massage therapy have also been found helpful in the early stages of lymphedema to spread the fluid into surrounding tissues for reabsorption.

Mononucleosis is also known as *mono*. Because it frequently affects teenagers and is a highly contagious viral infection spread through the saliva of the infected person, it has earned the nickname "the kissing disease." Mono is also spread through coughing and sneezing.

- **Causes.** Mononucleosis is caused by either the Epstein-Barr virus or the cytomegalovirus (CMV).
- **Signs and symptoms.** Unexplained fever, extreme fatigue, and sore throat are common. Other symptoms include weakness, headache, and swollen, tender lymph nodes.
- **Treatment.** Rest, proper nutrition, and antibiotics to prevent secondary infections usually result in recovery from acute symptoms in a week or two, although complete recovery may take a month or longer.

Systemic lupus erythematosus (SLE), commonly referred to as lupus, is an autoimmune disorder that affects a few or, sometimes, many organ systems of the body. In this condition, people produce antibodies that target their own cells and tissues. As with many autoimmune disorders, lupus affects women much more often than men. Although the reason is unknown, autoimmune disorders affect women almost 75% of the time, often during childbearing years.

- **Causes.** This disorder may be caused by some drugs or by bacterial infections, but except for its autoimmune component, its actual cause is unknown.
- **Signs and symptoms.** The list of signs and symptoms is extensive and may include any or all of the following:
  - Fatigue
  - General body aches
  - Fever
  - Weight loss (anorexia)
  - Hair loss
  - Arthritis
  - Numbness of the fingers and toes
  - "Butterfly" rash on the face
  - Sensitivity to sunlight (photophobia)
  - Vision problems
  - Nausea

continued ⟶

Common Diseases and Disorders of the Immune System *(concluded)*

- Nosebleeds (epistaxis)
- Headaches
- Mental disorders
- Seizures
- Abnormal blood clots
- Chest pains
- Inflammation of heart tissues (carditis)
- Anemia
- Shortness of breath

- Fluid accumulation around the lungs
- Renal failure
- Blood in the urine (hematuria)
- **Treatment.** Treatment options include anti-inflammatory medications, including steroids, as well as protective clothing and creams to prevent damage from sunlight. Dialysis, immunosuppressive medications, and kidney transplants may be necessary for more serious cases.

Summary

The body's major line of defense is the immune system. The primary function of the immune system is to protect the body against infection, toxins, and cancer. Its major organs include the spleen, thymus, and lymph nodes. The lymph vessels transport the immune fluid, called lymph, throughout the body. The two major lymphatic collecting ducts are the thoracic duct and the right lymphatic duct.

The defenses of the immune system can be either nonspecific or specific. Lymphocytes are the major types of cells in the immune system and are classified as either B cells or T cells. When the body is first exposed to an antigen, a primary immune response occurs. This response is less specific and slower than a secondary immune response, which occurs the next time the body is exposed to the same antigen.

An intact immune system is important because the body is attacked by numerous invaders every day. In order to effectively perform aseptic technique and infection control, the medical assistant must have a working knowledge of the immune system in order to best educate patients about protecting their bodies from pathogens.

CASE STUDY QUESTIONS

Now that you have completed this chapter, review the case study at the beginning of the chapter and answer the following questions:

1. Is it likely that this patient has a life-threatening illness?
2. What test should be done to diagnose this patient?
3. Based on her symptoms, what disease or disorder is this patient more likely to have?
4. Is the patient contagious? What precautions should she take to avoid spreading her illness?

Discussion Questions

1. What are the two major lymphatic collecting ducts? From what part of the body does each duct collect lymph fluid?
2. What are nonspecific body defenses? Give examples.
3. Explain how each of the four types of acquired immunity occur.
4. Discuss how B cells and T cells are activated.

Critical Thinking Questions

1. Describe what is meant by cancer staging. Explain each stage.
2. What is an allergy? Why are some allergies life-threatening and what is this type of allergic reaction called?
3. How do vaccines produce favorable effects?

Application Activities

1. Give an example of each of the following nonspecific defense mechanisms:
   a. Species resistance
   b. Chemical barrier
   c. Phagocytosis

2. Describe what produces the following signs of inflammation:
   a. Redness
   b. Swelling
   c. Heat
   d. Pain
3. Give the functions of each of the following defensive proteins or cells:
   a. Complement proteins
   b. Macrophages
   c. Helper T cells
   d. Memory cells
   e. Plasma cells
4. What is a pathogen?

Virtual Fieldtrip

Visit the McGraw-Hill Higher Education Medical Assisting website at www.mhhe.com/medicalassisting3 to complete the following activity:

Use the U.S. DHHS (Department of Health and Human Services) website for Women's Health, accessing information on autoimmune diseases. Answer the following questions from the webpage:

1. What is an autoimmune disease?
2. Who is at risk for getting autoimmune diseases?
3. What are the most common symptoms of autoimmune diseases?
4. Are CFS (chronic fatigue syndrome) and fibromyalgia autoimmune diseases?
5. What are flare-ups?
6. Are there medications to treat autoimmune diseases?
7. How can I manage my life now that I have an autoimmune disease?
8. What are some things I can do to feel better?
9. What kinds of doctors/therapists will I need to treat my autoimmune disease?

Open the CD and complete this chapter's practice activities, play the games, listen to the key terms, and test yourself with the interactive review. E-mail, print, and/or save your results to document your proficiency.

CHAPTER 11

The Digestive System

KEY TERMS

- acinar cells
- adenoids
- alimentary canal
- anal canal
- appendicitis
- ascending colon
- bicuspids
- bile
- bolus
- carboxypeptidase
- cardiac sphincter
- cecum
- cellulose
- chief cells
- chyme
- chymotrypsin
- cirrhosis
- colitis
- common bile duct
- cuspids
- cystic duct
- defecation reflex
- descending colon
- disaccharide
- diverticulitis
- diverticulosis
- duodenum
- esophageal hiatus
- feces
- gastric juice
- gastritis
- gastroesophageal reflux disease (GERD)
- glycogen
- hemorrhoids

CHAPTER OUTLINE

- Characteristics of the Alimentary Canal
- The Mouth
- The Pharynx
- The Esophagus
- The Stomach
- The Small Intestine
- The Large Intestine
- The Rectum and Anal Canal
- The Liver
- The Gallbladder
- The Pancreas
- The Absorption of Nutrients

LEARNING OUTCOMES

After completing Chapter 11, you will be able to:

11.1 List the functions of the digestive system.
11.2 Trace the pathway of food through the alimentary canal.

KEY TERMS (Concluded)

- hepatic duct
- hepatic lobule
- hepatic portal vein
- hepatitis
- hepatocytes
- hernia
- idiopathic
- ileocecal sphincter
- ileum
- incisors
- intestinal lipase
- intrinsic factor
- jejunum
- lactase
- laryngopharynx
- lingual frenulum
- lingual tonsils
- linoleic acid
- maltase
- mesentery
- microvilli
- molars
- monosaccharide
- mucosa
- mucous cells
- nasopharynx
- nucleases
- oropharynx
- palate
- palatine tonsils
- pancreatic amylase
- pancreatic lipase
- parietal cells
- parietal peritoneum
- parotid glands
- pepsin
- pepsinogen
- peptidases
- pharyngeal tonsils
- polysaccharide
- pyloric sphincter
- rectum
- serosa
- serous cells
- sigmoid colon
- sublingual gland
- submandibular gland
- submucosa
- sucrase
- transverse colon
- triglyceride
- trypsin
- uvula
- vermiform appendix
- visceral peritoneum

11.3 Describe the structure and functions of the mouth, teeth, tongue, and salivary glands.

11.4 Describe the structure and function of the pharynx.

11.5 Describe the swallowing process.

11.6 Describe the structure of the esophagus and tell how it propels food into the stomach.

11.7 Describe the structure and functions of the stomach.

11.8 List the substances secreted by the stomach and give their functions.

11.9 Describe the structure and functions of the small intestine.

11.10 List the substances secreted by the small intestine and describe the importance of each.

11.11 Describe the structure and functions of the large intestine, including the anal canal and rectum.

11.12 Explain the structures and functions of the liver, gallbladder, and pancreas.

11.13 List the substances released by the liver, gallbladder, and pancreas into the small intestine and give the function of each secretion.

11.14 Tell what types of nutrients are absorbed by the digestive system and where they are absorbed.

11.15 Describe the causes, signs and symptoms, and treatments of various diseases and disorders of the digestive system.

Introduction

Digestion is the mechanical and chemical breakdown of foods into forms that your body cells can absorb. The organs of the digestive system carry out digestion and can be divided into two categories—those of the alimentary canal and accessory organs. Organs of the alimentary canal extend from the mouth to the anus. They are the mouth, pharynx, esophagus, stomach, small intestine, large intestine, and anal canal. The accessory organs include the teeth, tongue, salivary glands, liver, gallbladder, and pancreas (Figure 11-1). You may find it helpful to review Figure 1-7 in Chapter 1 to review the abdominal regions and quadrants while studying the organs of this chapter.

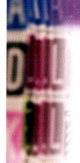

CASE STUDY

Yesterday afternoon, a 55-year-old female came to the gastroenterologist's office complaining of severe pain in her upper-right abdomen. She was nauseated and stated that for several months—and especially following meals—she had been having periodic abdominal pain. After several tests, she was diagnosed as having gallstones and was scheduled for the surgical removal of her gallbladder.

As you read this chapter, consider the following questions:

1. What is the function of the gallbladder?
2. How does the gallbladder empty bile into the small intestine?
3. What conditions can result if gallstones are not removed?
4. Will this patient need to change her diet once her gallbladder is removed?

Characteristics of the Alimentary Canal

The wall of the **alimentary canal,** also known as the digestive tract, consists of four layers:

1. Mucosa. The **mucosa** is the innermost layer of the wall and is mostly made of epithelial tissue that secretes enzymes and mucus into the lumen, or passageway, of the canal. This layer also is very active in absorbing nutrients.

2. Submucosa. The **submucosa** is the layer just inferior to the mucosa. It contains loose connective tissue, blood vessels, glands, and nerves. The blood vessels in this layer carry away absorbed nutrients.

3. Muscular layer. This layer is just outside the submucosa. It is made of layers of smooth muscle tissue and contracts to move materials through the canal.

4. Serosa. The **serosa** is the double-walled outermost layer of canal and is also known as the peritoneum. The innermost wall of the serosa is known as the **visceral peritoneum.** It secretes serous fluid to keep the outside of the canal moist, preventing it from sticking to other organs or to its outer layer, the **parietal peritoneum,** also called the abdominal lining.

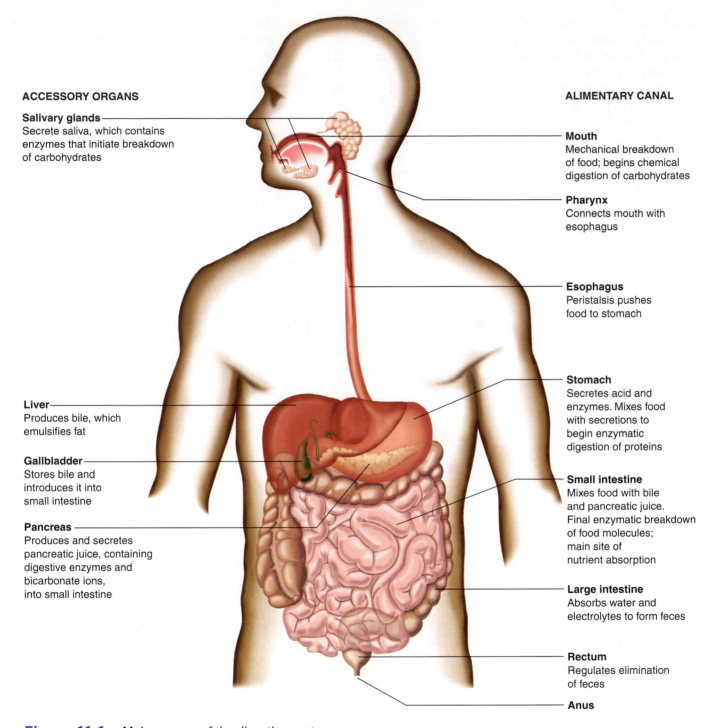

ACCESSORY ORGANS

Salivary glands
Secrete saliva, which contains enzymes that initiate breakdown of carbohydrates

Liver
Produces bile, which emulsifies fat

Gallbladder
Stores bile and introduces it into small intestine

Pancreas
Produces and secretes pancreatic juice, containing digestive enzymes and bicarbonate ions, into small intestine

ALIMENTARY CANAL

Mouth
Mechanical breakdown of food; begins chemical digestion of carbohydrates

Pharynx
Connects mouth with esophagus

Esophagus
Peristalsis pushes food to stomach

Stomach
Secretes acid and enzymes. Mixes food with secretions to begin enzymatic digestion of proteins

Small intestine
Mixes food with bile and pancreatic juice. Final enzymatic breakdown of food molecules; main site of nutrient absorption

Large intestine
Absorbs water and electrolytes to form feces

Rectum
Regulates elimination of feces

Anus

Figure 11-1. Major organs of the digestive system.

Smooth muscle in the wall of the canal can contract to produce two basic types of movements—churning and peristalsis. Churning mixes substances in the canal. Peristalsis propels substances through the tract (Figure 11-2).

The Mouth

The mouth, which is also known as the buccal cavity, takes in food and reduces its size through chewing. This process is known as mechanical digestion. The mouth also starts to chemically digest food because saliva (spit) contains the enzyme amylase, which breaks down carbohydrates.

The cheeks consist of skin, adipose tissue, skeletal muscles, and an inner lining of moist stratified squamous epithelium. The cheeks act to hold food in the mouth. The lips contain a lot of sensory nerve fibers that can judge the temperature of food before it enters the mouth. The tongue is mostly made of skeletal muscles and is covered by a mucous membrane. The body of the tongue is

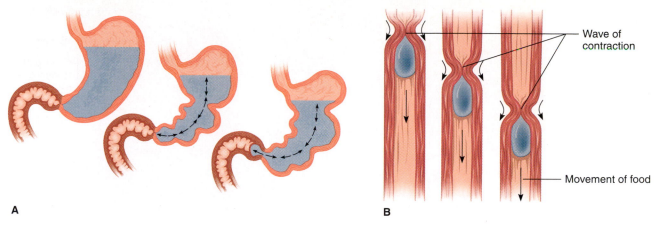

A

B

Figure 11-2. Movements through the alimentary canal: (A) Churning movements move substances back and forth to mix them. (B) Peristalsis moves contents along the canal.

held to the floor of the oral cavity by a flap of mucous membrane called the **lingual frenulum.** The tongue acts to mix food in the mouth and to hold the food between teeth. It also contains taste buds. The back of the tongue contains two lumps of lymphatic tissue called **lingual tonsils.** Lingual tonsils act to destroy bacteria and viruses on the back of the tongue.

The **palate** is the roof of the mouth. It functions to separate the oral cavity from the nasal cavity. The front of the palate, the hard palate, is rigid because it has bony

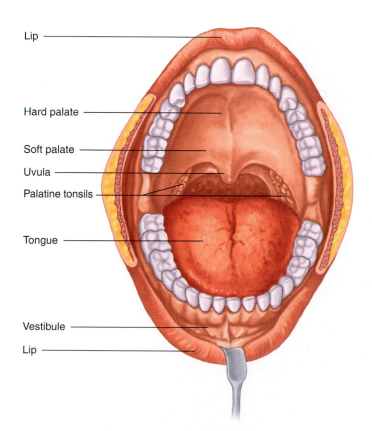

Figure 11-3. Structures of the mouth.

Lip

Hard palate

Soft palate

Uvula

Palatine tonsils

Tongue

Vestibule

Lip

plates in it. The back of the palate, soft palate, lacks bony material and therefore is not rigid. The back of the soft palate hangs down into the throat, and this portion of the soft palate is called the **uvula.** The uvula acts to prevent food and liquids from entering the nose during swallowing.

At the back of the mouth, where the oral cavity joins the pharynx in the area known as the oropharynx, are two masses of lymphatic tissue called **palatine tonsils.** Just above the palatine tonsils, in the area known as the nasopharynx (the nasal cavity joins the pharynx here), are two more masses of lymphatic tissue called the **pharyngeal tonsils (adenoids).** These masses of lymphatic tissue act to protect the area from bacteria and viruses (Figure 11-3).

Teeth act to decrease the size of food particles, and different types of teeth are adapted to handle food in different ways. The most medial teeth, called **incisors,** act as chisels to bite off food pieces. Teeth called **cuspids,** also known as the canines, are the sharpest teeth and they act to tear tough food (Figure 11-4). The back teeth, called **bicuspids** and **molars,** are flat. They are designed to grind food (Figure 11-5).

Salivary glands secrete saliva, which is a mixture of water, enzymes, and mucus. Salivary glands are made of two types of cells—**serous cells** and **mucous cells.** Serous cells secrete a fluid made mostly of water and they also secrete amylase. Mucous cells secrete mucus. The mass created by food mixed with the saliva and mucus mixture is called a **bolus.**

All major salivary glands are paired (Figure 11-6):

- **Parotid glands:** the largest of the salivary glands, located beneath the skin just in front of the ears
- **Submandibular glands:** located in the floor of the mouth just inside the surface of the mandibles (jaws)
- **Sublingual glands:** the smallest of the salivary glands, located in the floor of the mouth beneath the tongue

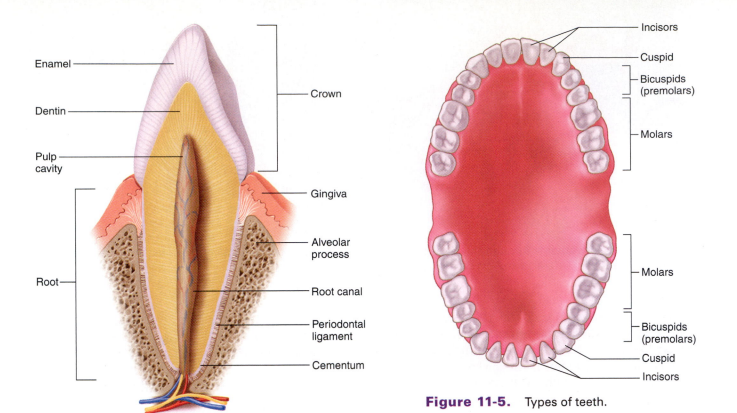

Figure 11-4. Structure of a cuspid tooth.

Figure 11-5. Types of teeth.

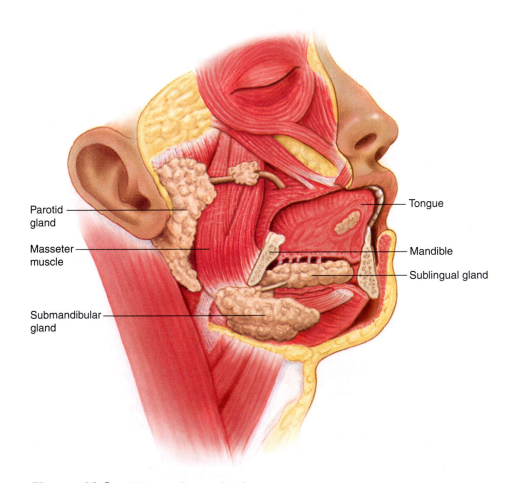

Figure 11-6. Major salivary glands.

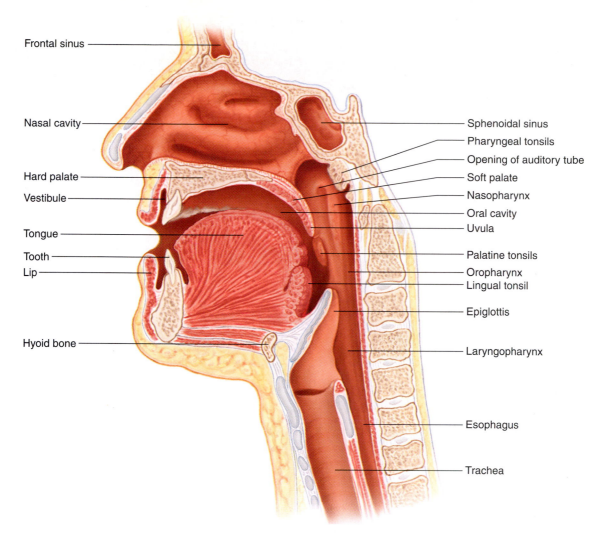

Frontal sinus

Nasal cavity

Hard palate

Vestibule

Tongue

Tooth

Lip

Hyoid bone

Sphenoidal sinus

Pharyngeal tonsils

Opening of auditory tube

Soft palate

Nasopharynx

Oral cavity

Uvula

Palatine tonsils

Oropharynx

Lingual tonsil

Epiglottis

Laryngopharynx

Esophagus

Trachea

Figure 11-7. Sagittal section of the mouth, nasal cavity, and pharynx.

The Pharynx

The pharynx is more commonly called the throat. It is a long, muscular structure that extends from the area behind the nose to the esophagus. It acts to connect the nasal cavity with the oral cavity for breathing through the nose. It also acts to push food into the esophagus (Figure 11-7).

The divisions of the pharynx are:

- **Nasopharynx:** the portion behind the nasal cavity.
- **Oropharynx:** the portion behind the oral cavity.
- **Laryngopharynx:** the portion behind the larynx. The laryngopharynx continues as the esophagus.

Swallowing is largely a reflex. In other words, it is an automatic response that does not require much thought. The following events occur during swallowing:

1. The soft palate rises, causing the uvula to cover the opening between the nasal cavity and the oral cavity.
2. The epiglottis covers the opening of the larynx so that food does not enter it (see Figure 11-7).
3. The tongue presses against the roof of the mouth, forcing food into the oropharynx.

4. The muscles in the pharynx contract, forcing food toward the esophagus.
5. The esophagus opens.
6. Food is pushed into the esophagus by the muscles of the pharynx.

The Esophagus

The esophagus is a muscular tube that connects the pharynx to the stomach (Figures 11-7 and 11-8). It descends through the thoracic cavity, through the diaphragm, and into the abdominal cavity where it joins the stomach. The hole in the diaphragm that the esophagus goes through is called the **esophageal hiatus.** This hiatus is a common place for hernias to occur. A **hernia** develops when an organ pushes through a wall that contains it. A hiatal hernia occurs when the stomach gets pushed up into the thoracic cavity through the esophageal hiatus. The **cardiac sphincter,** also known as the esophageal sphincter, controls the movement of food into the stomach. Sphincters are circular bands of muscle located at the openings of many tubes in the body. They open and close to allow or prevent the movement of substances out of a tube.

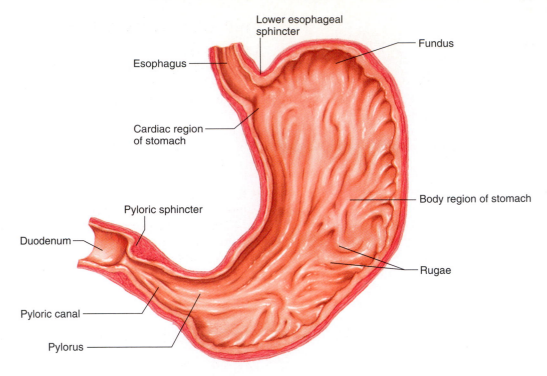

Figure 11-8. Regions of the stomach.

The Stomach

The stomach lies below the diaphragm in the left upper quadrant of the abdominal cavity. The folds of the inner lining of the stomach are called rugae. The stomach functions to receive the food bolus from the esophagus, mix food with **gastric juice** (secretions of the stomach lining), start protein digestion, and move food into the small intestine.

The beginning portion of the stomach that is attached to the esophagus is called the cardiac region. The portion of the stomach that balloons over the cardiac region is called the fundus. The main part of the stomach is called the body, and the narrow portion that is connected to the small intestine is called the pylorus. The **pyloric sphincter** controls the movement of substances from the pylorus of the stomach into the small intestine (Figure 11-8).

The lining of the stomach contains gastric glands. These glands are made of the following cell types:

- **Mucous cells.** These cells secrete mucus to protect the lining of the stomach.
- **Chief cells.** These cells secrete **pepsinogen,** which becomes **pepsin** in the presence of acid. Pepsin digests proteins.
- **Parietal cells.** These cells secrete hydrochloric acid, which is necessary to convert pepsinogen to pepsin. They also secrete **intrinsic factor,** which is necessary for vitamin B_{12} absorption.

When a person smells, tastes, or sees appetizing food, the parasympathetic nervous system stimulates the gastric

glands to secrete their products. A hormone called gastrin, made by the stomach, also stimulates the gastric glands to become active. A hormone called cholecystokinin (CCK) made by the small intestine inhibits gastric glands. The stomach does not absorb many substances but it can absorb alcohol, water, and some fat-soluble drugs. The mixture of food and gastric juices is called **chyme.** Once chyme is well mixed, stomach contractions push it into the small intestine a little at a time. It takes 4 to 8 hours for the stomach to empty following a meal.

If a patient is unable to swallow for any reason, a tube called a gastrostomy tube or G tube may be inserted into the patient's stomach so he can be fed liquid meals, such as Ensure®, through this tube.

The Small Intestine

The small intestine is a tubular organ that extends from the stomach to the large intestine. It fills most of the abdominal cavity and is coiled. The small intestine carries out most of the digestion in the body and is responsible for absorbing most of the nutrients into the bloodstream.

The beginning of the small intestine is called the **duodenum.** It is C-shaped and relatively short. The middle portion of the small intestine is called the **jejunum.** It is coiled and forms the majority of the small intestine. If a patient's stomach is diseased or removed, a jejunostomy or J tube may be inserted into the jejunum to allow her to receive nutrition.

The last portion of the small intestine is called the **ileum,** and it is directly attached to the large intestine. The jejunum

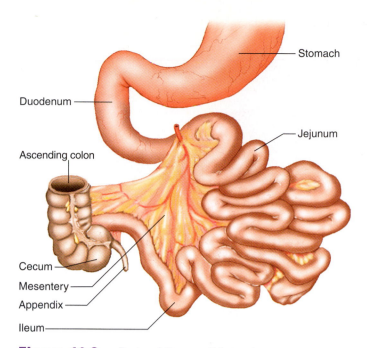

Figure 11-9. Parts of the small intestine.

and ileum are held in the abdominal cavity by a fan-like tissue called the **mesentery** that attaches to the posterior wall of the abdomen (Figure 11-9).

The lining of the small intestine contains cells that have **microvilli.** Microvilli greatly increase the surface area of the small intestine so that it can absorb many nutrients. The lining of the small intestine also contains intestinal glands that secrete various substances. The secretions of the small intestine include mucus and water. Water aids in digestion but some toxins cause the secretion of too much water, and this leads to diarrhea—which in turn aids the body in eliminating the toxins. Mucus protects the lining of the small intestine. The following are the major enzymes secreted by the small intestine:

- **Peptidases.** These enzymes digest proteins.
- **Sucrase, maltase,** and **lactase.** These enzymes digest sugars. A person who cannot produce lactase will not be able to digest lactose, which is the sugar in dairy products. This causes a condition called lactose intolerance.
- **Intestinal lipase.** This enzyme digests fats.

The parasympathetic nervous system and the stretching of the small intestine wall are the primary factors that trigger the small intestine to secrete its products. Almost all nutrients (water, glucose, amino acids, fatty acids, glycerol, and electrolytes) are absorbed by the small intestine. The wall of the small intestine contracts to mix chyme and to propel it toward the large intestine. If chyme moves too quickly through the small intestine, nutrients are not absorbed and diarrhea results. The **ileocecal sphincter** controls the movement of chyme from the ileum to the **cecum,** which is the beginning of the large intestine.

The Large Intestine

The large intestine extends from the ileum of the small intestine to where it opens to the outside of the body as the anus. The beginning of the large intestine is the cecum. Projecting off the cecum is the **vermiform appendix.** The appendix is made mostly of lymphoid tissue and has no significant function in humans. The cecum eventually gives rise to the **ascending colon,** which is the portion of the large intestine that runs up the right side of the abdominal cavity. If you remember that the appendix is in the right lower quadrant (RLQ), it will be easy to remember that the ascending colon also goes up the right side of the abdomen. The ascending colon becomes the **transverse colon** as it crosses the abdominal cavity; from there it becomes the **descending colon** as it descends the left side of the abdominal cavity. In the pelvic cavity, the descending colon then forms the S-shaped tube called the **sigmoid colon.**

The Rectum and Anal Canal

Eventually the sigmoid colon straightens out to become the **rectum.** The last few centimeters of the rectum is known as the **anal canal,** and the opening of the anal canal to the outside of the body is called the anus (Figure 11-10).

The lining of the large intestine only secretes mucus to aid in the movement of substances. As chyme leaves the small intestine and enters the large intestine, the proximal portion of the large intestine absorbs water and a few electrolytes from it. The leftover chyme is then called **feces.** Feces are made of undigested solid materials, a little water, ions, mucus, cells of the intestinal lining, and bacteria.

The contractions of the large intestine propel feces forward, but these contractions normally occur periodically and as mass movements. Mass movements trigger the **defecation reflex,** which allows anal sphincters to relax and feces to move through the anus in the process of elimination. The squeezing actions of the abdominal wall muscles also aid in the emptying of the large intestine.

The Liver

The liver is quite large and fills most of the upper-right abdominal quadrant. Part of its function is to store vitamins and iron. It is reddish-brown in color and is enclosed by a tough capsule. This capsule divides the liver into a large right lobe and a small left lobe (Figure 11-11). Each lobe is separated into smaller divisions called **hepatic lobules.** Branches of the **hepatic portal vein** carry blood from the digestive organs to the hepatic lobules. The hepatic lobules contain macrophages that destroy bacteria and viruses in the blood. Each lobule contains many cells called **hepatocytes.** Hepatocytes process the nutrients in blood and make **bile,** which is used in the digestion of fats. Bile leaves the liver through the **hepatic duct.** The hepatic duct merges with the **cystic duct** (the duct from the gallbladder) to form the **common bile duct.** This duct delivers bile to the duodenum.

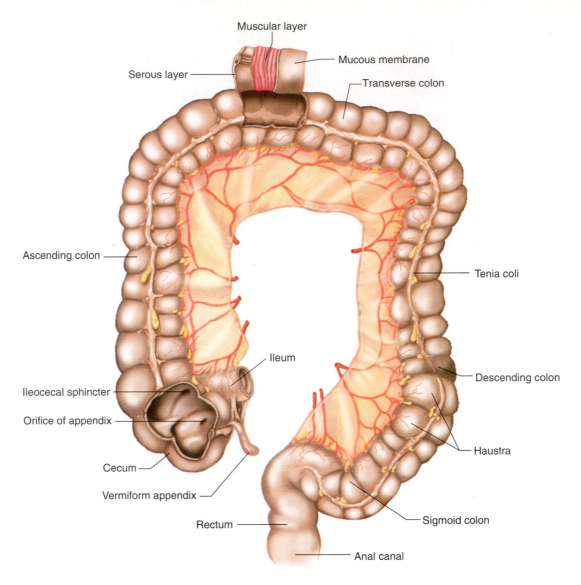

Figure 11-10. Parts of the large intestine.

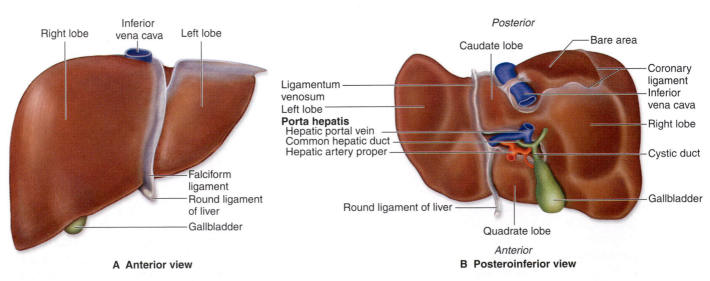

A Anterior view

B Posteroinferior view

Figure 11-11. Gross anatomy of the liver—the liver is in the right upper quadrant of the abdomen. (A) Anterior and (B) posteroinferior views show the four lobes of the liver, as well as the gallbladder and porta hepatis.

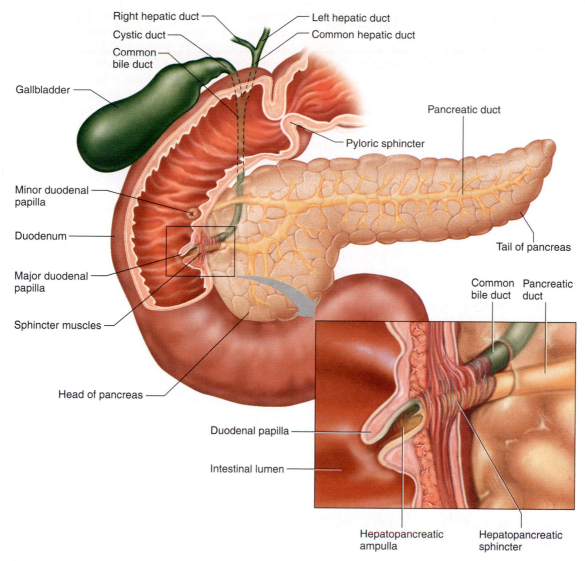

Figure 11-12. Pancreas and its connections to the gallbladder and duodenum.

The Gallbladder

The gallbladder is a small, sac-like structure located beneath the liver (Figures 11-11 and 11-12). Its only function is to store bile. Bile leaves the gallbladder through the cystic duct. The hormone cholecystokinin causes the gallbladder to release bile. The salts in bile break large fat globules into smaller ones so that they can be more quickly digested by the digestive enzymes. Bile salts also increase the absorption of fatty acids, cholesterol, and fat-soluble vitamins into the bloodstream.

The Pancreas

The pancreas is located behind the stomach. Pancreatic **acinar cells** produce pancreatic juice, which ultimately flows through the pancreatic duct to the duodenum

(Figure 11-12). Pancreatic juice contains the following enzymes:

- **Pancreatic amylase.** This enzyme digests carbohydrates.
- **Pancreatic lipase.** This enzyme digests lipids.
- **Nucleases.** These enzymes digest nucleic acids.
- **Trypsin, chymotrypsin,** and **carboxypeptidase.** These enzymes digest proteins.

The pancreas also secretes bicarbonate ions into the duodenum. These ions neutralize the acidic chyme arriving from the stomach. The parasympathetic nervous system stimulates the pancreas to release its enzymes. The hormones secretin and cholecystokinin also stimulate the pancreas to release digestive enzymes. Secretin and cholecystokinin come from the small intestine.

The Absorption of Nutrients

Nutrients are defined as necessary food substances. They include carbohydrates, proteins, lipids, vitamins, minerals, and water.

Three types of carbohydrates that humans ingest are starches (**polysaccharides**), simple sugars (**monosaccharides** and **disaccharides**), and **cellulose.** Starches come from foods such as pasta, potatoes, rice, and breads. Monosaccharides and disaccharides are obtained from sweet foods and fruits. Cellulose is a type of carbohydrate found in many vegetables that cannot be digested by humans. Therefore, cellulose provides fiber or bulk for the large intestine. This fiber helps the large intestine empty more regularly.

Harvard Medical International states a connection has been made between higher fiber diets and a decrease in colon diseases, including cancer. This may be because fiber increases water absorption and bulk, causing more rapid emptying of the colon and decreasing the production of benign growths such as adenomas or polyps, which increase the risk of cancer. Fiber may also neutralize toxins produced by GI (gastrointestinal) tract bacteria.

Most body cells use the monosaccharide glucose to make ATP. When a person has an excess of glucose, it can be stored in the liver and skeletal muscle cells as **glycogen.** Lipids (fats) are obtained through various foods. The most abundant dietary lipids are **triglycerides.** They are found in meats, eggs, milk, and butter. Cholesterol is another common dietary lipid and is found in eggs, whole milk, butter, and cheeses. Lipids are used by the body primarily to make energy when glucose levels are low. Excess triglycerides are stored in adipose tissue. Cholesterol is essential to cell growth and function; cells use it to make cell membranes and some hormones. People should have the essential fatty acid **linoleic acid** in their diet since the body cannot make it. This fatty acid is found in corn and sunflower oils. People also need a certain amount of fat to absorb fat-soluble vitamins.

Foods rich in protein include meats, eggs, milk, fish, chicken, turkey, nuts, cheese, and beans. Protein requirements vary from individual to individual, but all people must take in proteins that contain certain amino acids (called essential amino acids) because the body cannot make them. Proteins are used by the body for growth and the repair of tissues.

The fat-soluble vitamins are vitamins A, D, E, and K, and the water-soluble vitamins are all the B vitamins and vitamin C. Vitamins have many functions; they are summarized in Table 11-1.

Minerals make up about 4% of total body weight. They are primarily found in bones and teeth. Cells use minerals to make enzymes, cell membranes, and various proteins such as hemoglobin. The most important minerals to the human body are calcium, phosphorus, sulfur, sodium, chlorine, and magnesium. Trace elements are elements needed in very small amounts by the body. They include iron, manganese, copper, iodine, and zinc.

TABLE 11-1	Common Vitamins and Their Importance in the Body
Vitamin	**Function**
Vitamin A	Needed for the production of visual receptors, mucus, the normal growth of bones and teeth, and the repair of epithelial tissues
Vitamin B_1 (thiamine)	Needed for the metabolism of carbohydrates
Vitamin B_2 (riboflavin)	Needed for carbohydrate and fat metabolism and for the growth of cells
Vitamin B_6	Needed for the synthesis of protein, antibodies, and nucleic acid
Vitamin B_{12} (cyanocobalamin)	Needed for myelin production and the metabolism of carbohydrates and nucleic acids
Biotin	Needed for the metabolism of proteins, fats, and nucleic acids
Folic acid	Needed for the production of amino acids, DNA, and red blood cells
Pantothenic acid	Needed for carbohydrate and fat metabolism
Niacin	Needed for the metabolism of carbohydrates, proteins, fats, and nucleic acids
Vitamin C (ascorbic acid)	Needed for the production of collagen, amino acids, and hormones and for the absorption of iron
Vitamin D	Needed for the absorption of calcium
Vitamin E	Antioxidant that prevents the breakdown of certain tissues
Vitamin K	Needed for blood clotting

Aging and the Digestive System

Changes related to aging are evident throughout all body systems and the digestive system is no exception. In general, the mucus lining thins and the blood supply and number of smooth muscle cells within the alimentary canal decreases, which leads to decreased motility. The decreasing motility often causes gastro-esophageal reflux disease (GERD) and constipation. The decreasing blood supply also affects the patient's ability to absorb medications and nutrients. Gastric secretions from the stomach, liver, and pancreas decrease and the ability of the liver to detoxify the blood also lessens. This makes adjusting medication dosages more difficult until it is clear (through lab tests or patient response) how rapidly and how much medication the patient's body is absorbing. If the patient drinks alcohol, he may notice a difference in the way alcohol affects him. Advancing age also leaves the patient more likely to develop ulcerations and cancers of the GI system, including colorectal cancer, which is the second-leading cause of cancer deaths in the United States, according to the American Cancer Society.

Many elderly people state their sense of taste is altered and that food loses some of its enjoyment. If loneliness and/or isolation as a result of the patient's social situation is present, his diet will likely change because "it is no fun or too much work to cook just for myself." If depression is a component, the patient's diet will likely change. The medical assistant should be aware of these possibilities, looking for clues such as weight loss, depression, or patient comments, and should relate information to the health-care provider with a goal of securing social service assistance for the patient if needed.

Pathophysiology

Common Diseases and Disorders of the Digestive System

Appendicitis is an inflammation of the appendix. If not treated promptly, it can be life-threatening.

- **Causes.** This disorder may be caused by blockage of the appendix with feces or a tumor, infection, or other unknown (**idiopathic**) cause.
- **Signs and symptoms.** The signs and symptoms include lack of appetite, pain in the RLQ that may radiate throughout the abdomen and even down the right leg, nausea, slight fever, and an increased white blood cell count.
- **Treatment.** The primary treatments are antibiotics to prevent infection and surgery to remove the appendix, known as an appendectomy.

Cirrhosis is a chronic liver disease in which normal liver tissue is replaced with nonfunctional scar tissue.

- **Causes.** This disease is often an autoimmune disease. It may also be caused by some medications and alcohol consumption. Hepatitis B and C infections can also contribute to the development of cirrhosis.
- **Signs and symptoms.** There are many symptoms to this disease. They include anemia, fatigue, mental confusion, fever, vomiting, blood in the vomit, an enlarged liver, jaundice, unintended weight loss, swelling of the legs or abdomen, abdominal pain, a decreased urine output, and pale feces.
- **Treatment.** Alcohol consumption should be discontinued. A patient with cirrhosis may be given various medications, including antibiotics and diuretics. A liver transplant may be needed for the most seriously ill patients.

Colitis is defined as inflammation of the large intestine. This condition can be chronic or short-lived, depending on the cause.

- **Causes.** Colitis can be caused by a viral or bacterial infection or the use of antibiotics. Ulcers in the large intestine, Crohn's disease, various other diseases, and stress may also contribute to the development of this disorder.
- **Signs and symptoms.** The primary symptoms are abdominal pain, bloating, and diarrhea.
- **Treatment.** The first goal of therapy is to treat the underlying causes. Changing antibiotics, treating existing ulcers, and drinking plenty of fluids are other treatment options. In advanced cases, surgery to remove the affected area of the colon, known as a colectomy, may be recommended. If too much of the colon is

continued ⟶

Common Diseases and Disorders of the Digestive System *(continued)*

affected, a colostomy may be performed. In this procedure, the majority of the colon is removed and the opening to the outside of the body is moved to the abdomen where an appliance known as an ostomy, usually with a collecting device, commonly called a bag, collects fecal material.

Colorectal cancer usually comes from the lining of the rectum or colon. This type of cancer is curable if treated early.

- **Causes.** The causes are mostly unknown, although research is putting some blame on high fat/low fiber diets. Polyps in the colon or rectum can become cancerous, leading to this disease. Colorectal cancer may be prevented through regular screenings for polyps, which is done with a procedure known as a colonoscopy.
- **Signs and symptoms.** Anemia, unintended weight loss, abdominal pain, blood in the feces, narrow feces, or changes in bowel habits are all common symptoms.
- **Treatment.** Chemotherapy is the first line of treatment. Surgery to remove a cancerous tumor or the affected portions of colon or rectum (colectomy or colostomy) may be needed in more advanced cases.

Constipation is the condition of difficult defecation, which is the elimination of feces.

- **Causes.** The primary causes are a lack of physical activity, a lack of fiber and adequate water in the diet, the use of certain medications, and thyroid and colon disorders.
- **Signs and symptoms.** Common signs and symptoms include infrequent bowel movements (for example, no bowel movement for 3 days), bloating, abdominal pain and pain during bowel movements, hard feces, and blood on the surface of feces.
- **Treatment.** Treatment includes an increase in dietary fiber, adequate fluid intake, regular exercise, and the use of stool softeners, laxatives, and enemas (for extreme cases only).

Crohn's disease is a common type of disorder called inflammatory bowel disease. It typically affects the end of the small intestine.

- **Causes.** This disease is an autoimmune disorder.
- **Signs and symptoms.** The signs and systems of Crohn's disease include fever, tender gums, joint pain, GI ulcers, abdominal pain and gas, constipation or diarrhea, abnormal abdominal sounds, weight loss, intestinal bleeding, and blood in the feces.
- **Treatment.** The first treatment is to change the patient's diet. Other treatments include medications to reduce inflammation, including steroids, as well as antibiotics and bowel rest in which IV (intravenous) feedings are given so the patient's digestive system is

not used and so "rests." For the most serious cases, surgery to remove the affected part of the intestine may be needed (enterectomy).

Diarrhea is the condition of watery and frequent feces. Many cases of diarrhea do not require treatment because they usually stop within a day or two.

- **Causes.** The causes of diarrhea include bacterial, viral, or parasitic infections of the digestive system. It may also be caused by the ingestion of toxins; food allergies, including lactose intolerance; ulcers; Crohn's disease; laxative use; antibiotics; chemotherapy; and radiation therapy. Diarrhea related to infections may be prevented by thoroughly washing hands and cooking food properly.
- **Signs and symptoms.** The symptoms include abdominal cramps, watery feces, and the frequent passage of feces.
- **Treatment.** Patients should drink fluids to prevent dehydration. The underlying causes, if known, should be treated. Medications and dietary changes are the primary treatment options. In severe cases, antidiarrheal medications such as Lomotil® may be prescribed.

Diverticulitis is inflammation of diverticuli in the intestine. Diverticuli are abnormal dilations or pouches in the intestinal wall. When the diverticuli are not inflamed, the condition is known as **diverticulosis.**

- **Causes.** The causes are mostly unknown. Lack of fiber in the diet and a bacterial infection of the diverticuli can cause this disorder. Patients have found that certain foods, such as peanuts and seeds, aggravate this disorder.
- **Signs and symptoms.** Signs and symptoms include fever, nausea, abdominal pain, constipation or diarrhea, blood in the feces, and a high white blood cell count.
- **Treatment.** Treatments include a diet high in fiber, antibiotics, and keeping a food diary to track foods that cause flare-ups. Surgery to remove the affected portion of the intestine (colectomy) may be necessary in severe cases.

Gastritis is an inflammation of the stomach lining. It is often referred to as an "upset stomach."

- **Causes.** Gastritis can be caused by bacteria or viruses, some medications, the use of alcohol, spicy foods, excessive eating, poisons, and stress. Cooking food properly to kill harmful bacteria and viruses can help to prevent this condition.
- **Signs and symptoms.** Symptoms include nausea, lack of appetite, heartburn, vomiting, and abdominal cramps. An upper endoscopy may be done to confirm the diagnosis and rule out more serious conditions, such as an ulcer or cancer.

continued ⟶

Common Diseases and Disorders of the Digestive System *(continued)*

- **Treatment.** Lifestyle changes should be implemented to avoid foods or medications that irritate the stomach lining. Treatment with various medications to reduce the production of stomach acids such as Pepcid® and Nexium® can provide relief from the symptoms of this disorder.

Heartburn is also called **gastroesophageal reflux disease (GERD).** It occurs when stomach acids are pushed into the esophagus.

- **Causes.** Alcohol, some foods, a defective cardiac sphincter, pregnancy, obesity, a hiatal hernia, and repeated vomiting can contribute to the development of this disease.
- **Signs and symptoms.** Common symptoms include frequent burping, difficulty swallowing, a sore throat, a burning sensation in the chest following meals and when lying down, nausea, and blood in the vomit.
- **Treatment.** Treatment includes weight loss, making dietary changes, reducing the consumption of alcohol, taking medications such as Pepcid® and Nexium®, and elevating the head, neck, and chest when lying down.

Hemorrhoids are varicose veins of the rectum or anus.

- **Causes.** Hemorrhoids are caused by constipation, excessive straining during bowel movements, liver disease, pregnancy, and obesity.
- **Signs and symptoms.** Signs and symptoms include itching in the anal area, painful bowel movements, bright red blood on feces, and veins that protrude from the anus.
- **Treatment.** Constipation can be avoided or improved by eating a high-fiber diet. Other treatments include stool softeners, medications to reduce the inflammation of hemorrhoids, and the surgical removal of hemorrhoids (hemorrhoidectomy).

Hepatitis is defined as inflammation of the liver. There are many different types of hepatitis.

- **Causes.** Causes include bacteria, viruses, parasites, immune disorders, the use of alcohol and drugs, and an overdose of acetaminophen. Preventive measures include getting hepatitis B (HBV) vaccinations, practicing safer sex, avoiding undercooked food (especially seafood), and using prescription or over-the-counter drugs (especially those containing acetaminophen) at their recommended dosages or as prescribed by a physician.
- **Signs and symptoms.** Symptoms include mild fever, bloating, lack of appetite, nausea, vomiting, abdominal pain, weakness, jaundice, the itching of various body parts, an enlarged liver, dark urine, and breast development in males.
- **Treatment.** Patients should avoid using alcohol and drugs. Various medications may be prescribed.

A *hiatal hernia* occurs when a portion of the stomach protrudes into the chest through an opening in the diaphragm.

- **Causes.** The causes are mostly unknown, although obesity and smoking are considered risk factors. Eating small meals can be an effective preventive measure.
- **Signs and symptoms.** Signs and symptoms include excessive burping, difficulty swallowing, chest pain, and heartburn.
- **Treatment.** Treatments are weight reduction, medications to reduce the production of stomach acid, and surgical repair of the hernia.

Inguinal hernias occur when a portion of the large intestine protrudes into the inguinal canal, which is located where the thigh and the body trunk meet. In males, the hernia can also protrude into the scrotum.

- **Causes.** The causes are mostly unknown, although these hernias may be caused by weak muscles in the abdominal walls.
- **Signs and symptoms.** A lump in the groin or scrotum, or pain in the groin area that gets worse when bending or straining are the common symptoms.
- **Treatment.** Pain medications may be prescribed. Surgery to repair the hernia is needed where the large intestine is pushed back into the abdominal cavity.

Oral cancer usually involves the lips or tongue but can occur anywhere in the mouth. This type of cancer tends to spread rapidly to other organs.

- **Causes.** The causes are mostly unknown, although the use of tobacco products and alcohol are known risk factors. Poor oral hygiene and ulcers in the mouth can also cause oral cancer.
- **Signs and symptoms.** Signs and symptoms include difficulty tasting, problems swallowing, and ulcers on the tongue, lip, or other mouth structures. Leukoplakia or hardened white patches in the mucus membrane of the mouth are considered precancerous lesions. They should be examined by a health-care professional and biopsied if suspicious.
- **Treatment.** Radiation therapy, chemotherapy, and surgical removal of the malignant area are the treatment options.

Pancreatic cancer is the fourth leading cause of cancer death in the United States.

- **Causes.** Causes are mostly unknown, although smoking and alcohol consumption are considered risk factors.
- **Signs and symptoms.** Common signs and symptoms include depression, fatigue, lack of appetite, nausea or vomiting, abdominal pain, constipation or diarrhea, jaundice, and unintended weight loss.
- **Treatment.** Treatment includes radiation therapy, chemotherapy, and surgical removal of the tumor.

continued ⟶

Common Diseases and Disorders of the Digestive System *(concluded)*

Stomach cancer most commonly occurs in the uppermost or cardiac portion of the stomach. It appears to occur more frequently in Japan, Chile, and Iceland than in the United States.

- **Causes.** The causes are mostly unknown, although stomach ulcers may contribute to the development of stomach cancer.
- **Signs and symptoms.** Signs and symptoms include frequent bloating, lack of appetite, feeling full after eating small amounts, nausea, vomiting (with or without blood), abdominal cramps, excessive gas, and blood in the feces.
- **Treatment.** Treatment includes radiation therapy, chemotherapy, and surgical removal of the tumor.

Stomach ulcers occur when the lining of the stomach breaks down.

- **Causes.** Stomach ulcers can be caused by bacteria (particularly *Helicobacter pylori*), smoking, alcohol, excessive aspirin use, and hypersecretion of stomach acid. They may be prevented by stopping smoking and avoiding aspirin, certain foods, and alcohol.
- **Signs and symptoms.** Symptoms include nausea, abdominal pain, vomiting (with or without blood), and weight loss. Diagnosis can be confirmed by an upper endoscopy.
- **Treatment.** Treatment options include antibiotics, medications to reduce stomach acid production, surgery to remove the affected portion of the stomach (partial gastrectomy), and a vagotomy (cutting the vagus nerve) in order to reduce the production of stomach acid.

Summary

The purpose of the digestive system is to provide nutrients to the body. This is accomplished by taking in food, mechanically and chemically breaking it down, and absorbing the digested molecules. The organs of the alimentary canal primarily responsible for this process are the mouth, teeth, salivary glands, pharynx, esophagus, stomach, small intestine, and large intestine. The accessory organs that assist in this process are the pancreas, liver, and gallbladder. An additional function of this system is to eliminate the waste products of digestion. A healthy digestive system is important for the health of all other body systems. Understanding this system is essential when assisting with procedures such as endoscopic exams and when teaching a patient about diet and nutrition.

CASE STUDY QUESTIONS

Now that you have completed this chapter, review the case study at the beginning of the chapter and answer the following questions:

1. What is the function of the gallbladder?
2. How does the gallbladder empty bile into the small intestine?
3. What conditions can result if gallstones are not removed?
4. Will this patient need to change her diet once her gallbladder is removed?

Discussion Questions

1. List the path of the alimentary canal, beginning with the mouth and ending with the anus. Don't forget to include the sphincters and the individual parts of organs where applicable.
2. What substances are normally digested in the small intestine? What substances are normally absorbed through the wall of the small intestine?
3. Explain the difference between mechanical and chemical digestion and where each process begins.

Critical Thinking Questions

1. Describe how the digestive system processes a piece of pepperoni pizza so the body can use it.
2. What complications might a person encounter after the removal of his gallbladder?
3. a. List the names and locations for each of the three sets of tonsils.
   b. What is the purpose of the tonsils?
   c. Why do you believe physicians are in less of a hurry to remove tonsils than they were in the past?

Application Activities

1. Give the locations of each of the following digestive organs:
   a. Salivary glands
   b. Gallbladder
   c. Pharynx
   d. Esophagus
   e. Small intestine
   f. Large intestine
   g. Pancreas
2. Give the functions of the following enzymes or chemicals:
   a. Amylase
   b. Lipase
   c. Lactase
   d. Pepsin
   e. Hydrochloric acid
3. List the four types of teeth in the mouth, giving the purpose and location for each type.

Virtual Fieldtrip

Visit the McGraw-Hill Higher Education Medical Assisting website at www.mhhe.com/medicalassisting3 to complete the following activity:

Access the USDA website. You will find the most recent food pyramid from the U.S government. The front page includes an area where visitors are encouraged to answer three questions: age, gender, and activity level. Complete this questionnaire using your own information. Compare results with your classmates.

Based on the information given to you on this website, create a day's diet based on your individual information that is workable and realistic for you.

 Open the CD and complete this chapter's practice activities, play the games, listen to the key terms, and test yourself with the interactive review. E-mail, print, and/or save your results to document your proficiency.

CHAPTER 12

The Endocrine System

KEY TERMS

acromegaly

Addison's disease

adrenocorticotropic hormone (ACTH)

antidiuretic hormone (ADH)

atrial natriuretic peptide

calcitonin

cortisol

Cushing's disease

diabetes insipidus

diabetes mellitus

dwarfism

epinephrine

exophthalmos

feedback loop

gigantism

glucagon

goiter

gonads

G-protein

Graves' disease

growth hormone (GH)

hormone

insulin

islets of Langerhans

melanocyte-stimulating hormone (MSH)

melatonin

myxedema

nonsteroidal hormone

optic chiasm

parathyroid glands

pineal body

CHAPTER OUTLINE

- Hormones
- Negative and Positive Feedback Loops
- The Hypothalamus
- The Pituitary Gland
- The Thyroid Gland and Parathyroid Glands
- The Adrenal Glands
- The Pancreas
- Other Hormone-Producing Organs
- The Stress Response

LEARNING OUTCOMES

After completing Chapter 12, you will be able to:

12.1 Define the term endocrine glands.

12.2 Describe the general functions of the endocrine system.

12.3 Define the term hormone.

12.4 Explain the difference in hormone control by positive and negative feedback loops.

12.5 Describe the locations of the hypothalamus, pituitary gland, pineal body, thyroid gland, parathyroid glands, adrenal glands, pancreas, thymus, and gonads.

12.6 List the hormones released by the pituitary gland and give the functions of each.

12.7 List the hormones released by the thyroid gland and parathyroid glands and give the functions of each.

12.8 List the hormones released by the adrenal glands and give the functions of each.

12.9 List the names of the endocrine cells of the pancreas, the hormones released by them, and the function of each hormone.

12.10 List the hormones released by the pineal body, thymus, and gonads, and give the function of each.

12.11 Name the hormones produced by the kidneys and heart, listing which organ produces the hormone and the hormone's function.

12.12 Describe stressors and their effect on the body.

12.13 Describe the causes, signs and symptoms, and treatments of various endocrine disorders.

KEY TERMS (Concluded)

prolactin (PRL)	thymosin	thyroid-stimulating hormone (TSH)
steroidal hormone	thymus gland	
stressor	thyroid hormone	

Introduction

The endocrine (*endo,* meaning *within,* and *crine,* meaning *to secrete*) system includes the organs of the body that secrete hormones directly into body fluids such as blood. Hormones help to regulate the chemical reactions within cells. They therefore control the functions of the organs, tissues, and other cells that comprise these cells. In this chapter you will learn about the processes and organs of the endocrine system. See Figure 12-1 for an illustration of the organs of the endocrine system, as well as the heart and kidney, both of which secrete a hormone, although hormone secretion is not the primary function of either of them.

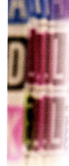

CASE STUDY

A 45-year-old woman comes to the office today complaining of feeling "odd." Among her symptoms are weight loss for no apparent reason, "jitteriness" with a feeling like her heart is racing, and overall irritability. You notice that the patient's eyes appear more prominent than normal.

As you read this chapter, consider the following questions:

1. What gland is likely to be causing this woman's problems?
2. Where is this gland located?
3. What is the patient's likely diagnosis?
4. What treatment options are available?

Hormones

Endocrine glands are ductless glands. This means that they release their hormones directly into the tissues where they act or to the bloodstream where they are carried to their target cells. As you study each gland discussed within this chapter, refer to Figure 12-1 for the location of each gland. **Hormones** can be defined as chemicals secreted by a cell that affect the functions of other cells. Once released, most hormones enter the bloodstream where they are carried to their target cells. The target cells of a hormone are the cells that contain the receptors for the hormone. A hormone cannot affect a cell unless the cell has receptors for it, in much the same way that a locked door needs the key specifically cut to open its lock. Table 12-1 outlines the endocrine glands, the hormone(s) secreted by each, and the action resulting from each hormone.

Many hormones in the body are derived from steroids. Steroids are soluble in lipids and can therefore cross cell membranes very easily. Once a **steroidal hormone** is inside a cell, it binds to its receptor, which is commonly in the nucleus of the cell. The hormone-receptor complex turns a gene on or off. When new genes are turned on or off, the cell begins to carry out new functions, and this is ultimately how steroidal hormones affect their target cells. Examples of steroidal hormones are estrogen, progesterone, testosterone, and **cortisol.**

Nonsteroidal hormones are those that are made of amino acids or proteins. Proteins cannot cross the cell membrane easily. Therefore, these hormones bind to receptors on the surface of the cell. The hormone-receptor complex in the membrane usually activates a **G-protein.**

The G-protein causes enzymes inside the cell to be turned on. Different chemical reactions then begin inside the cell. The cell now takes on new functions.

Prostaglandins are local hormones, also known as tissue hormones. They are derived from lipid molecules and typically do not travel in the bloodstream to find their target cells. Instead, their target cells are located close by. They have the same effects as other hormones and are produced by many body organs, including the kidneys, stomach, uterus, heart, and brain.

Negative and Positive Feedback Loops

Hormone levels are controlled by a mechanism known as a **feedback loop,** which can be either negative or positive (Figure 12-2). In a negative feedback loop, a stimulus such as eating raises blood sugar levels. This increase is detected by the beta cells of the islets of Langerhans in the pancreas and the cells secrete the hormone insulin in response. As cells of the liver take up glucose to store it as glycogen and the body cells take up glucose for energy, the blood glucose levels decline and the insulin release stops as blood glucose levels normalize. In a positive feedback loop, a stimulus also begins the process, as when a nursing infant suckles at the mother's breast. The suckling sends an impulse to the hypothalamus, which in turn signals the posterior pituitary to release oxytocin. The oxytocin stimulates milk production and ejection from the mammary glands. Milk continues to be released as long as the infant continues to nurse.

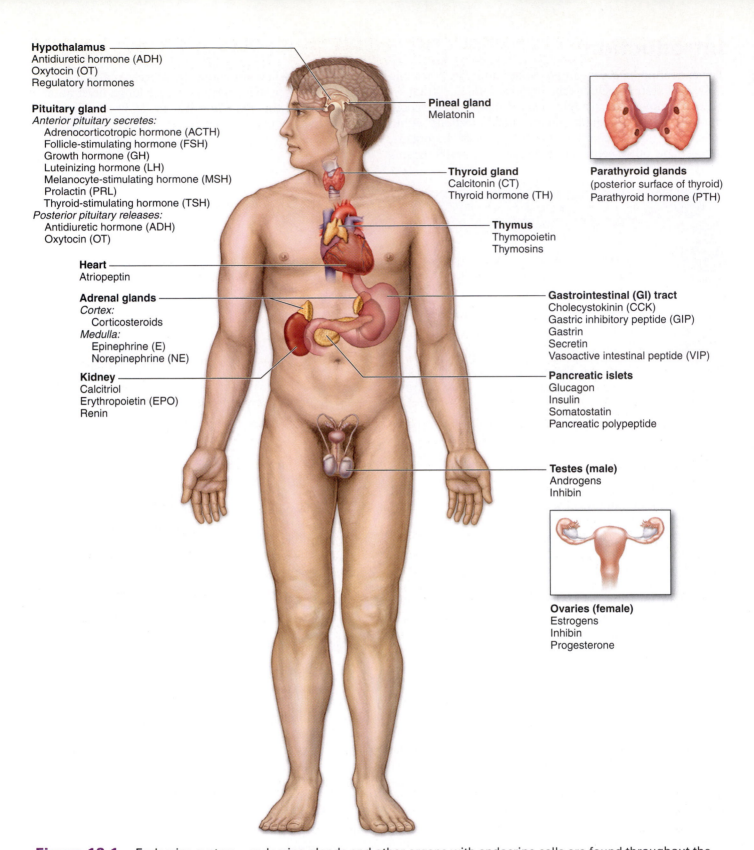

Hypothalamus
Antidiuretic hormone (ADH)
Oxytocin (OT)
Regulatory hormones

Pituitary gland
Anterior pituitary secretes:
    Adrenocorticotropic hormone (ACTH)
    Follicle-stimulating hormone (FSH)
    Growth hormone (GH)
    Luteinizing hormone (LH)
    Melanocyte-stimulating hormone (MSH)
    Prolactin (PRL)
    Thyroid-stimulating hormone (TSH)
Posterior pituitary releases:
    Antidiuretic hormone (ADH)
    Oxytocin (OT)

Heart
Atriopeptin

Adrenal glands
Cortex:
    Corticosteroids
Medulla:
    Epinephrine (E)
    Norepinephrine (NE)

Kidney
Calcitriol
Erythropoietin (EPO)
Renin

Pineal gland
Melatonin

Thyroid gland
Calcitonin (CT)
Thyroid hormone (TH)

Thymus
Thymopoietin
Thymosins

Gastrointestinal (GI) tract
Cholecystokinin (CCK)
Gastric inhibitory peptide (GIP)
Gastrin
Secretin
Vasoactive intestinal peptide (VIP)

Pancreatic islets
Glucagon
Insulin
Somatostatin
Pancreatic polypeptide

Testes (male)
Androgens
Inhibin

Parathyroid glands
(posterior surface of thyroid)
Parathyroid hormone (PTH)

Ovaries (female)
Estrogens
Inhibin
Progesterone

Figure 12-1. Endocrine system—endocrine glands and other organs with endocrine cells are found throughout the body. They produce various types of hormones.

TABLE 12-1   Endocrine Glands: Their Hormones and Actions

Gland	Hormone	Action Produced
Hypothalamus (produces)	Antidiuretic hormone (ADH)	Stored and released by posterior pituitary
	Oxytocin (OT)	Stored and released by posterior pituitary
Anterior pituitary	Growth hormone (GH)	Promotes growth and tissue maintenance
	Melanocyte stimulating hormone (MSH)	Stimulates pigment regulation in epidermis
	Adrenocorticotropic hormone (ACTH)	Stimulates adrenal cortex to produce its hormones
	Thyroid stimulating hormone (TSH)	Stimulates the thyroid to produce its hormones
	Follicle stimulating hormone (FSH)	(F) Stimulates ovaries to produce ova and estrogen (M) Stimulates testes to produce sperm and testosterone
	Luteinizing hormone (LH)	(F) Stimulates ovaries for ovulation and estrogen production (M) Stimulates testes to produce testosterone
	Prolactin (PRL)	(F) Stimulates breasts to produce milk (M) Works with and complements LH
Posterior pituitary (releases)	Antidiuretic hormone (ADH)	Stimulates kidneys to retain water
	Oxytocin (OT)	Stimulates uterine contractions for labor and delivery
Pineal body	Melatonin	Regulates biological clock; linked to onset of puberty
Thyroid	T3 and T4	Protein synthesis and increased energy production for all cells
	Calcitonin	Increases bone calcium and decreases blood calcium
Parathyroid	Parathyroid hormone (PTH)	Agonist to Calcitonin; decreases bone calcium/increases blood calcium
Thymus	Thymosin & Thymopoietin	Both hormones stimuate the production of T lymphocytes
Adrenal cortex	Aldosterone	Stimulates body to retain sodium and water
	Cortisol	Decreases protein synthesis; decreases inflammation
Adrenal medulla	Epinephrine & Norepinephrine	Prepares body for stress; increases heart rate, respiration, and BP
Pancreas (islets of Langerhans)	Alpha cells—Glucagon	Increases blood sugar; decreases protein synthesis
	Beta cells—Insulin	Decreases blood sugar; increases protein synthesis
Gonads: Ovaries (female)	Estrogen and Progesterone	Secondary sex characteristics; female reproductive hormone
Testes (male)	Testosterone	Secondary sex characteristics; male reproductive hormone

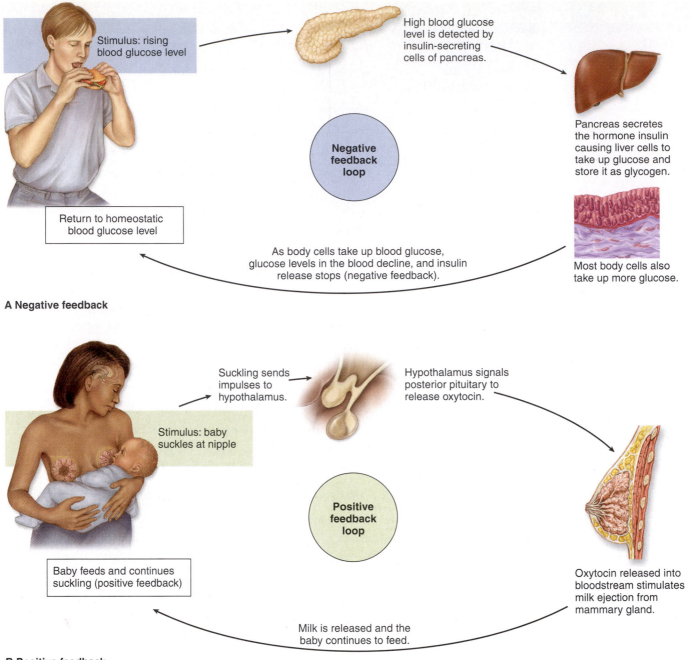

Stimulus: rising blood glucose level

High blood glucose level is detected by insulin-secreting cells of pancreas.

Negative feedback loop

Pancreas secretes the hormone insulin causing liver cells to take up glucose and store it as glycogen.

Return to homeostatic blood glucose level

As body cells take up blood glucose, glucose levels in the blood decline, and insulin release stops (negative feedback).

Most body cells also take up more glucose.

A Negative feedback

Suckling sends impulses to hypothalamus.

Hypothalamus signals posterior pituitary to release oxytocin.

Stimulus: baby suckles at nipple

Positive feedback loop

Baby feeds and continues suckling (positive feedback)

Oxytocin released into bloodstream stimulates milk ejection from mammary gland.

Milk is released and the baby continues to feed.

B Positive feedback

Figure 12-2. Positive and negative feedback loops in the endocrine system—the initial step in any feedback pathway is the stimulus. (A) A negative feedback loop occurs when the end product of a pathway acts to turn off or slow down the pathway, whereas (B) a positive feedback loop is involved when the end product of a pathway stimulates further pathway activity.

The Hypothalamus

The hypothalamus is located in the diencephalon of the brain (Chapter 7) and produces the hormones oxytocin and antidiuretic hormone (ADH). These hormones are transported to the posterior pituitary, where they are stored and released as directed by the hypothalamus.

The Pituitary Gland

The pituitary gland, also known as the hypophysis, is located at the base of the brain and is controlled by the hypothalamus. This gland is well protected by a bony structure called the sella turcica. Just superior to the gland is the **optic chiasm,** which carries visual information to

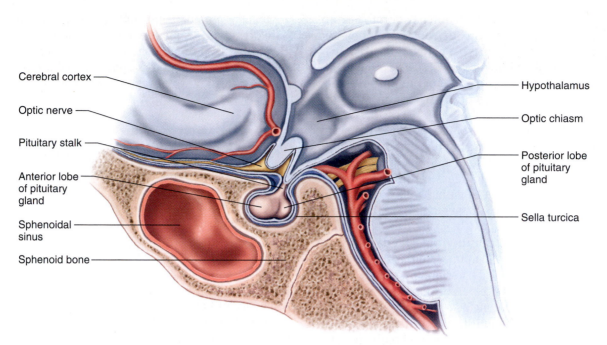

Figure 12-3. Location of the pituitary gland.

the brain for interpretation. The pituitary is divided into two lobes—the anterior and the posterior (see Figures 12-1 and 12-3).

The Anterior Lobe of the Pituitary Gland

The anterior lobe of the pituitary gland, also known as the adenohypophysis, secretes the following hormones:

- **Growth hormone (GH).** As its name suggests, this hormone stimulates an increase in the size of the muscles and bones in the body. It is very important in childhood for growth. It also stimulates the repair of tissues. Growth hormone is also known by the name somatotropin.
- **Melanocyte-stimulating hormone (MSH).** This hormone stimulates synthesis of melanin and its disbursement to the skin cells of the epidermis.
- **Adrenocorticotropic hormone (ACTH).** This hormone stimulates the adrenal cortex to release its hormones.
- **Thyroid-stimulating hormone (TSH).** This hormone stimulates the thyroid gland to release its hormones.
- Follicle-stimulating hormone (FSH). In females, this hormone stimulates the production of estrogen by the ovaries. More significantly, FSH stimulates maturation of the ova (eggs) before ovulation. In males, it stimulates sperm production.
- Luteinizing hormone (LH). In females, this hormone stimulates ovulation (the release of an egg from the

ovaries) and the production of estrogen. In males, it stimulates the production of testosterone.
- **Prolactin (PRL).** In females, this hormone stimulates milk production by the mammary glands. Because of this function, it is sometimes called the lactogenic hormone. In males, prolactin is known to enhance the functioning of LH.

The Posterior Lobe of the Pituitary Gland

The posterior lobe of the pituitary gland, also known as the neurohypophysis, secretes the following hormones:

- **Antidiuretic hormone (ADH).** This hormone stimulates the kidneys to conserve water. It therefore decreases urine output and helps to maintain blood pressure.
- Oxytocin (OT). In females, this hormone causes contractions of the uterus during childbirth. It also causes the ejection of milk from mammary glands during breast-feeding. In males, oxytocin stimulates the contraction of the prostate and vas deferens during sexual arousal.

The Thyroid Gland and Parathyroid Glands

The thyroid gland consists of two lobes and sits below the voice box or larynx. It is covered by a capsule and is divided into follicles. The follicles store some of the hormones produced by the thyroid gland. Two major hormones produced by the thyroid gland are **thyroid hormones** and **calcitonin.** There are two main types of thyroid hormones—triiodothyronine (T_3) and thyronxine (T_4). The T stands for thyroid, and the numeral refers to the number of iodine atoms that are needed for each of these hormones to work properly.

Thyroid hormones increase energy production by cells, stimulate protein synthesis, and speed up the repair of damaged tissues. In children, they are important for normal growth and the development of the nervous system. Calcitonin lowers blood calcium levels by activating osteoblasts. Osteoblasts use excess blood calcium to build new bone tissue.

Most people have four **parathyroid glands.** They are small glands that are embedded into the posterior surface of the thyroid gland. The only hormone secreted by the parathyroid glands is called parathormone or parathyroid hormone (PTH). This hormone acts as an agonist to calcitonin by raising blood calcium levels through the activation of osteoclasts. Osteoclasts are bone-dissolving cells. When they dissolve bone, calcium levels in bone decrease as calcium is released into the bloodstream. This action raises blood calcium levels.

The Adrenal Glands

An adrenal gland sits on top of each kidney. It is divided into two portions—the adrenal medulla and the adrenal cortex. The adrenal medulla is the central portion of the gland and secretes **epinephrine** and norepinephrine. These hormones produce the same effects that the sympathetic nervous system produces. They increase heart rate, breathing rate, blood pressure, and all the other actions that prepare the body for stressful situations.

The adrenal cortex is the outermost portion of the adrenal gland. It secretes many hormones but the two major ones are aldosterone and cortisol. Aldosterone stimulates the body to retain sodium, which helps it to retain water. It is important for maintaining blood pressure. Cortisol is released when a person is stressed. It decreases protein synthesis, so it slows down the repair of tissues. Its advantage is that is also decreases inflammation, which decreases pain.

The Pancreas

The pancreas is located behind the stomach. It is an endocrine gland as well as an exocrine gland. It is considered an exocrine gland because it secretes digestive enzymes into a duct that leads to the small intestine. It is considered an endocrine gland because it contains structures known as **islets of Langerhans** that secrete hormones into the bloodstream. The islets of Langerhans consist of two types of cells: alpha cells, which secrete **glucagon,** and beta cells, which secrete **insulin.**

Insulin promotes the uptake of glucose by cells. It therefore reduces glucose concentrations in the bloodstream. It also promotes the transport of amino acids into cells and increases protein synthesis. Glucagon increases glucose concentrations in the bloodstream and slows down protein synthesis.

Other Hormone-Producing Organs

The **pineal body** is a small gland located between the cerebral hemispheres. It secretes a hormone called **melatonin.** Melatonin helps to regulate your circadian rhythms, which are more commonly known as your biological clock. Your biological clock helps you decide when you should be awake or asleep. Melatonin is also thought to play a role in the onset of puberty.

The **thymus gland** lies between the lungs. It secretes a hormone called **thymosin.** Thymosin promotes the production of certain lymphocytes known as T lymphocytes. Refer to Chapter 10 for further information on thymosin and the function of T cells.

Sometimes referred to as the **gonads,** the ovaries and testes are reproductive organs that secrete hormones. The ovaries release estrogen and progesterone, and the testes produce testosterone. The functions of these hormones are provided in Chapter 9.

The stomach and small intestines also secrete hormones. The stomach produces gastrin, and the small intestine releases secretin and cholecystokinin. These hormones are discussed in Chapter 11.

The heart secretes a hormone called **atrial natriuretic peptide,** which regulates blood pressure. The kidneys secrete a hormone called erythropoietin, which stimulates blood cell production.

The Stress Response

Any stimulus that produces stress is termed a **stressor.** Stressors include physical factors such as extreme heat or cold, infections, injuries, heavy exercise, and loud sounds. Stressors can also include psychological factors such as personal loss, grief, anxiety, depression, and guilt. Even positive stimuli such as sexual arousal, joy, and happiness can be stressors.

The body's physiologic response to stress consists of a group of reactions called the general stress syndrome, which is primarily caused by the release of hormones. This syndrome results in an increase in the heart rate, breathing rate, and blood pressure. Glucose and fatty acid concentrations also increase in the blood, which leads to weight loss. Prolonged stress causes the release of cortisol. Cortisol slows down body repair because it prevents protein synthesis and inhibits immune responses, which is why a person under stress becomes more susceptible to being sick.

Pathophysiology

Common Diseases and Disorders of the Endocrine System

TABLE 12-2	Endocrine System Diseases/Conditions: Quick Reference Guide	
Hormone	**Hypo or Hyper Secretion**	**Disease or Condition**
GH (Somatotropin)	Hyposecretion (children)	Dwarfism
	Hypersecretion (children)	Gigantism
	Hypersecretion (adults)	Acromegaly
ACTH	Hyposecretion (adrenal cortex—cortisol)	Addison's disease
	Hypersecretion (adrenal cortex—cortisol)	Cushing's syndrome
ADH	Hyposecretion	Diabetes insipidus (dehydration)
	Hypersecretion	Edema, hypertension
T3/T4	Hyposecretion (congenital/children) Hyposecretion (adults)—*severe cases* Hypersecretion (adults or children)	Cretinism Hypothyoidism and *Myxedema* Graves' disease (hyperthyroidism)
Glucagon	Hyposecretion Hypersecretion	Hypoglycemia Hyperglycemia
Insulin	Hyposecretion Hypersecretion	Hyperglycemia (Diabetes mellitus) Hypoglycemia (hyperinsulinism)

Refer to Table 12-2, which provides a quick reference to diseases and disorders of the endocrine system. The table lists hormones according to the hyposecretion or hypersecretion of individual hormones. They are listed in "head-to-toe" order by the organ from which the hormone comes.

Acromegaly is a disorder in which too much growth hormone is produced in adults (Figure 12-4).

- **Causes.** This disorder is caused by an increased production of growth hormone or by a tumor of the pituitary gland.
- **Signs and symptoms.** The primary signs and symptoms include enlargement of the bones in the entire skull as well as in the hands and feet, and thickening of the skin. Other symptoms include headache, fatigue, profuse sweating, pain (especially in the arms and legs), gaps between the teeth, weight gain, excessive hair production, cardiovascular diseases, arthritis, and vision problems.
- **Treatment.** Treatment includes medications to lower the production of growth hormone, radiation therapy to reduce the size of a pituitary tumor, or surgery to remove a pituitary tumor.

Addison's disease is a condition in which the adrenal glands fail to produce enough corticosteroids. It affects about 1 in every 25,000 people (Figure 12-5).

- **Causes.** The cause of this disease is most often unknown. It may be caused by an autoimmune dysfunction. It can be caused by cancer and other serious diseases that damage the adrenal glands.
- **Signs and symptoms.** The signs and symptoms may begin long before a diagnosis is made. They include weakness, fatigue, and dizziness after rising from a sitting or reclining position. Other symptoms include weight loss, muscle pain, lack of appetite, nausea, vomiting, diarrhea, and dehydration.
- **Treatment.** Because this disease can be life-threatening, the first treatment is to administer corticosteroids. Medications or other hormones may be prescribed to help balance the levels of sodium and potassium.

Cretinism is an extreme form of hypothyroidism present prior to or soon after birth (Figure 12-6).

- **Causes.** The cause is hypothyroidism at birth related to absence or malformation of the thyroid gland, abnormal formation of thyroid hormones, or pituitary failure that results in a lack of thyroid stimulation.
- **Signs and symptoms.** Stunted growth, abnormal bone formation, mental retardation, low body temperature, and overall sluggishness are the primary signs and symptoms.

continued ⟶

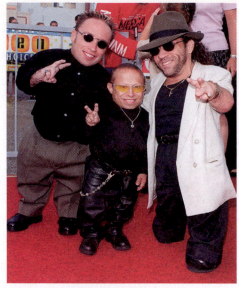

A Pituitary dwarfism

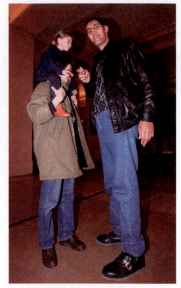

B Gigantism

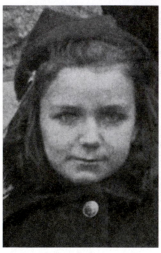

Age 9

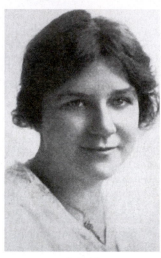

Age 16

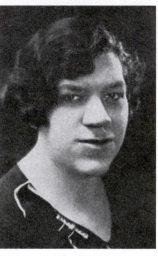

Age 33

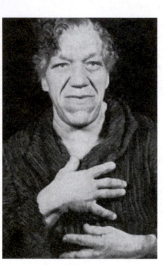

Age 52

C Acromegaly

Figure 12-4. (A) Pituitary dwarfism is caused by hyposecretion of GH. (B) Gigantism results from hypersecretion of GH. (C) Acromegaly is caused by secretion of excessive growth hormone (GH) in adulthood. The face and hands are most notably affected, as seen in an individual with acromegaly at ages 9, 16, 33, and 52.

- **Treatment.** The treatment is thyroid hormone replacement.

Cushing's disease is also known as hypercortisolism. In this condition, a person produces too much cortisol (see Figure 12-5).

- **Causes.** This disease is caused by an excessive production of ACTH (a hormone that increases the production of cortisol), a tumor of the adrenal gland (the source of cortisol), a tumor of the pituitary gland (the source of ACTH), or the long-term use of steroidal hormones.

- **Signs and symptoms.** Common symptoms include a round or full face ("moon face"), a hump of fat between the shoulders ("buffalo hump"), thin arms and legs with a large abdomen, fatigue, thin skin, acne, frequent thirst, frequent urination, mental disabilities, a loss of menstrual cycle in females, high blood pressure, high glucose blood levels, and body aches in the muscles, back, or head.

- **Treatment.** The first treatment is lifestyle changes, especially stopping the use of steroidal hormones. Radiation therapy or surgery may be needed to treat any tumors.

continued ⟶

Common Diseases and Disorders of the Endocrine System *(continued)*

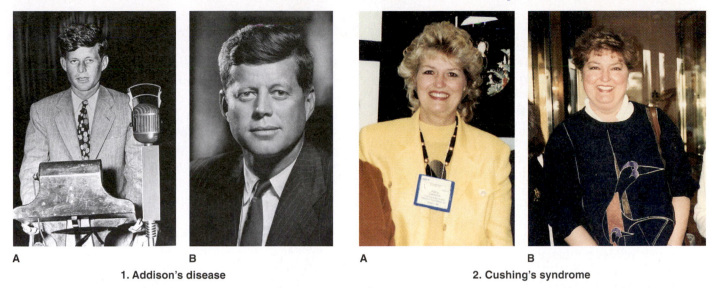

A   B
1. Addison's disease

A   B
2. Cushing's syndrome

Figure 12-5. 1. Addison's disease: (A) John F. Kennedy prior to being treated for Addison's disease. (B) In 1960, facial swelling was one of the effects of cortisone treatment for Kennedy's Addison's disease. 2. Cushing's syndrome: (A) Photo prior to the onset of Cushing's syndrome. (B) Symptoms resulting from the excessive glucocorticoid secretion in Cushing's syndrome include "buffalo hump" and "moon face."

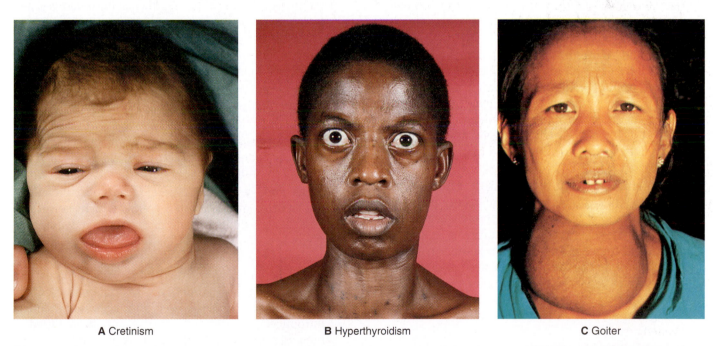

A Cretinism   **B** Hyperthyroidism   **C** Goiter

Figure 12-6. (A) Cretinism is the result of an underactive thyroid gland during infancy and childhood. (B) Hyperthyroidism with protruding eyes. (C) An iodine deficiency causes simple (endemic) goiter and results in high levels of TSH.

Diabetes insipidus is a condition where the kidneys fail to reabsorb water, causing excessive urination.

- **Causes.** The primary cause is the hyposecretion of ADH.
- **Signs and symptoms.** These include excessive thirst, even with a more-than-adequate fluid intake. Other signs and symptoms include excessive urination and, in severe cases, muscle cramps and cardiac arrhythmias

related to electrolyte imbalances caused by the excessive fluid loss.

- **Treatment.** The primary treatment is increased fluid intake. Other treatments include surgery for any tumor of the pituitary that may cause the inadequate secretion of ADH. Changes in diet and medication help increase water retention.

continued ⟶

Common Diseases and Disorders of the Endocrine System *(continued)*

Diabetes mellitus is a chronic disease that is characterized by high glucose levels in the blood. There are at least three different types of diabetes mellitus. Type 1 is referred to as early onset diabetes or insulin-dependent diabetes mellitus, and usually develops during childhood. Type 2 is the most common type and is often called late-onset diabetes or noninsulin-dependent diabetes mellitus because, historically, it is primarily diagnosed in adults. Of concern in recent years is a national surge in the number of adolescents and teens being diagnosed with type 2 diabetes. This is being directly linked to a lack of exercise and excessive weight gain in this age group. Gestational diabetes occurs only in pregnant women and is usually temporary, although a history of gestational diabetes has been found to put the patient at higher risk of developing type 2 diabetes later in life. Women with gestational diabetes should be monitored closely for type 2 diabetes. African Americans, Hispanics, and Native Americans are more likely to develop diabetes than any other ethnic groups.

- **Causes.** This disease is caused by the production of too little or no insulin by the pancreas. Other causes include body cells having too few insulin receptors, obesity, high blood pressure, pregnancy, and high cholesterol levels in the blood.
- **Signs and symptoms.** There are many signs and symptoms of this disease. They include high levels of glucose in the blood, excessive thirst, frequent urination, fatigue, increased appetite, unexplained weight loss, blurry vision, impotence in men, nausea, skin wounds that heal slowly, high glucose and ketone levels in the urine, and lower extremity problems (due to poor circulation).
- **Treatment.** Treatment includes daily injections of insulin, oral medications to increase insulin production, oral medications to increase the body's sensitivity to insulin, frequent monitoring of glucose levels in the blood, and frequent monitoring of ketone levels in the urine. Lifestyle changes are important and should include reducing weight (especially if obese), changing eating habits, and getting regular exercise. Lifestyle changes to prevent injury to legs and feet may also be needed.
- **Complications.** Left untreated, diabetes can result in long-term and life-threatening complications. Blood vessels become thickened, which can damage vital organs including the kidneys, eyes, heart, and brain. Long-term damage can result in kidney disease, blindness, and atherosclerosis (the buildup of fatty deposits in blood vessels). Circulation worsens, which not only affects organs but may result in slower overall healing and ulcers that develop in the lower extremities,

particularly the feet. Because of the body's decreased ability to heal, these ulcers may require the amputation of the affected foot and possibly part of the leg (below-knee amputation or BKA).

Dwarfism is a condition in which too little growth hormone (somatotropin) is produced in childhood (see Figure 12-4).

- **Causes.** This condition can be caused by an underproduction of the growth hormone during childhood, trauma to the pituitary gland, or a pituitary tumor.
- **Signs and symptoms.** Symptoms include short height, abnormal facial features, cleft lip or palate, delayed puberty, headaches, frequent urination, and excessive thirst.
- **Treatment.** Treatment is the administration of supplemental growth hormone.

Gigantism is a condition in which too much growth hormone is produced during childhood (see Figure 12-4).

- **Causes.** This condition is caused by overproduction of the growth hormone during childhood. It can also be caused by a tumor in the pituitary gland.
- **Signs and symptoms.** Very tall height, delayed sexual maturity, thick facial bones, thick skin, weakness, and vision problems are common symptoms.
- **Treatment.** Treatment includes medications to reduce growth hormone levels, radiation therapy, and surgery to remove the tumor.

Goiter is an enlargement of the thyroid gland causing (sometimes disfiguring) swelling of the neck (see Figure 12-6).

- **Causes.** Typically, a simple goiter is caused by deficiency of iodine in the diet. Iodine is needed for the thyroid to produce thyroid hormone.
- **Signs and symptoms.** These include overgrowth of the follicles of the thyroid gland, which causes enlargement of the gland and of the neck, and abnormal thyroid function tests (TFTs).
- **Treatment.** The most common treatment is iodine supplementation in the diet. In the United States, salt contains iodine, so goiters are seldom seen. Because a goiter may not shrink even after adequate iodine is introduced into the diet, surgery may be required to remove some or most of the enlarged gland.

Graves' disease is a disorder in which a person develops antibodies that attack the thyroid gland (see Figure 12-6). This attack causes the thyroid to produce too many thyroid hormones. Graves' disease is the most common type of hyperthyroidism in the United States.

- **Causes.** This disease is caused by an overproduction of thyroid hormones. It is also considered an autoimmune disorder.

continued ⟶

Common Diseases and Disorders of the Endocrine System *(concluded)*

- **Signs and symptoms.** The most common signs and symptoms include **exophthalmos** (protrusion of the eyes) and goiter (thyroid enlargement). Other symptoms include insomnia, unexplained weight loss, anxiety, muscle weakness, increased appetite, excessive sweating, vision problems, and an increased heart rate.

- **Treatment.** Treatment includes medications to reduce heart rate, sweating, and nervousness; radiation to destroy the thyroid gland; surgery to remove the thyroid gland (thyroidectomy); and supplemental thyroid hormones if the gland is destroyed or removed.

Myxedema is a disorder in which the thyroid gland does not produce adequate amounts of thyroid hormone. It is a severe type of hypothyroidism that is most common in females over age 50.

- **Causes.** Causes include the removal of the thyroid, radiation treatments to the neck area, and obesity. This disorder may be congenital.

- **Signs and symptoms.** Signs and symptoms include weakness, fatigue, weight gain, depression, general body aches, dry skin and hair, hair loss, puffy hands or feet, a decreased ability to taste food, abnormal menstrual periods, pale or yellow skin, a slow heart rate, low blood pressure, anemia, an enlarged heart, high cholesterol levels, or coma.

- **Treatment.** Treatment consists of giving supplemental thyroid hormones intravenously or orally and closely monitoring the levels of thyroid hormones.

Summary

The endocrine system regulates all chemical reactions in cells. The substances responsible for this regulation are known as hormones. Hormones are produced by endocrine glands. They are released directly into the affected tissues or into the bloodstream to create a response. The major endocrine glands are the hypothalamus, pituitary, pineal body, thyroid, parathyroid, thymus, adrenals, and pancreas. An understanding of this system can help medical assistants be aware of the signs and symptoms of common endocrine system disorders and to be more effective when helping patients learn about the advantages and disadvantages of hormone replacement therapy.

REVIEW

CHAPTER 12

CASE STUDY QUESTIONS

Now that you have completed this chapter, review the case study at the beginning of the chapter and answer the following questions:

1. What gland is likely to be causing this woman's problems?
2. Where is this gland located?
3. What is the patient's likely diagnosis?
4. What treatment options are available?

Discussion Questions

1. Define the term endocrine gland and describe its general function.
2. Name the major endocrine organs of the body and give their locations.
3. Explain how the body responds to stress.
4. Explain why the testes and ovaries are described as both endocrine organs and reproductive organs.

Critical Thinking Questions

1. Patients who are on hemodialysis due to end-stage renal disease are often anemic. Explain how renal disease can cause or worsen this problem.
2. List the organs and hormones that cause the unrelated diseases of diabetes mellitus and diabetes insipidus. What is at least one consequence of the progression of each of these diseases?
3. Why is hyposecretion (insufficient secretion) of thyroid hormone in newborns more serious than hyposecretion in adults?

Application Activities

1. Tell which endocrine gland secretes the following hormones:
   a. ACTH
   b. ADH
   c. Calcitonin
   d. PTH
   e. Cortisol

2. Describe the effects the following hormones produce:
   a. Oxytocin
   b. Calcitonin
   c. LH and FSH
   d. Epinephrine and norepinephrine
   e. Melatonin
3. For each of the following diseases, name the hormone that is involved:
   a. Acromegaly
   b. Myxedema
   c. Diabetes insipidus
   d. Diabetes mellitus
   e. Cushing's disease
4. Define what a stressor is and give an example.

Virtual Fieldtrip

Visit the McGraw-Hill Higher Education Medical Assisting website at www.mhhe.com/medicalassisting3 to complete the following activity:

Access the Diabetes Association homepage. Click the *All about Diabetes* tab and then choose the topic *prediabetes.*

1. On a piece of paper, define *prediabetes.*
2. Back on the home page, click the link titled *How to tell if you have prediabetes.* What patient populations are most at risk?
3. What are the two blood tests to check for prediabetes?
4. On the same page is a link for the *Diabetes Risk Test.* Click the link and take the test. How did you do?
5. Now, choose the topic that discusses the link among diabetes, heart disease, and stroke. What is the link?
6. Click the *Make the Link* area. List the ABCs of taking care of your heart.

Open the CD and complete this chapter's practice activities, play the games, listen to the key terms, and test yourself with the interactive review. E-mail, print, and/or save your results to document your proficiency.

Special Senses

CHAPTER OUTLINE

- The Nose and the Sense of Smell
- The Tongue and the Sense of Taste
- The Eye and the Sense of Sight
- The Aging Eye
- Vision Testing
- Treating Eye Problems
- The Ear and the Senses of Hearing and Equilibrium
- The Aging Ear
- Hearing Loss
- Hearing and Diagnostic Tests
- Treating Ear and Hearing Problems

LEARNING OUTCOMES

After completing Chapter 13, you will be able to:

13.1 Describe the anatomy of the nose and the function of each part.

13.2 Describe how smell sensations are created and interpreted.

13.3 Describe the anatomy of the tongue and the function of each part.

13.4 Describe how taste sensations are created and interpreted.

13.5 Name the four primary taste sensations and the acknowledged fifth taste sensation.

13.6 Describe the anatomy of the eye and the function of each part, including the accessory structures and their functions.

13.7 Trace the visual pathway through the eye and to the brain for interpretation.

KEY TERMS *(Concluded)*

lens	orbit	semicircular canals
limbus	organ of Corti	sensorineural hearing loss
macular degeneration	otologist	
malleus	otosclerosis	sensory adaptation
Meniere's disease	oval window	stapes
myopia	papillae	strabismus
nasolacrimal duct	perilymph	taste bud
nystagmus	presbyopia	tinnitus
olfactory	pupil	tympanic membrane
ophthalmologist	refraction	umami
optician	retina	vertigo
optometrist	rods	vestibule
orbicularis oculi	sclera	vitreous humor

KEY TERMS

- accommodation
- amblyopia
- aqueous humor
- astigmatism
- audiologist
- audiometer
- auricle
- bone conduction
- cataracts
- cerumen
- chemoreceptor
- choroid
- ciliary body
- cochlea
- conductive hearing loss
- cones
- conjunctiva
- conjunctivitis
- cornea
- decibels
- ectropion
- endolymph
- entropion
- eustachian tube
- external auditory canal
- extrinsic eye muscles
- frequency
- glaucoma
- gustatory receptors
- hyperopia
- incus
- iris
- labyrinth
- lacrimal apparatus
- lacrimal gland

13.8 Identify ways that patients can practice preventive eye care.

13.9 State ways that vision changes with age.

13.10 List the medical professionals involved in diagnosis and treatment of visual disorders, including the roles that each plays in patient care.

13.11 List treatments for visual disorders.

13.12 Describe the causes, signs and symptoms, and treatments of various diseases and conditions of the eye.

13.13 Describe the anatomy of the ear and the function of each part.

13.14 Explain the role of the ear in maintaining equilibrium.

13.15 Explain how sounds travel through the ear and are interpreted in the brain.

13.16 State ways that hearing changes with age.

13.17 List the types of hearing loss and how they differ.

13.18 Describe treatments for ear and hearing disorders.

13.19 Explain how patients can be educated about preventive ear care.

13.20 Describe the causes, signs and symptoms, and treatments of various disorders of the ear and hearing.

Introduction

The special senses are smell, taste, vision, hearing, and equilibrium. They are called special senses because their sensory receptors are located within relatively large sensory organs in the head—the nose, tongue, eyes, and ears. Although the skin is also considered a sense organ, in fact it is the largest sense organ, touch is not considered a special sense but a generalized one (refer to Ch. 2, The Integumentary System). As you read this chapter, keep in mind that no matter how a stimulus starts, it is sent, via the nervous system, to the brain for interpretation (and then reaction, if necessary). This chapter introduces the structure and function of the special sense organs.

As a medical assistant, it is likely that you will be asked to assist with or perform examinations and treatments for common disorders of the eyes and ears. Therefore, you will need to understand the functioning of these important sense organs.

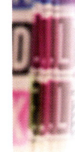

CASE STUDY

A 42-year-old man comes to the doctor's office complaining of dizziness, nausea, and a loud ringing in his left ear. He is diagnosed with Meniere's disease. The doctor explains to him that this disorder is caused by the buildup of fluid in the inner ear.

As you read this chapter, consider the following questions:

1. Why is the patient experiencing dizziness and difficulty hearing?
2. What is the clinical term for ringing in the ear?
3. What precautions should this patient take because of his dizziness?
4. A diuretic is a drug that decreases fluids in the body. Why might the doctor prescribe a diuretic?

The Nose and the Sense of Smell

Smell receptors are also called **olfactory** receptors and are **chemoreceptors.** This means that they respond to changes in chemical concentrations. Chemicals that activate smell receptors must be dissolved in the mucus of the nose. This explains why a person with either a "dry nose" or excessive mucus related to an upper respiratory tract infection or allergies, has trouble smelling.

Smell receptors are located in the olfactory organ, which is in the upper part of the nasal cavity. Humans have a relatively poor sense of smell compared to animals because chemicals must diffuse all the way up the nasal cavity in order to activate smell receptors.

Once smell receptors are activated, they send their information to the olfactory nerves. The olfactory nerves send the information along olfactory bulbs and tracts to different areas of the cerebrum. The cerebrum interprets the information as a particular type of smell (Figure 13-1). An interesting fact about our sense of smell is that it undergoes **sensory adaptation,** which means that the same chemical can stimulate smell receptors for only a limited amount of time. In a relatively short period of time, the smell receptors fatigue and no longer respond to the same (odor) chemical, and it can no longer be smelled. Sensory adaptation explains why you smell perfume when you first encounter it, but after a few minutes you cannot smell it or may be less aware of it.

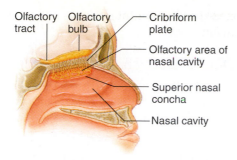

Figure 13-1. The olfactory area (organ) is located in the superior part of the nasal cavity.

The Tongue and the Sense of Taste

Taste or **gustatory receptors** are located on taste buds. **Taste buds** are found on the **papillae** (bumps) of the tongue. Taste buds are microscopic structures on the papillae and cannot be seen with the naked eye. Some taste buds are also scattered on the roof of the mouth and in the walls of the throat.

Each taste bud is made of taste cells and supporting cells. The taste cells function as taste receptors, and the supporting cells simply fill in the spaces between the taste cells. Like the olfactory cells of smell, taste cells are types of chemoreceptors because they are activated by chemicals found in food and drink that must be dissolved in saliva as part of the digestive process (Figure 13-2).

There are four types of taste cells, and each type is activated by a particular group of chemicals. Therefore, the following four primary taste sensations are produced:

1. Sweet. Taste cells that respond to "sweet" chemicals are concentrated at the tip of the tongue.
2. Sour. Taste cells that respond to "sour" chemicals are concentrated on the sides of the tongue.
3. Salty. Taste cells that respond to "salty" chemicals are concentrated on the tip and sides of the tongue.
4. Bitter. Taste cells that respond to "bitter" chemicals are concentrated at the back of the tongue.

In addition to these four well-known taste sensations, in the 1980s, science recognized a taste known as **umami.** In 1908, a Japanese scientist discovered that glutamic acid found in kelp produced a savory taste that he named umami. This unique taste is found most notably in tomatoes, and also in meats, fish, and dairy products, including mothers' breast milk. Although discovered and named in the early 1900s, it was not until the 1980s that studies found that glutamate, the substance responsible for this unique taste, created a fifth basic taste that has become universally recognized.

When taste cells are activated, they send their information to several cranial nerves. The information eventually reaches the gustatory cortex in the parietal lobe of the cerebrum. The gustatory cortex interprets the information as a particular taste. Although not an actual taste sensation, eating spicy foods activates pain receptors on the tongue that are then interpreted by the brain as "spicy."

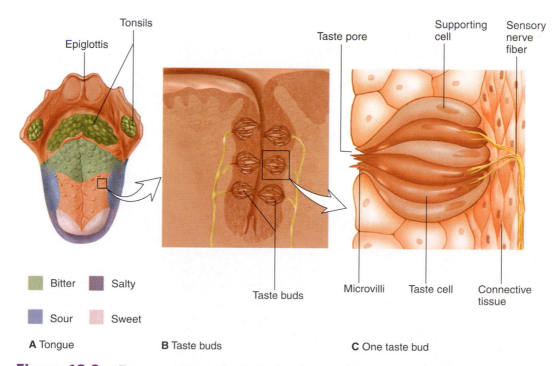

Figure 13-2. Tongue and taste buds. (A) Areas of the tongue are sensitive to different tastes, as indicated. (B) Taste buds are on and in papillae. (C) Taste buds are composed of taste cells and supporting cells.

The Eye and the Sense of Sight

The sense of sight comes from the eyes and is also supported by visual accessory organs.

Vision

A person's visual system consists of the eyes; the optic nerve, which connects the eye to the vision center of the brain; and several accessory structures. If these parts of the system are healthy and normal, the individual is able to see normally.

The Eye

The eye is a complex organ that processes light to produce images. It is made up of three main layers, two chambers, and a number of specialized parts, as shown in Figure 13-3.

The Outer Layer. The white of the eye, called the **sclera**, is the tough, outermost layer of the eye. This layer, through which light cannot pass, covers all except the

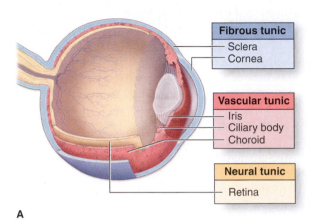

A

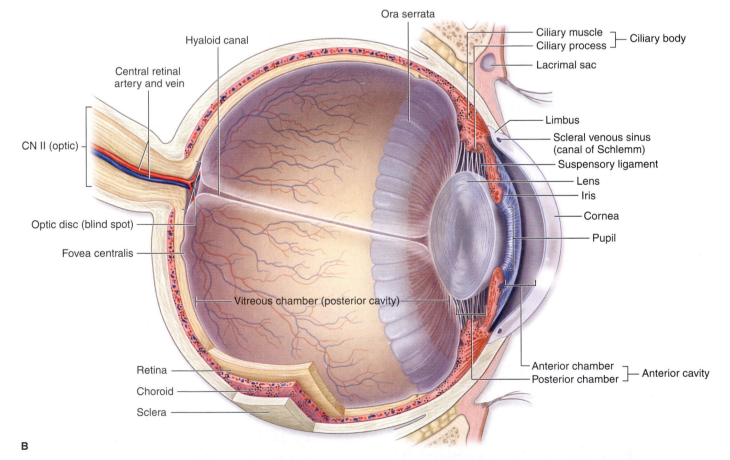

B

Figure 13-3.   Anatomy of the internal eye—sagittal views depict (A) the three tunics of the eye, and (B) internal eye structures.

front of the eye. Here the sclera gives way to the cornea in an area known as the **limbus** or corneal-scleral junction. The **cornea** is a transparent area on the front of the eye that acts as a window to let light into the eye. There are no blood vessels in the sclera. However, there are numerous sense receptors to detect even the smallest particles on the surface of the eyeball.

The Middle Layer.
The **choroid** is the middle layer of the eye, which contains most of the eye's blood vessels. In the anterior part of the choroid are the iris and the ciliary body. The **iris** is the colored part of the eye. It is made of muscular tissue. As this tissue contracts and relaxes, an opening at its center grows larger or smaller. This opening is the **pupil.** The size of the pupil regulates the amount of light that enters the eye. In bright light the pupil becomes constricted (smaller). In dim light it becomes dilated (larger).

The **ciliary body** is a wedge-shaped thickening in the middle layer of the eyeball. Muscles in the ciliary body control the shape of the lens—making the lens more or less curved for viewing either near or distant objects. The **lens** is a clear, circular disk located just posterior to the iris. Because the lens can change shape, it helps the eye focus images of objects that are near or far away. This process is called **accommodation** (Figure 13-4). Clouding and hardening of the lens, which often occurs with aging, leads to visual changes in a condition known as cataracts. This condition will be discussed in more detail later in this chapter.

The Inner Layer.
The inner layer of the eye consists of the **retina.** Nerve cells at the posterior of the retina sense light. The area where the optic nerve enters the retina is known as the optic disk. This area contains no sensory nerves itself and is referred to as the blind spot. There are

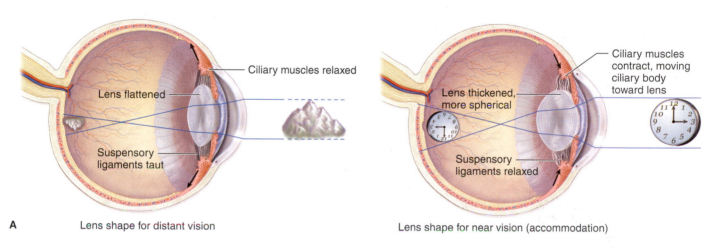

A — Lens shape for distant vision

Lens shape for near vision (accommodation)

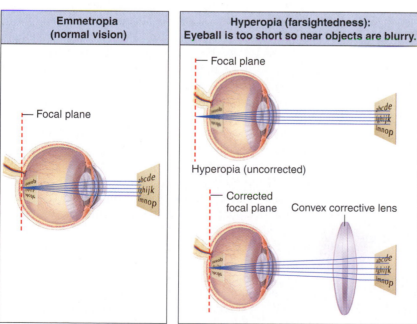
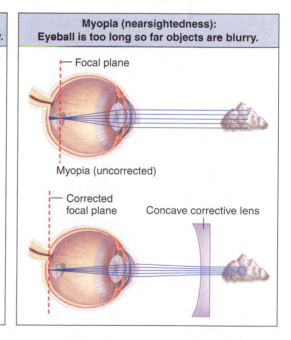

B Vision correction using (*center*) convex and (*right*) concave lenses.

Figure 13-4. (A) Lens shape for distant vision and lens shape for near vision (accommodation). (B) Emmetroia, hyperopia, and myopia.

two types of nerve cells, each named for its shape. **Rods** are highly sensitive to light. They function in dim light but do not provide a sharp image or detect color, only black, white, and shades of gray. They give us our limited "night vision" as well as peripheral vision. **Cones** function best in bright light. They are sensitive to color and provide sharper images. They are responsible for our ability to differentiate different tones and hues of color. Deficiencies in the number or types of cones are responsible for the various types of color blindness, which is generally an inherited condition.

The Chambers of the Eye.
Each eyeball is divided into two chambers—the anterior and the posterior.

The Anterior Chamber. The anterior chamber is in front of the lens and is filled with a watery fluid called **aqueous humor.** Aqueous humor provides nutrients to and bathes the structures in the anterior chamber of the eyeball. When there is an accumulation of aqueous humor, a person develops a visual condition known as **glaucoma.** This disorder will be discussed later in the chapter.

The Posterior Chamber. The posterior chamber of the eyeball is behind the lens and is filled with a very thick, jelly-like fluid called **vitreous humor.** Vitreous humor keeps the retina flat and helps to maintain the shape of the eye.

Visual Accessory Organs

Visual accessory organs assist and protect the eyeball. They include the orbits, eyebrows, eyelids and eyelashes, conjunctivas, the lacrimal apparatus, and extrinsic eye muscles.

Eye Orbits.
The eye sockets, or **orbits,** form a protective shell around the eyes. Eyebrows serve to protect the eyes by reducing the chances that sweat and direct sunlight will enter the eyes.

Eyelids.
Each eyelid is composed of skin, muscle, and dense connective tissue. The muscle in the eyelid is called the **orbicularis oculi** and is responsible for blinking and squinting. Blinking the eyelids prevents the mucus membrane surface of the eyeball from drying. A moist eyeball surface is much less likely to grow bacteria than a dry one is. Blinking also protects the eyes, keeping foreign material from entering the eyes with the assistance of the eyelashes, which catch foreign substances, including perspiration and dust, and keep those substances from getting into the eye.

Conjunctivas.
Conjunctivas are mucous membranes that line the inner surfaces of the eyelids and cover the anterior surface of each eyeball. They are called mucous membranes because they produce mucus that keeps the surface of the eyeballs moist.

The Lacrimal Apparatus.
The **lacrimal apparatus** consists of lacrimal glands and nasolacrimal ducts (Figure 13-5). **Lacrimal glands** are located on the lateral edge of each eyeball and produce tears. Tears are mostly water, but they also contain enzymes (lysozymes) that can destroy bacteria and viruses as part of the body's system to protect itself. Tears also have an outer oily layer that prevents them

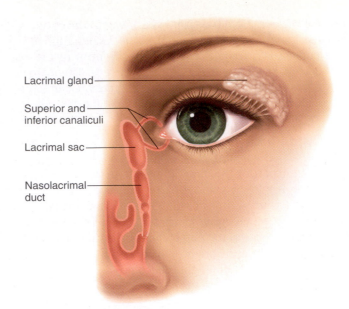

Figure 13-5. Lacrimal apparatus.

Labels: Lacrimal gland; Superior and inferior canaliculi; Lacrimal sac; Nasolacrimal duct

from evaporating. **Nasolacrimal ducts** are located on the medial aspect of each eyeball. They drain tears into the nose. When a person cries, the abundance of tears entering the nose produces the "runny nose" associated with crying.

Extrinsic Eye Muscles.
Extrinsic eye muscles are skeletal muscles that move the eyeball. Each eyeball has six extrinsic eye muscles attached to it that move the eyeball superiorly, inferiorly, laterally, or medially.

Visual Pathways

The eye works much like a camera. Light reflected from an object, or produced by one, enters the eye from the outside and passes through the cornea, pupil, lens, and fluids in the eye. The cornea, lens, and fluids help focus the light onto the retina by bending it, in a process known as **refraction.** As in a camera, an image of an object is carried by light patterns. The image is projected upside down—on film in a camera and on the retina in an eye. The retina converts the light into nerve impulses. These impulses are transmitted along the optic nerve to the brain. This nerve, which consists of about a million fibers, serves as a flexible cable connecting the eyeball to the brain.

Parts of the optic nerve cross at a structure called the optic chiasm, located at the base of the brain. The visual area in the occipital lobes of the cerebrum is responsible for interpreting vision. Because visual information crosses in the optic chiasm, about half of the visual information detected in each eye is interpreted on the opposite side of the brain. Therefore, half of what a person sees in the right eye is interpreted in the left side of the brain and vice versa, where it is brought together as one image. The brain interprets these impulses, turns the image right-side up, and "develops" a picture of the object from which the light originally came. See Table 13-1 for a summary of the parts of the eye and their functions.

TABLE 13-1	The Functions of the Parts of the Eye
Structure	**Function**
Aqueous humor	Nourishes and bathes structures in the anterior eye cavity
Vitreous humor	Holds the retina in place; maintains the shape of the eyeball
Sclera	Protects the eye
Cornea	Allows light to enter the eye; bends light as it enters the eye (refraction)
Choroid	Supplies nutrients and provides a blood supply to the eye
Ciliary body	Holds the lens; controls the shape of the lens for focusing
Iris	Controls the amount of light entering the eye
Lens	Focuses light onto the retina (accommodation)
Retina	Contains visual receptors
Rods	Allow vision in dim light; detect black, white, and gray images; detect broad outlines of images
Cones	Allow vision in bright light; detect colors; detect details
Optic nerve	Carries visual information (stimuli) from rods and cones toward the brain

Educating the Patient

Eye Safety and Protection

Almost 90% of all eye injuries could be prevented by eye safety practices or proper protective eyewear. You can educate patients about preventing eye injuries in the home, at work, and during recreational activities.

Eye Safety in the Home

Patients should follow these suggestions to protect their eyes in the home:

- Pad or cushion the sharp corners and edges of furniture and home fixtures.
- Make sure adequate lighting and handrails are available on stairs.
- Keep personal use items (for example, cosmetics and toiletries), kitchen utensils, and desk supplies out of the reach of children.
- Keep toys with sharp edges out of the reach of children. Also, make sure toys intended for older children are kept away from younger children.
- Before mowing the lawn, remove dangerous debris.
- Wear safely goggles when operating any type of power equipment.
- Keep dangerous solvents, paints, cleaners, fertilizers, and other chemicals out of the reach of children.
- Never mix cleaning agents.

Eye Safety at Work

Approximately 15% of eye injuries in the workplace lead to temporary or permanent vision loss. Eye injuries at work can be diminished if patients take the following precautions:

- Safety eyewear should be chosen according to the type of work being performed and the type of eye protection that is needed.
- Safety eyewear should be worn whenever there is a chance of flying objects from machines.
- Safety eyewear should be worn whenever there is possible exposure to harmful chemicals, body fluids, or radiation.

Eye Safety During Sports and Recreational Activities

Common eye injuries that occur while playing a sport include scratched corneas, inflamed irises and retinas, bleeding in the anterior chamber of the eye, traumatic cataracts, and fractures of the eye socket. Wearing sports eye guards can prevent most sports eye injuries. These guards are recommended for baseball, basketball, soccer, football, rugby, and hockey. Virtually any type of contact sport requires appropriate eye protection.

The Aging Eye

With age, a number of changes occur in the structure and function of the eye.

- The amount of fat tissue diminishes; this loss may cause the eyelids to droop
- The quality and quantity of tears decrease
- The conjunctiva becomes thinner and may be drier because of a decrease in tear production
- The cornea begins to appear yellow, and a ring of fat deposits may appear around it
- The sclera may develop brown spots
- Changes in the iris cause the pupil to become smaller, limiting the amount of light entering the eye
- The lens becomes denser and more rigid; this trend reduces the amount of light that reaches the retina and makes focusing more difficult
- Yellowing of the lens causes problems in distinguishing colors
- Changes in the retina may make vision fuzzy
- The ability of the eye to adapt to changes in light intensities may be reduced; glare can become painful as this ability diminishes
- Night vision may be impaired

- Peripheral vision is reduced, limiting the area a person can see and reducing depth perception
- The vitreous humor breaks down, producing tiny clumps of gel or cellular material that cause floaters—dark spots or lines—that appear in a person's field of vision
- Rubbing of the vitreous humor on the retina produces flashes of light or "sparks"

Because of changes that impair vision—such as reductions in the field of vision, in depth perception, and in visual clarity—elderly people may fall more often than younger people. See Educating the Patient section for some tips for preventing such falls.

Vision Testing

When doctors perform complete physical examinations, they usually screen patients for vision problems and for the general health of the eyes. An **ophthalmologist** (a medical doctor who is an eye specialist) usually performs a thorough eye examination. She tests the external as well as internal structures of the eyes, along with eye movement and coordination. The kinds of testing you will perform or help perform will depend on where you work. You will, however, be expected to assist the doctor and ensure that the patient is comfortable.

Educating the Patient

Preventing Falls in the Elderly

Falls can occur at any age, but in the elderly they can have especially serious consequences. Bones become brittle with age, and falls can cause breaks in major bones, such as the hip and wrist. Complications from falls and bone fractures can lead to death in individuals in this age group.

The elderly are prone to falling because of vision problems, possible poor health, slowing reflexes, and changes in the ear that cause equilibrium problems. In addition, medications can increase the risk of falls because they may make the patient less alert. Discuss a safety checklist with elderly patients and their families. Point out that by taking the precautions listed, elderly patients can reduce the risk of falling. Make sure patients and their families understand these instructions.

- Remove reading glasses before getting up and walking around.
- Make sure that potentially hazardous areas, such as stairs and doorway entrances, are well lit.
- Use night-lights in the bedroom and bathroom to help prevent falls at night.

- When getting up from a reclining or recumbent position, sit at the edge of the bed for a few minutes before trying to stand to allow blood flow and blood pressure to adjust.
- Wear well-fitting shoes with low heels and slippers with nonslip soles.
- Use a cane or walker if you are unsteady on your feet.
- Secure rugs and floor coverings to the floor to prevent slippage.
- Attach all electrical cords to the walls or floor moldings.
- Place sturdy banisters along all stairs inside and outside the home.
- Install secure handrails near the bathtub and toilet.
- Use nonslip mats in the bathtub and shower.
- Minimize clutter in the home.
- Store frequently used items within easy reach.

Other eye professionals include **optometrists** and **opticians.** The optometrist is not an M.D. but an O.D., or optometric doctor. An optometrist often works with or under the direction of an ophthalmologist, providing vision screenings and diagnostic testing. If disease or further workup is needed, the patient will be referred to an ophthalmologist. The optician is responsible for filling the vision prescriptions for glasses and contacts written by the ophthalmologist and optometrist.

Types of Vision Screening Tests

Screening tests are used to detect a number of common visual problems. Some problems may involve the ability to see clearly, known as hyperopia, presbyopia, and myopia. Others may involve the ability to distinguish shades of gray or colors. When you record the results of vision tests, you will use the following abbreviations:

- O.D. (right eye)
- O.S. (left eye)
- O.U. (both eyes)
- $\overline{cc}$ (with correction)

Distance Vision. Impairment of distance vision is known as **myopia** (see Figure 13-4B). In myopia, the eyeball is too "long," resulting in the light being focused anterior to the retina. To test the distance vision of adults, the Snellen letter chart is commonly used. This chart has several rows of letters of the alphabet. Within each row, letter size is the same, but from row to row, letter size decreases from top to bottom. Patients are asked to read the letters from larger to smaller. A chart such as the Snellen E chart, the Landolt C chart (similar to Snellen E, using the letter C), or a pictorial chart is used for children and adults who do not know the alphabet.

When distance vision is tested, normal vision is referred to as 20/20. This number means that at the standard testing distance of 20 feet (first number), a patient can see what a person with normal vision can see at 20 feet (second number). A patient who has 20/80 vision can see at 20 feet what a person with normal vision sees at 80 feet.

The first number (20) always stays the same because a patient always stands 20 feet away from the chart. The second number, however, changes with a patient's visual acuity. If a patient misses only one or two letters on a line during vision testing, record the results with a minus sign. For example, one letter missed with the right eye would be O.D. 20/30 –1. Two letters would be O.D. 20/30 –2.

Near Vision. Refractive error in close vision is called **hyperopia.** In hyperopia, the eyeball is shorter than normal, resulting in objects being focused posterior to the retina (see Figure 13-4B). To test for near vision, special handheld charts are used. These cards contain letters, numbers, or paragraphs in various sizes of print. They may be held and read at a normal reading distance or mounted in a plastic and metal frame and read through optical lenses. **Presbyopia** is visual impairment as a result of aging and is caused by the loss of lens elasticity, resulting in difficulty seeing items close to you. The combination of myopia and presbyopia occurring together is the reason that many people require bifocal lenses as they age.

Contrast Sensitivity. To test for the ability to distinguish shades of gray (contrast sensitivity), the Pelli-Robson contrast sensitivity chart, the Vistech Consultants vision contrast test system, or another testing system is used. Newer systems use special equipment to provide contrast variations in a projected image. These tests can detect cataracts or problems of the retina even before the sharpness of the patient's vision is impaired.

Color Vision. To test color vision, illustrations such as those of the Ishihara color system or the Richmond pseudoisochromatic color test are used. These illustrations contain numbers or symbols made up of colored dots that appear among other colored dots. The patient is asked to identify what he sees. A patient who is color-blind will not be able to report seeing the numbers or symbols. Color blindness may be inherited; it occurs more commonly in males. Changes in one's ability to see colors, however, may indicate a disease of the retina or optic nerve.

Career Opportunities

Ophthalmic Assistant

To gain medical assistant credentials, you must fulfill the requirements of either the American Association of Medical Assistants (Certified Medical Assistant) or the American Medical Technologists (Registered Medical Assistant). After obtaining your medical assistant certification or registration, you may wish to acquire additional skills in specialty areas through course work or on-the-job training. Although this course work or training may not lead to an additional certification or degree, it will enable you to expand your role in the medical office and advance your career as the demand for skilled health professionals increases.

continued ⟶

Ophthalmic Assistant *(concluded)*

Skills and Duties

An ophthalmic assistant provides administrative and clinical support for an ophthalmologist. The assistant works with patients, assists with surgery, and keeps instruments and equipment in proper working order.

The ophthalmic assistant works with patients in a number of ways. Taking the medical history is basic to the ophthalmic assistant's job. She must gather information about the patient's ocular history, family medical history, past and present systemic illnesses, medications, and allergies. As with any medical specialty, she needs to preserve patient confidentiality and use proper recording techniques.

An ophthalmic assistant may conduct tests that evaluate aspects of vision, such as distance acuity, near acuity, and color perception. She must understand how these tests work and how to run them and be prepared to help patients with special needs as she conducts the tests. Tonometry, the measurement of fluid pressure in the eyeball with a machine called a tonometer, may also be the responsibility of an ophthalmic assistant.

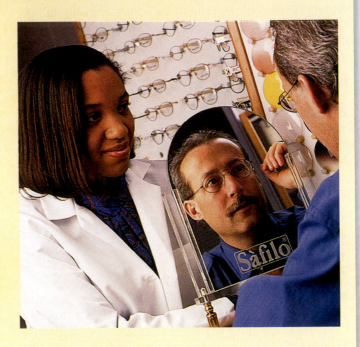

When patients need help with their eyeglasses, the ophthalmic assistant is often the person who records prescriptions, adjusts and repairs damaged frames and lenses, and instructs patients in the care of their eyeglasses. The assistant is trained to administer eye medications to patients in the form of drops, ointments, and irrigating solutions.

The ophthalmic assistant may also assist the ophthalmologist with minor surgery. She prepares the room and instruments, instructs the patient before and after the procedure, and assists the doctor during the surgical procedure.

The operation and care of specialized ophthalmologic instruments, such as ophthalmoscopes, retinoscopes, tonometers, and slitlamps, are often the responsibility of an ophthalmic assistant. She must maintain infection control in the office or operating room, including sanitization, disinfection, and sterilization of instruments and surfaces.

Workplace Settings

The ophthalmic assistant always works under the supervision of an ophthalmologist. She may work in a private office, clinic, or hospital setting.

Education

Certification as an ophthalmic assistant requires a high school diploma or equivalency, followed by a clinical program approved by the Joint Review Committee for Ophthalmic Medical Personnel (JRCOMP). After completing the program, the student must pass an examination that tests seven basic content areas: history taking, basic skills and lensometry, patient services, basic tonometry, instrument maintenance, general medical knowledge, and special studies. She must also provide a current CPR card (such as those issued by the Red Cross or the American Heart Association) and an endorsement from her supervising ophthalmologist. After passing the examination, the student gains the title of Certified Ophthalmic Assistant (COA). Certification must be renewed every 3 years.

Where to Go for More Information

American Academy of Ophthalmology
PO Box 7424
San Francisco, CA 94120

Association of Technical Personnel in
  Ophthalmology (ATPO)
2025 Woodlane Dr.
St. Paul, MN 55125

Joint Commission on Allied Health Personnel
  in Ophthalmology
2025 Woodlane Dr.
St. Paul, MN 55125

Treating Eye Problems

Some common eye problems include **conjunctivitis** (inflammation of the conjunctiva), blepharitis (inflammation of the eyelid), and corneal abrasions (scratching of the cornea). The eye is an extremely delicate organ. Even what seems to be a minor injury or infection can have lasting consequences. Therefore, you must use the greatest caution as well as proper (sterile) techniques when treating a patient's eyes. You should also provide patients with information on how to routinely care for their eyes. See the Educating the Patient section for specific guidelines to follow when presenting preventive eye-care information.

Administration of Medications to the Eye

Your responsibilities as a medical assistant may include dispensing medications and explaining their use. Some medications are used to diagnose conditions, whereas others are used to treat conditions. Only medications for ophthalmic use should be used in the eye. You should teach patients to check medication labels carefully before administering them at home. Optic medications for use in the eye could easily be confused with otic medications for the ear. Medications other than optic medications may be too concentrated or may contain substances that will injure sensitive eye tissue.

Educating the Patient

Preventive Eye-Care Tips

You can help patients take care of their eyes and protect their vision by providing them with guidelines to follow. Go over each item slowly and carefully. Ask whether the patient has questions before moving on to the next item. Answer all the patient's questions, and make sure the patient understands the answers. Eye-care tips include the following.

1. Get regular health checkups. Patients may not appreciate the connection between their general health and their eyes. Point out that high blood pressure and diabetes can cause eye problems.

2. Get regular eye examinations. Most people need eye examinations every 1 to 2 years. Patients with diabetes should see their eye-care specialists more frequently.

3. Be alert for the warning signs of eye disease. Tell patients to call their eye-care specialist immediately if they experience any of these signs:
   - Eye pain
   - Loss of vision
   - Double or blurred vision
   - Headache with blurred vision
   - Redness of the eye or eyelid
   - A gritty or sticky feeling around the eye
   - Excessive tearing
   - Difficulty seeing in the dark
   - Flashes of light
   - Halos around lights
   - Sensitivity to light
   - Loss of color perception

4. Wear sunglasses with ultraviolet protection to shield the eyes from bright sunlight, even in the winter. Recommend that patients ask to have ultraviolet protection added when purchasing new distance prescription glasses. Explain to patients that the cornea can get sunburned, which can be painful and damaging. Also tell patients that excessive exposure to the sun is a contributing factor in the development of cataracts and malignant melanoma of the eye—a dangerous type of skin cancer that may spread through the bloodstream or lymphatic system.

5. Wear protective eye equipment to prevent eye injury. Indicate to patients that they should wear protective eyewear every time they participate in sports, work with chemicals, or encounter a situation in which they may be exposed to flying debris.

6. Use nonprescription eye medications properly. Show patients how to use eye drops, emphasizing that the tip of the dropper should never touch the eye. Explain to patients that medications should be used only as indicated on the label and discarded after the condition has cleared up.

7. Patients should also be told to never share eye make up because bacterial infections can be passed via the applicators. Patients should also take care of the applicators to minimize contamination of any applicators.

If you administer eye medications as part of your job, avoid touching a dropper or ointment tube tip to the eye. Such touching can injure the eye, cause an infection, and contaminate the medication.

Eye Irrigation

When foreign materials enter the eye, they must be flushed out. Flushing (or irrigation) should be done with a sterile solution especially formulated for this purpose. Someone's eye may also need to be irrigated to relieve discomfort from irritating substances, such as smog, pollen, chemicals, or chlorinated water.

The Ear and the Senses of Hearing and Equilibrium

The organ of hearing is the ear. In addition to providing the sense of hearing, the ear aids the body in maintaining balance, or equilibrium.

Pathophysiology

Common Diseases and Disorders of the Eyes

Amblyopia is more commonly called lazy eye and occurs when a child does not use one eye regularly. A child with this disorder does not have normal depth perception and often also has concurrent strabismus, a condition in which the eyes do not focus in unison.

- **Causes.** Amblyopia can be caused by any disorder of the eyes that affects normal eye development and use, including hyperopia, myopia, strabismus, cataracts, and astigmatism.
- **Signs and symptoms.** The most common symptoms are blurred vision and an eye that appears to turn inward or outward.
- **Treatment.** Treating the underlying conditions, placing a patch over the normal eye to strengthen the lazy eye, and using corrective lenses are the primary treatment options.

Astigmatism occurs when the cornea or lens has an abnormal shape, which causes blurred images during near or distant vision.

- **Causes.** This is normally considered to be a congenital condition.
- **Signs and symptoms.** There are no symptoms with this condition other than blurred vision. However, it can be diagnosed during an ophthalmic (eye) exam.
- **Treatment.** Treatment includes corrective lenses or surgery, such as photorefractive keratectomy (PRK) or, more commonly now, laser-assisted in situ keratomileusis (LASIK) to reshape the cornea (Figure 13-6).

Cataracts are opaque structures within the lens that prevent light from going through the lens. Over time, images begin to look fuzzy and, if left untreated, may cause blindness (Figure 13-7).

- **Causes.** Aging is the most significant risk factor associated with this disorder. Cataracts can also be caused by eye injuries, some medications, and certain underlying diseases. Excessive exposure to damaging UV rays from sunlight is also felt to be a risk factor for developing cataracts.

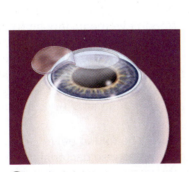 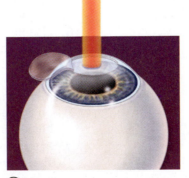 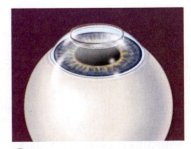

① Cornea is sliced with a sharp knife. Flap of cornea is reflected, and deeper corneal layers are exposed.

② A laser removes microscopic portions of the deeper corneal layers, thereby changing the shape of the cornea.

③ Corneal flap is put back in place, and the edges of the flap start to fuse within 72 hours.

Figure 13-6. LASIK laser vision correction procedure.

continued ⟶

Common Diseases and Disorders of the Eyes *(continued)*

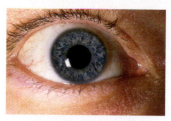

Eye without a cataract

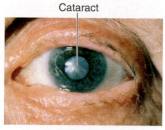

Cataract

Eye with a cataract

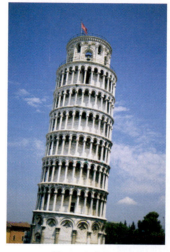

Normal vision

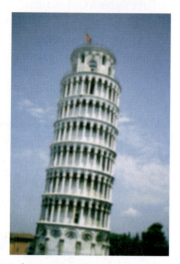

Image seen through cataract

Figure 13-7. Cataracts.

- **Signs and symptoms.** The primary symptom is poor or impaired vision with a "milky" spot over the lens.
- **Treatment.** Treatment includes the use of eyeglasses, medications to dilate the pupils, or surgery, such as phakoemulsification, to remove the cataracts followed by implantation of an artificial intraocular lens.

Conjunctivitis is commonly called pink eye and is highly contagious when the cause is bacterial in nature.

- **Causes.** This disease is caused by bacteria, viruses, or allergies.
- **Signs and symptoms.** The signs and symptoms are red, itchy eyes; swollen eyelids; a watery discharge when caused by viruses and allergies; and a sticky, purulent discharge when the cause is bacterial. The allergic type usually affects both eyes, whereas viral and bacterial conjunctivitis more commonly begins in one eye and spreads to the other.
- **Treatment.** Cool compresses and anti-inflammatory drugs are used to treat conjunctivitis caused by viruses and allergies, with antihistamines being added for those caused by allergies. The bacterial type is best treated with antibiotics.

Dry eye syndrome is one of the most common eye problems treated by physicians. This syndrome results from a decreased production of the oil within tears, which normally occurs with age.

- **Causes.** Dry eye can be caused by cigarette smoke; air conditioning; eye strain created by long hours at a computer monitor; some medications; contact lenses; hormonal changes associated with menopause; and hot, dry, or windy climates.
- **Signs and symptoms.** The common eye symptoms include burning, irritation, redness, itching, and excessive tearing.
- **Treatment.** Artificial tears may provide relief to many patients and newer drugs such as Restasis have helped patients with this condition make more of their own tears. People with this condition should drink 8 to 10 glasses of water a day and make a conscious effort to blink more frequently and avoid rubbing their eyes. In addition, punctual plugs can be inserted to trap tears on the eyes, which prevents the tears from entering the nasolacrimal duct and being drained.

Ectropion is characterized by eversion of the lower eyelid.

- **Causes.** Aging and skin relaxation or scar tissue may cause this condition.
- **Signs and symptoms.** Common signs and symptoms include redness, irritation, and drying of the conjunctiva. Poor tear drainage through the nasolacrimal system may also be present.
- **Treatment.** Surgery to repair the defect may be needed if the condition is bothersome to the patient.

Entropion is characterized by an inversion of the lower eyelid.

- **Causes.** Aging and scar tissue may cause this condition.
- **Signs and symptoms.** Signs include irritation of the sclera as the lashes brush against it, which may lead to corneal ulceration or scarring.
- **Treatment.** Surgery is the only treatment option to correct this problem

Glaucoma is indicated by an increase in intraocular pressure, caused by a buildup of aqueous humor in the anterior chamber. If untreated, this excess pressure can lead to permanent damage of the optic nerves, resulting in blindness.

- **Causes.** *Open-angle glaucoma* progresses relatively slowly; it can be caused by slowing of the drainage of aqueous humor from the anterior chamber of the eye. *Angle closure* or *narrow-angle glaucoma* is a more serious type of glaucoma; it results when the space between the iris and the cornea, which is more narrow than usual, is suddenly blocked so that the humor cannot be drained. Certain medications, trauma, and tumors may all cause secondary glaucoma.

continued ⟶

Common Diseases and Disorders of the Eyes *(continued)*

- **Signs and symptoms.** There are usually no symptoms of open-angle glaucoma. Common symptoms of angle closure glaucoma include nausea, vomiting, extreme eye pain, headache, and a sudden loss of vision related to the sudden buildup of the aqueous humor.

- **Treatment.** Treatments include medications and eye-drops such as Timoptic® and pilocarpine to control pressure in the anterior segment of the eye. In the case of angle closure glaucoma, surgery to correct the blockage may be needed.

Hyperopia is commonly called farsightedness (see Figure 13-4B). It occurs when light entering the eye is focused behind the retina. Common causes include flat corneas or shortened eyeballs. Treatments include corrective lenses, contact lenses, and surgery such as LASIK to alter the shape of the cornea.

Macular degeneration is a progressive disease that usually affects people over the age of 50. It occurs when the retina no longer receives an adequate blood supply. It is the most common cause of vision loss in the United States.

- **Causes.** Genetics, age, smoking, and exposure to ultraviolet radiation (from sunlight) are known risk factors. In most cases that are not age-related, underlying conditions such as diabetes mellitus, ocular infection, and trauma are causative agents. Nutrition may play a role in preventing this disease; diets high in fruits and vegetables that contain vitamins A, C, and E, as well as diets low in saturated fats are recommended. However, there is no current definitive data on the effectiveness of nutrition in prevention or slowing the progression of this disease.

- **Signs and symptoms.** Common symptoms include loss of central vision (may be gradual or sudden), distortions in vision (straight lines begin to look wavy, for example), and difficulty seeing details (Figure 13-8).

- **Treatment.** In most cases, there are no treatments. Laser treatments may repair the damaged blood vessels of the retina.

Myopia is commonly called nearsightedness (see Figure 13-4B). It occurs when light entering the eye is focused in

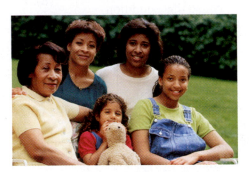
Normal vision

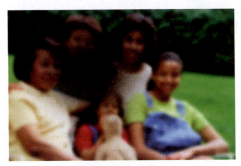
The same scene as viewed by a person with macular degeneration

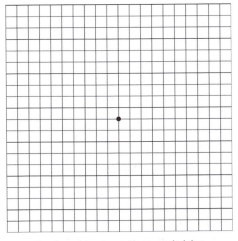
Amsler grid, seen with normal vision

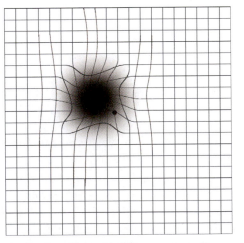
Amsler grid, as viewed by a person with macular degeneration

Figure 13-8. Photos and Amsler grids show the differences between *(left)* normal vision and *(right)* the vision of a person with macular degeneration.

continued ⟶

Common Diseases and Disorders of the Eyes *(concluded)*

front of the retina. Treatments include corrective lenses or surgery to alter the shape of the cornea (LASIK).

Nystagmus is rapid, involuntary eye movements.

- **Causes.** Alcohol and some drug use may cause nystagmus. Inner ear disturbances may also result in involuntary eye movements. Brain lesions and injury (including those that may occur during birth), and cerebrovascular accidents (CVA) or strokes, may also cause nystagmus.
- **Signs and symptoms.** Rapid, irregular eye movements that may be horizontal, vertical, or rotary, depending on the underlying cause of the nystagmus.
- **Treatment.** Treatment will be focused on the underlying cause of the disorder.

Presbyopia is a common eye disorder that results in the loss of lens elasticity (see Figure 13-4B). It develops with age and causes a person to have difficulty seeing objects close up. Treatments include contact lenses, eyeglasses, and eye surgery such as conductive keratoplasty (CK).

Retinal detachment occurs when the layers of the retina separate. It is considered a medical emergency and if not treated right away leads to permanent vision loss.

- **Causes.** This disorder is sometimes caused by fluids that seep between layers of the retina; this occurs most commonly in nearsighted people. In diabetics, vitreous body or scar tissue pulls the retina loose. Other causes include eye trauma that causes fluid to collect underneath the layers of the retina.

- **Signs and symptoms.** Signs and symptoms include light flashes, wavy vision, a sudden loss of vision, particularly of peripheral vision, and a larger amount of floaters.
- **Treatment.** The treatment measures include the following:
  - Pneumatic retinopexy, which involves injecting a gas bubble into the posterior segment of the eye. The pressure flattens the retina, and the retina is later fixed in place with a laser.
  - Scleral buckle, which involves using a silicone band to hold the retina in place.
  - Replacing the vitreous body with silicone oil to reattach the retina.

Strabismus is a misalignment of the eyes. Convergent strabismus is more commonly referred to as crossed eyes. In this condition, the eyes do not focus together, and one or both eyes turn inward. In divergent strabismus, sometimes called wall eyes, one or both eyes turn outward instead of focusing together.

- **Causes.** The causes are mostly unknown, although some known causes include eye and brain injuries, cerebral palsy, and various disorders of the retina.
- **Signs and symptoms.** Blurred vision and depth perception are the most common symptoms.
- **Treatment.** Treatment includes eyeglasses, eye exercises, patching the stronger eye to force the weaker eye to work, and surgery to realign the eyes.

Structure of the Ear

The ear is divided into three parts—external ear, middle ear, and inner ear (Figure 13-9).

External Ear. The external ear is composed of the **auricle** or pinna and the **external auditory canal.** The auricle is the flap of skin and cartilage that hangs off the side of the head. It functions to collect sound waves. The external auditory canal is more commonly called the ear canal and is lined with skin that contains hairs and glands that produce **cerumen,** a waxlike substance commonly known as earwax. Cerumen functions to lubricate the ear and protect it by trapping dirt, dust, and other microbes. This canal carries sound waves to the **tympanic membrane** or eardrum. The tympanic membrane is a fibrous partition located at the inner end of the external auditory canal and separates the external ear from the middle ear.

Middle Ear. The middle ear begins with the tympanic membrane. This membrane is relatively thin and vibrates when sound waves hit it. On the other side of the tympanic membrane are three tiny bones called ear ossicles—the **malleus** (hammer), **incus** (anvil), and **stapes** (stirrup).

When the tympanic membrane vibrates, it causes the ossicles to vibrate and hit a membrane called the oval window.

The middle ear is connected to the throat by a tube called the **eustachian** (auditory) **tube.** This tube helps maintain equal pressure on both sides of the eardrum, which is important for normal hearing. Because the middle ear is connected to the throat by this tube, any throat infection can easily spread to the ear and vice versa. The **oval window** ends the middle ear and marks the beginning of the inner ear.

Inner Ear. The inner ear is a very complex system of communicating chambers and tubes known as the **labyrinth.** It is divided into three portions—**semicircular canals,** a **vestibule,** and a **cochlea** (Figure 13-10). There are three semicircular canals per ear, and they function to detect the balance of the body. The cochlea is shaped like a snail's shell and contains hearing receptors, including the **organ of Corti,** which is known as the organ of hearing. The vestibule is the area between the semicircular canals and the cochlea. Like the semicircular canals, it also functions in equilibrium. When the head moves, fluids known as **perilymph** and **endolymph** in the semicircular canals and vestibule move, which activates equilibrium receptors

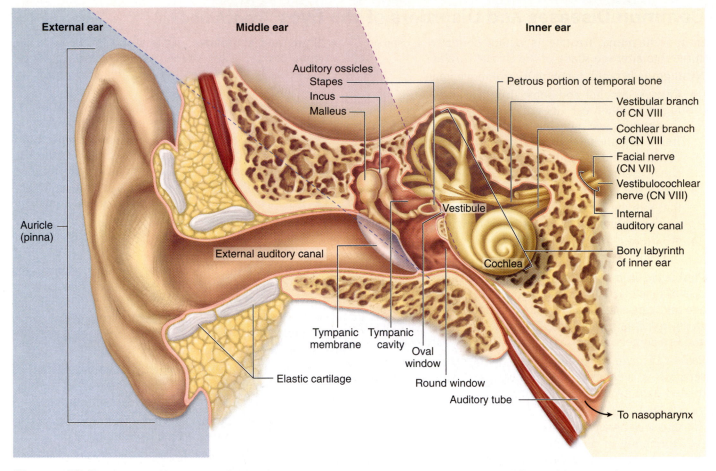

External ear | **Middle ear** | **Inner ear**

Auditory ossicles
Stapes
Incus
Malleus

Petrous portion of temporal bone

Vestibular branch of CN VIII

Cochlear branch of CN VIII

Facial nerve (CN VII)

Vestibulocochlear nerve (CN VIII)

Internal auditory canal

Bony labyrinth of inner ear

Vestibule

Cochlea

Auricle (pinna)

External auditory canal

Tympanic membrane

Tympanic cavity

Oval window

Round window

Auditory tube

To nasopharynx

Elastic cartilage

Figure 13-9. Anatomic regions of the right ear—the ear is divided into external, middle, and inner regions.

as well as hearing receptors. The equilibrium receptors send the information along vestibular nerves to the cerebrum for interpretation. The cerebrum can then advise the body if it needs to make any adjustments to prevent a fall.

When sound waves of different volumes and frequencies activate the hearing receptors in the cochlea, they send their information to auditory nerves. Auditory nerves (vestibulocochlear nerves) deliver the information to the auditory cortex in the temporal lobe of the cerebrum. The auditory cortex interprets the information as sounds.

The Hearing Process

A sound consists of waves of different frequencies that move through the air. The external ear initiates sound conduction when it collects these waves and channels them to the tympanic membrane. There the waves make the tympanic membrane vibrate. The vibrations, in turn, are amplified by the ossicles of the middle ear. The amplified waves enter the inner ear and the cochlea. These waves cause tiny hairs that line the cochlea to bend. Movements of the hairs trigger nerve impulses. The impulses are transmitted by the auditory nerve to the brain, where they are perceived as sound.

Sound waves are also conducted through the bones of the skull directly to the inner ear, a process called **bone**

conduction. This alternative pathway for sound bypasses the external and middle ears. When you hear your own voice, the sound has reached your inner ear mainly through bone conduction. By comparing a person's ability to sense sounds by bone conduction and through the entire ear, doctors can often identify what part of the ear is causing a hearing problem. For example, if bone conduction is normal, a hearing problem likely involves the middle or external ear rather than the inner ear.

The Aging Ear

As a person grows older, a number of changes occur in the ear. The external ear appears larger because of continued growth of cartilage and the loss of skin elasticity. The earlobe gets longer and may have a wrinkled appearance. The glands that produce cerumen become less efficient, producing earwax that is much drier and prone to impaction. The ear canal also becomes narrower.

In the middle ear, changes in the eardrum cause it to shrink and appear dull and gray. The joints between the bones of the middle ear degenerate, so they do not move as freely. In the inner ear, the semicircular canals become less sensitive to changes in position, and this reduced sensitivity affects balance.

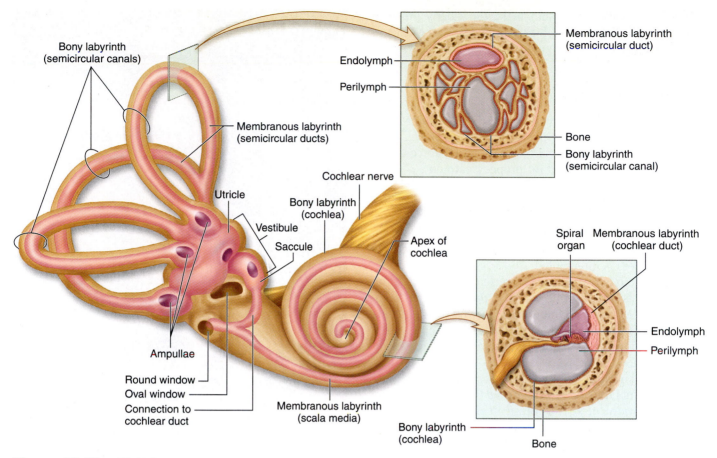

Figure 13-10. Right inner ear—the inner ear is composed of a bony labyrinth cavity that houses a fluid-filled membranous labyrinth. Within the bony labyrinth are the vestibular organs for equilibrium and balance, and the cochlea for hearing.

How to Recognize Hearing Problems in Infants

Hearing problems in infants are not easy to recognize. The following general guidelines can be used to teach parents how to identify normal hearing in infants. Any deviations from these guidelines may indicate a hearing loss.

- Infants up to 4 months old:
  - They should be startled by loud noises (barking dog, hand clap, etc.).
  - When sleeping in a quiet room, they should wake up at the sound of voices.
  - Around the fourth month of age, they should turn their head or move their eyes to follow a sound.
  - They should recognize the mother's or primary caregiver's voice better than other voices.

- Infants 4 to 8 months of age:
  - They should regularly turn their heads or move their eyes to follow sounds.
  - Their facial expressions should change at the sound of familiar voices or loud noises.
  - They should begin to enjoy certain sounds such as rattles or ringing bells.
  - They should begin to babble at people who talk to them.
- Babies 8 to 12 months of age:
  - They should turn quickly to the sound of their name.
  - They should begin to vary the pitch of the sounds they produce in their babbling.
  - They should begin to respond to music.
  - They should respond to the instruction "no."

Problems with equilibrium make the elderly prone to falls. Some ear disorders, such as hearing loss and Meniere's disease, are also more common in older individuals.

Hearing Loss

Hearing loss is actually a symptom of a disease, not a disease in itself. Contrary to what most people believe, hearing loss is not a normal part of the aging process and should always be evaluated for proper treatment.

Types of Hearing Loss

There are two types of hearing loss, conductive and sensorineural. The two types differ in the point at which the hearing process is interrupted.

A **conductive hearing loss** is caused by an interruption in the transmission of sound waves to the inner ear. Conditions that can cause conductive hearing loss include obstruction of the ear canal, as with cerumen impaction or tumor, infection of the middle ear, and reduced movement of the stirrup.

A **sensorineural hearing loss** occurs when there is damage to the inner ear, to the nerve that leads from the ear to the brain, or to the brain itself. In this kind of loss, sound waves reach the inner ear, but the brain does not perceive them as sound. This type of hearing loss can be hereditary, can be caused by repeated exposure to loud noises or viral infections, or can occur as a side effect of medications. **Tinnitus,** which is an abnormal ringing in the ear, suggests damage to the auditory nerve.

Sensorineural hearing loss can be differentiated from conductive hearing loss by hearing tests. It is also possible for both types of hearing loss to occur together.

Noise Pollution

Prolonged exposure to loud noises is a common cause of hearing loss because of damage to the sensitive cells in the cochlea. People who work around noisy equipment, including construction workers, aircraft personnel, and machine operators, are likely to suffer from this type of hearing loss unless they protect their ears (Figure 13-11). Repeatedly listening to loud music from a personal stereo or car radio set at too high a volume can also damage the ears.

Working With Patients With a Hearing Impairment

You may come in contact with patients of all ages who have hearing impairments. Many patients wear hearing aids to amplify normal speech. Some patients, however, may not admit they have a problem—out of fear, vanity, or misinformation. It is estimated that one-third of patients between the ages of 65 and 74 and one-half of

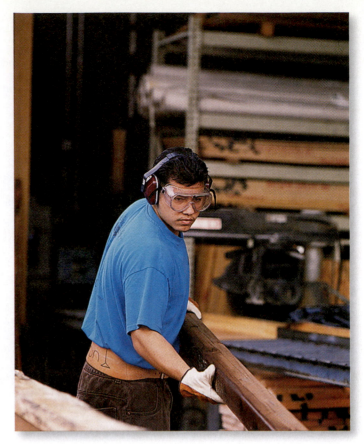

Figure 13-11. Loud noises, such as those produced by a jet engine, can damage hearing unless appropriate ear protectors are worn.

those between the ages of 75 and 79 suffer from some loss of hearing.

To improve communication with a patient whose hearing is impaired, you can do the following:

- Speak at a reasonable volume. Do not shout. Shouting can actually make your words harder to understand. A hearing aid filters out loud sounds, so the patient may not hear everything you say if you shout.
- Speak in clear, low-pitched tones. Elderly patients lose the ability to hear high-pitched sounds first.
- Avoid speaking directly into the patient's ear. Stand 3 to 6 feet away, and face the patient so she can see your lip movements and facial expressions. Avoid covering your mouth with your hands. Speak at a normal rate.
- Avoid overemphasizing your lip movements, which makes lip reading difficult.
- Avoid hand gestures unless they are appropriate.
- If the patient does not understand what you say, restate the message in short, simple sentences. Have the patient repeat the message to verify that your words were understood.
- Treat patients who have a hearing impairment with patience and respect.

Hearing and Diagnostic Tests

Various tests are performed to find out whether a person hears normally. If the tests reveal a problem, follow-up tests are performed to determine the cause of the problem.

Hearing Tests

As part of a general examination, physicians may perform a simple hearing test with one or more tuning forks. Physicians use the tuning forks to determine whether there is a hearing loss. Tuning forks can also be helpful in differentiating conductive from sensorineural hearing loss.

If you have the necessary training, you may help perform a test that uses an audiometer. An **audiometer** is an electronic device that measures hearing acuity by producing sounds in specific frequencies and intensities. A **frequency** is the number of complete fluctuations of energy per second in the form of waves. Frequency is best described as the pitch of sound. High frequency is high-pitched, and low frequency is low-pitched. The audiometer allows a physician or other health practitioner to test a person's hearing and to determine the nature and extent of a person's hearing loss.

Many types of audiometers are available. Some machines automatically generate the various tones at different **decibels** (units for measuring the relative intensity of sounds on a scale from 0 to 130) and print out the patient's responses. Others must be manually adjusted and the results charted by hand. During the test, the patient wears a headset to hear the sounds produced by the audiometer. Depending on the particular unit, the patient indicates hearing a sound by raising a finger or by pushing a button. In the former case the person administering the test records the response. In the latter case the response may be recorded automatically or by the test giver.

Adults and children who can understand directions and respond appropriately can be screened in this manner. If you work in a pediatrician's office, you may also help check an infant's response to sounds. These tests require special techniques because infants cannot understand directions.

Diagnostic Testing

A diagnostic test called tympanometry measures the eardrum's ability to move and thus gauges pressure in the middle ear. Tympanometry is used to detect diseases and abnormalities of the middle ear.

To perform the test, a small, soft-rubber cuff is placed over the external ear canal, producing an airtight seal. The tympanometer then automatically measures air pressure and prints out a graph of the results.

Treating Ear and Hearing Problems

Some common ear problems that you may encounter in the physician's office include cerumen impaction (a buildup of earwax in the ear canal), rupture of the eardrum, otitis media (inflammation of the middle ear), and otitis externa (inflammation of the outer ear). Physicians use various approaches and techniques with each problem to restore the health of a patient's ears. For a detailed description of the techniques used for patients with otitis media, see the Points on Practice and Pathophysiology sections.

Physicians also employ special techniques and devices to improve patients' hearing and maintain the health of their ears. As a medical assistant, you can provide patients with information on preventive ear-care techniques, as described in the Educating the Patient section.

Ear Medications and Irrigation

Part of your job may be to administer ear medications to patients. You may also teach patients how to administer ear medications at home.

Irrigating the ear may relieve inflammation or irritation of the ear canal and may help loosen and remove impacted cerumen (earwax) or a foreign body. This procedure is performed in the physician's office.

Hearing Aids

Hearing aids may be worn inside or outside the ear. If worn outside, they may be located behind the ear, mounted on eyeglasses, or worn on the body. Hearing aids consist of the following parts:

- A tiny microphone to pick up sounds
- An amplifier to increase the volume of sounds
- A tiny speaker to transmit sounds to the ear

You may need to teach patients how to obtain a hearing aid. You can also pass along tips to patients to help them take proper care of their hearing aids and to troubleshoot problems.

Obtaining a Hearing Aid. A patient with signs of hearing loss should be referred to an **otologist,** a medical doctor specializing in the health of the ear, or an **audiologist,** a specialist who focuses on evaluating and correcting hearing problems. Audiologists are not medical doctors and do not treat diseases of the ear. Instead, they evaluate the patient's hearing, fit hearing aids, give instruction in the use of hearing aids, and provide service for hearing aids if necessary. It is important for hearing aids to fit properly. If they do not, sounds may not be transmitted well into the ear.

Otitis Media: The Common Ear Infection

Otitis media, commonly referred to as an ear infection, affects almost all children by age 6. This inflammation of the middle ear accounts for 24.5 million doctor visits each year—second only to upper respiratory infections.

Ear infections typically start when fluid becomes trapped in the middle ear. The lining of the middle ear and **eustachian tube** is lined with a layer of fluid similar to that found in the nose. The normal flow of this fluid from the ear into the back of the nose helps keep the middle ear and the eustachian tube free of bacteria. When a child gets a cold or flu, the lining of the eustachian tube and middle ear can become inflamed and can trap the fluid, which becomes infected.

There are four distinct types of otitis media to be aware of. One or both (bilateral) ears may be affected.

1. Acute otitis media typically refers to a bacterial infection of the middle ear that comes on suddenly. This type is common in children and typically follows an upper respiratory tract infection. The symptoms include pain, a feeling of fullness in the ear, some loss of hearing, and possible fever. In severe cases the eardrum may rupture because of the fluid pressure. Acute infections are usually treated with oral antibiotics. If not treated, this type of otitis media can cause scarring of the tympanic membrane and associated hearing loss.

2. Recurrent otitis media is diagnosed when a child contracts acute otitis repeatedly, perhaps once or twice every month.

3. Otitis media with effusion, also known as OME, involves an accumulation of fluid in the middle ear. Children with OME do not exhibit any symptoms, and they may not experience any discomfort.

4. Chronic otitis media is diagnosed when fluid is present in the ear and fails to clear up after 3 months or more. Infection may or may not be present. Without treatment the undrained fluid thickens, resulting in possible changes in the shape of the eardrum. These changes may cause temporary hearing loss. Antibiotics and reconstructive surgery may be used to treat chronic otitis media.

If a child suffers from recurrent or chronic otitis media, myringotomy, the surgical insertion of tubes, commonly called "tubing," may be recommended to keep the fluid draining continuously. This procedure usually removes enough fluid so the infection clears up. Depending on the type of tube, it falls out on its own within 3 to 18 months of insertion.

Ear infections may be difficult to identify, especially in a young child who cannot talk. The following symptoms may be indications of a possible ear infection, particularly if more than one is present:

- Tugging or rubbing the ear
- Fever ranging from 100°F to 104°F
- Difficulty balancing
- Excessive crankiness
- Difficulty hearing or speaking
- An unwillingness to lie down (The pain may become more severe in a reclining position because of increased pressure against the eardrum.)

Care and Use of Hearing Aids. Hearing aids run on batteries that typically last about 2 weeks. Therefore, the patient must keep a fresh supply of batteries on hand. The hearing aid itself must be routinely cleaned, or the microphone, switches, or dials may not work properly. Moisture can damage the aid, so it must not get wet. Hair sprays can clog hearing aid openings or interfere with the operation of moving parts. For these reasons spray should be applied before a hearing aid is inserted. Cerumen often builds up behind hearing aids that are worn in the ear, reducing sound transmission. If buildup does occur, the cerumen plug should be removed by ear irrigation.

Other Devices and Strategies

People whose hearing cannot be substantially improved by hearing aids may need to use other devices or strategies to overcome the problem. These devices include appliances that light up as well as ring, such as telephones, doorbells, smoke detectors, alarm clocks, and burglar alarms. Patients can purchase amplifiers for the telephone, television set, and radio. Many closed-captioned television programs are also available. To benefit from closed captioning, the patient must have a television set with a decoder that translates the captioning and displays the captions on the screen.

Educating the Patient

Preventive Ear-Care Tips

You can help patients protect their ears and take care of their hearing by providing them with guidelines to follow. As with any patient education, go over items slowly, ask patients whether they have questions before moving on, and answer questions completely. Ear-care tips include the following.

1. **Get routine hearing exams.** Screening for hearing problems is often part of a comprehensive physical exam. Encourage patients who have not had their hearing screened or who suspect they have hearing problems to arrange for testing by their doctor. Older patients, who may not admit they have a problem, may need special encouragement.

2. **Avoid injury when cleaning the ears.** Instruct patients in proper ear care. Point out that they should not put objects in the ear that might injure the eardrum or ear canal, which includes vigorous probing with cotton-tipped swabs.

3. **Avoid injury from nonprescription ear-care products.** Tell patients to check with a doctor before using nonprescription products for softening earwax.

4. **Use proper ear protection.** Urge patients to wear ear protectors around loud work equipment and to avoid listening to loud music. It is especially important to keep the volume at a reasonable level when listening through earphones and through ear buds that fit directly into the external auditory canal.

5. **Use all medications properly.** Show patients how to use eardrops; emphasize that they must follow instructions precisely. Explain to patients that following instructions applies to all medications because many, including aspirin and some antibiotics, may cause hearing loss if used improperly.

6. **Be alert for warning signs.** Tell patients to call their doctor immediately if they experience any of these signs of ear problems:
   - Ear pain
   - Stuffiness
   - Discharge from the ear
   - Vertigo (dizziness)

   Also have patients notify the doctor if they have any of these signs of hearing problems:
   - Tinnitus (ringing)
   - Hearing others' speech as mumbled sounds
   - Speaking in a very loud voice without being aware of it

Pathophysiology

Common Diseases and Disorders of the Ears

Cerumen impaction. This condition refers to the build up of ear wax within the external auditory canal.

- **Causes.** Cerumen impaction may be caused by inadequate cleaning of cerumen from the ear canal, or by overactive ceruminous glands producing more than normal cerumen

- **Signs and symptoms.** The most common sign is some degree of hearing loss because of the blockage of sound waves. Some patients may also complain of ear pain.

- **Treatment.** Treatment includes ear irrigation to remove the blockage. Severely hardened cerumen may require an ear wax softener such as Debrox® to soften and loosen the cerumen before the impaction can be removed.

Hearing loss. Also known as deafness, hearing loss is the loss of the ability to hear sounds at normal levels.

- **Causes.** The two types of hearing loss are conductive and sensorineural. Conductive hearing loss is caused by a blockage of sound waves caused by cerumen impaction, a foreign body, otosclerosis (hardening of the stapes), or a tumor. Sensorineural hearing loss involves damage to the auditory nerve. Causes may include infection, medications, head trauma, and vascular disorders. In some cases, both types of hearing loss may be evident.

- **Signs and symptoms.** Patients may report gradual or sudden difficulty hearing voices, television, and other sounds within their environment. People around them may notice the need for increased volume when listening to television or the radio, or that the patient himself is speaking in a louder voice than necessary. Sudden hearing loss requires immediate medical attention.

continued ⟶

Common Diseases and Disorders of the Ears *(concluded)*

- **Treatment.** The treatment depends on the type of hearing loss involved. Any obstruction should be removed by irrigation or surgery if necessary. If hearing loss is a medication side effect, medication changes may be necessary. Hearing aids may be the answer for many patients. Cochlear implants may be an option for those not assisted adequately with hearing aids as long as the auditory nerve remains intact.

Meniere's disease is a disturbance in the equilibrium characterized by **vertigo** (dizziness), tinnitus (ringing in the ears), nausea, and progressive hearing loss

- **Causes.** The cause is not totally understood, but it is related to an accumulation of endolymph fluid within the membranous labyrinth of the inner ear
- **Signs and symptoms.** Patients often complain of episodes of tinnitus, vertigo, nausea, and balance disturbances. Hearing is affected by the tinnitus and, in the early periods of the disease, episodes of hearing loss are temporary. However, permanent hearing loss usually results as the disease progresses.
- **Treatment.** Antihistamines and fluid restrictions are commonly used to control fluid accumulation. Anti-nausea and anti-vertigo drugs may also be prescribed. Because tinnitus is often more bothersome at night (during quiet), mild sedatives are commonly used, especially at bedtime. Patients are often advised to avoid caffeine, alcohol, and cigarettes. Fatigue and stress may also aggravate the condition.

Otitis is inflammation of the ear. All three areas of the ear may be inflamed. *Otitis externa* is known as swimmers' ear, *otitis media* is a middle ear infection, and *otitis interna* (labyrinthitis) is an inner ear infection.

- **Causes.** Bacterial infections are often to blame for otitis externa. Otitis media often results from the spread of an upper respiratory infection from the throat that enters the eustachian tube and infects the middle ear. Labyrinthitis, especially the purulent or infective type, occurs from a spread of otitis media to the inner ear.
- **Signs and symptoms.** Pain in the ear with associated hearing loss is the primary symptom. Labyrinthitis also often causes vertigo and nausea. Purulent (pus-containing) drainage may also occur in some forms of otitis media.
- **Treatment.** Antibiotics are given to treat the causative agent, and pain medication and fever reducers may be given to make the patient more comfortable. Antihistamines and anti-nausea medications may also be used in the case of otitis interna.

Otosclerosis is the immobilization of the stapes within the inner ear, which is a common cause of conductive hearing loss.

- **Causes.** Genetics seems to play a role. This disease occurs more frequently in females than in males.
- **Signs and symptoms.** These include a slow and progressive hearing loss that may be accompanied by tinnitus.
- **Treatment.** Surgical removal of the stapes (stapedectomy) with insertion of a prosthetic stapes may result in at least a partial restoration of hearing.

Presbycusis is hearing loss because of the aging process.

- **Causes.** As part of the natural aging process, the auditory system deteriorates, resulting in a loss of hair cells in the organ of Corti.
- **Signs and symptoms.** Signs and symptoms include gradual, progressive hearing loss, usually of high-frequency sounds first. Tinnitus may accompany this loss and the patient may become depressed and frustrated at his developing inability to communicate well as a result of the hearing loss.
- **Treatment.** In most cases, hearing aids are prescribed to alleviate some of the hearing loss, although the condition itself is irreversible.

Summary

The ability to detect changes in the environment is critical to survival. The human body has various organs for this purpose. The nose senses odors in the environment and the tongue senses tastes. The eyes allow us to visualize our environment and our ears to hear. Each of these special senses works in concert with the nervous system to assist the body in coping with environmental changes experienced throughout the day.

You can help prevent, detect, and treat eye and ear problems in your work as a medical assistant. Because conditions that affect the eyes and ears can have an impact on vision, hearing, and balance, these conditions affect a patient's quality of life. Vision and hearing provide people with information about the world around them; balance allows people to move securely and effectively through their environment.

A basic understanding of the anatomy and physiology of the eyes and ears will help you provide good eye and ear care to patients. You must also become familiar with many health, medication, safety, and hygiene concerns to teach patients to care for their own eyes and ears properly.

Be sensitive to the needs of individual patients as you care for their eyes and ears. Learn all you can about how to meet the special needs of children, elderly patients, and patients with conditions that make preventing, detecting, and treating eye and ear problems a challenge.

CASE STUDY QUESTIONS

Now that you have completed this chapter, review the case study at the beginning of the chapter and answer the following questions:

1. Why is the patient experiencing dizziness and difficulty hearing?
2. What is the clinical term for ringing in the ear?
3. What precautions should this patient take because of his dizziness?
4. A diuretic is a drug that decreases fluids in the body. Why might the doctor prescribe a diuretic?

Discussion Questions

1. Explain the concept that the eye works like a camera.
2. How can you help elderly patients cope with the changes that occur in the eyes and ears as a result of aging?
3. Identify the four primary taste sensations and tell what part of the tongue is associated with each. What is the fifth acknowledged taste sensation?
4. Discuss the difference between sensorineural and conductive hearing loss, and give an example of how each might be caused.

Critical Thinking Questions

1. Explain why smell and taste are affected when a patient has an upper respiratory infection (URI) with excess mucus production.
2. How are the signs and symptoms of cataracts, glaucoma, and macular degeneration different?
3. Explain why listening to music, music videos, and video games with ear buds for prolonged periods of time may be cause for concern.

Application Activities

1. Give the functions of the following:
   a. Retina
   b. Cornea
   c. Aqueous humor
   d. Choroid
   e. Vitreous humor

2. State if the following structures are part of the outer, middle, or inner ear. Also give the function of each.
   a. Labyrinth
   b. Cochlea
   c. Eustachian tube
   d. Ear ossicles
   e. Tympanic membrane
3. What are the two ways hearing occurs? Explain the difference between the two
4. Shop around for a hearing aid. Find out how much different types of aids cost, what sizes and types are available, the cost of a fitting, how to change the batteries, and how to clean a hearing aid properly. Present your findings to the class, remarking on the service you received and whether you would recommend the place or places where you shopped.

Virtual Fieldtrip

Visit the McGraw-Hill Higher Education Medical Assisting website at www.mhhe.com/medicalassisting3 to complete the following activity:

Access the Medline Plus website for eye diseases. Scroll to the *Seniors* area and choose the subject *Aging and Your Eyes.* Answer the following questions:

1. What are five steps you can use to protect your eyesight?
2. Explain the term *low vision.* What are the symptoms of low vision?
3. Can low vision be corrected? What are some suggestions for patients suffering from low vision to help them have a better quality of life even with their visual difficulties?

Open the CD and complete this chapter's practice activities, play the games, listen to the key terms, and test yourself with the interactive review. E-mail, print, and/or save your results to document your proficiency.

APPENDIX I
AAMA/CAAHEP Competencies for the Medical Assistant

The Entry-Level Competencies for the medical assistant include, but are not limited to:

a. Administrative Competencies:

1. Perform Clerical Functions
   a. Schedule and manage appointments
   b. Schedule inpatient and outpatient admissions and procedures
   c. Organize a patient's medical record
   d. File medical records

2. Perform Bookkeeping Procedures
   a. Prepare a bank deposit
   b. Post entries on a daysheet
   c. Perform accounts receivable procedures
   d. Perform billing and collection procedures
   e. Post adjustments
   f. Process credit balance
   g. Process refunds
   h. Post NSF checks
   i. Post collection agency payments

3. Process Insurance Claims
   a. Apply managed care policies and procedures
   b. Apply third party guidelines
   c. Perform procedural coding
   d. Perform diagnostic coding
   e. Complete insurance claim forms

b. Clinical Competencies:

1. Fundamental Procedures
   a. Perform hand washing
   b. Wrap items for autoclaving
   c. Perform sterilization techniques
   d. Dispose of biohazardous materials
   e. Practice Standard Precautions

2. Specimen Collection
   a. Perform venipuncture
   b. Perform capillary puncture
   c. Obtain specimens for microbiological testing
   d. Instruct patients in the collection of a clean-catch midstream urine specimen
   e. Instruct patients in the collection of fecal specimens

3. Diagnostic Testing
   a. Perform electrocardiography
   b. Perform respiratory testing
   c. CLIA Waived Tests:
      (i) Perform urinalysis
      (ii) Perform hematology testing
      (iii) Perform chemistry testing
      (iv) Perform immunology testing
      (v) Perform microbiology testing

4. Patient Care
   a. Perform telephone and in-person screening
   b. Obtain vital signs
   c. Obtain and record patient history
   d. Prepare and maintain exam and treatment areas
   e. Prepare patient for and assist with routine and specialty exams
   f. Prepare patient for and assist with procedures, treatments, and minor office surgeries
   g. Apply pharmacology principles to prepare and administer oral and parenteral (excluding IV) medications
   h. Maintain medication and immunization records
   i. Screen and follow-up test results

c. General Competencies

1. Professional Communications
   a. Respond to and initiate written communications
   b. Recognize and respond to verbal communications
   c. Recognize and respond to nonverbal communications
   d. Demonstrate telephone techniques

2. Legal Concepts
   a. Identify and respond to issues of confidentiality
   b. Perform within legal and ethical boundaries
   c. Establish and maintain the medical record
   d. Document appropriately
   e. Demonstrate knowledge of federal and state health-care legislation and regulations

3. Patient Instruction
   a. Explain general office policies
   b. Instruct individuals according to their needs
   c. Provide instruction for health maintenance and disease prevention
   d. Identify community resources

4. Operational Functions
   a. Perform an inventory of supplies and equipment
   b. Perform routine maintenance of administrative and clinical equipment
   c. Utilize computer software to maintain office systems
   d. Use methods of quality control

General Competencies may be addressed in clinical, administrative, or both areas.

APPENDIX II

AMT Registered Medical Assistant (RMA) Certified Examination Topics Correlation Chart

Examination Topics

I. GENERAL MEDICAL ASSISTING KNOWLEDGE

  A. *Orientation*
   1. Introduction and review of program
   2. Employment outlook
   3. General responsibilities

  B. *Anatomy and Physiology*
   1. Anatomy and Physiology
   2. Diet and nutrition
   3. Study of diseases and etiology
   4. All body systems
   5. Diagnostic/treatment modalities

  C. *Medical Terminology*
   1. Basic structure of medical words (roots, prefixes, suffixes, spelling, and definitions)
   2. Combining word elements to form medical words
   3. Medical specialties and short forms
   4. Medical abbreviations

  D. *Medical Law and Ethics*
   1. Ethical decisions, medical jurisprudence, and confidentiality
   2. Legal terminology pertaining to office practice
   3. Medical/ethical issues in today's society
   4. Risk management

  E. *Psychology of Human Relations*
   1. Dealing with difficult patients with normal/abnormal behavior
   2. Caring for patients with special and specific needs
   3. Caring for cancer and terminally ill patients
   4. Emotional crisis/patients and/or family
   5. Various treatment protocols
   6. Basic principles
   7. Developmental stages of the life cycle
   8. Hereditary, cultural, and environmental influences on behavior standards

  F. *Career Development*
   1. Instruction regarding internship rules, regulations
   2. Job search, professional development, and success
   3. Goal setting, time management, and employment opportunities
   4. Resume writing, interviewing techniques, and follow-up
   5. Dress for success
   6. Professionalism

II. ADMINISTRATIVE MEDICAL ASSISTING

  A. *Medical Office Business Procedures/Management*
   1. Manual and computerized records management
    (1) Patient case histories (confidentiality)
    (2) Filing
    (3) Appointments and scheduling
    (4) Inventory/Control
   2. Financial Management
    (1) Basic bookkeeping
    (2) Billing and collections
    (3) Purchasing
    (4) Banking and payroll
   3. Insurance (including HMOs, PPOs, co-pays, CPT coding, etc.)
   4. Equipment and Supplies (including ordering/maintaining/storage/inventory)
   5. Reception, public, and interpersonal relations
    (1) Telephone techniques
    (2) Professional conduct and appearance
    (3) Professional office environment and safety
   6. Office safety and security

  B. *Basic Keyboarding*
   1. Office machines, transcriptions, computerized systems/medical data processing
   2. Transcribing medical correspondence and medical reports
   3. Medical terminology review

III. CLINICAL MEDICAL ASSISTING

  A. *Medical Office Clinical Procedures*
   1. Basic clinical skills (e.g., vital signs)
   2. Basic skills and procedures used in medical emergencies
   3. Patient exam
    (1) Patient histories
    (2) Patient preparation
    (3) Physical exam
    (4) Instruments
    (5) Assisting the physician
    (6) Housekeeping
   4. Medical Equipment
    (1) Electrocardiogram, centrifuge, etc.
    (2) Physical therapy
    (3) Radiology
     (a) Safety
     (b) Patient preparation
     (c) Radiography of chest and extremities
    (4) Medical asepsis/sterilization and minor office surgery
    (5) Specialties
    (6) First Aid, CPR
    (7) Injections (dosage calculations)
     (a) IM
     (b) Subq
     (c) ID
    (8) Universal precautions in the medical office

  B. *Medical Laboratory Procedures*
   1. Orientation
    (1) Laboratory equipment and maintenance
    (2) Safety

(3) Storage of chemicals and supplies
(4) Fire safety
(5) Care of microscope (introduction)
2. Urinalysis
(1) Specimen collection
(2) Physical exam
(3) Chemical analysis
(4) Microscopic exam
3. Hematology
(1) Personal protection equipment
(2) Specimen collection
(a) Venipuncture
(b) Finger puncture
(3) Hemoglobin
(4) Hematocrit
(5) WBC
(6) RBC
(7) Slide preps
(8) Serology
(a) Blood typing
(b) Blood morphology
(9) Quality control
4. Basic blood chemistries
5. HIV/AIDS and blood-borne pathogens
6. OSHA compliance rules and regulations
C. *Pharmacology*
1. Occupational math and metric conversions (drug calculations)
2. Use of PDRs and medication books
3. Common abbreviations used in prescription writing
4. Legal aspects of writing prescriptions
5. FDC and state laws
6. Medications prescribed for the treatment of illness and disease based on a systems method

APPENDIX III

National Healthcareer Association (NHA)
Medical Assisting Duty/Task List

Duties:

A. DISPLAY PROFESSIONALISM

B. APPLY COMMUNICATION SKILLS

C. DEMONSTRATE KEYBOARDING SKILLS AND COMPUTER AWARENESS

D. PERFORM BUSINESS SOFTWARE APPLICATIONS

E. WORK WITHIN COMPUTER OPERATING ENVIRONMENTS

F. PERFORM ADMINISTRATIVE DUTIES

G. PERFORM CLINICAL DUTIES

H. APPLY LEGAL, ETHICAL, AND CONFIDENTIALITY CONCEPTS TO PRACTICE

I. MANAGE THE OFFICE

J. PROVIDE PATIENT INSTRUCTION

K. MANAGE PRACTICE FINANCES

Duty A: Display Professionalism

A. 01 Project a Positive Attitude

A. 02 Demonstrate Ethical Behavior

A. 03 Practice Within the Scope of Education, Training and Personal Capabilities

A. 04 Maintain Confidentiality

A. 05 Work as a Team Member

A. 06 Conduct Oneself in a Courteous and Diplomatic Manner

A. 07 Adapt to Change

A. 08 Show Initiative and Responsibility

A. 09 Promote the Profession

A. 10 Apply Critical Thinking Skills to Workplace Situations

A. 11 Manage stress

Duty B: Apply Communication Skills

B. 01 Listen and Observe

B. 02 Treat all Patients with Empathy and Impartiality

B. 03 Adapt Communication to Individual's Abilities to Understand

B. 04 Recognize and Respond to Verbal and Nonverbal Communication

B. 05 Serve as Liaison Between Physician and Others

B. 06 Evaluate Understanding of Communication

B. 07 Receive, Organize, Prioritize and Transmit Information

B. 08 Use Proper Telephone Technique

B. 09 Interview Effectively

B. 10 Use Medical Terminology Appropriately

B. 11 Compose Written Communication Using Correct Grammar, Spelling and Format

Duty C: Demonstrate Keyboarding Skill and Computer Awareness

C. 01 Perform Keyboarding by Touch on a Microcomputer

C. 01 Use Basic Terminology Common in the Computer Industry

C. 02 Demonstrate Care and Routine Maintenance of Computer Systems

C. 03 Identify the Types and Functions of Hardware and Peripheral Components

C. 04 Identify the Types of Operating Systems

C. 05 Define Differences in the Application of Microcomputer Software

Duty D: Perform Business Software Applications

D. 01 Explain the Characteristics and Components of Word Processing

D. 02 Start Up Word Processing Software

D. 03 Produce and Format Common Business Documents Such as Letters, Memos, and Reports

D. 04 Edit a Document

D. 05 Print a Document

D. 06 Retrieve a Document

D. 07 Enhance a Document

D. 08 Utilize Software Reference/Documentation

D. 09 Explain the Uses of Database Management Concepts and Applications

D. 10 Perform Basic Database Operations

D. 12 Index and/or Sort Databases

D. 13 Link Databases

D. 14 Design Reports

D. 15 Integrate Software Applications

D. 16 Utilize Software Reference/Documentation

Duty E: Work Within Computer Operating Environments

E. 01 Use Operating System Commands

E. 02 Work with Directories and Subdirectories

E. 03 Demonstrate File Naming Conventions

E. 04 Understand the Basic Function of Batch Files

E. 07 Explain the Characteristics and Components of Graphical User Interface Software

E. 08 Start Up Graphical User Interface Software

E. 09 Utilize the Programs in the Standard Graphical User Interface Software Groups

E. 10 Build and Use Icons

E. 11 Perform Basic File Commands on Network Drive

E. 12 Print Using a Network Printer

Duty F: Perform Administrative Duties

F. 01 Perform Records Management

F. 02 Use and Maintain Office Equipment

F. 03 Handle Incoming Mail

F. 04 Schedule and Monitor Appointments

F. 05 Prepare and Maintain Medical Records

F. 06 Implement a Health Care Software System

F. 07 Operate a Health Care Software System

F. 08 Information for Patients and Employers

F. 11 Manage Calendar/Itineraries

F. 12 Organize Meetings and Presentations

Duty G: Perform Clinical Duties

G. 01 Apply Principles of Aseptic Technique

G. 02 Apply Principles of Infection Control

G. 03 Vital Signs

G. 04 Recognize Emergencies

G. 05 Perform First-Aid and CPR

G. 06 Prepare and Maintain Examination and Treatment Area

G. 07 Interview and Take Patient History

G. 08 Prepare Patients for Procedures

G. 09 Assist Physician with Examinations and Treatments

G. 10 Use Quality Control

G. 11 Collect and Process Specimens

G. 12 Perform Selected Tests That Assist With Diagnosis and Treatment

G. 13 Perform Immunological Tests and Record Results

G. 14 Perform Microbiological Tests and Record Results

G. 15 Perform Tuberculosis Screen and Record Results

G. 16 Run an Electrocardiogram and Record Results

G. 17 Perform Vision Testing and Record Results

G. 18 Screen and Follow Up Patient Test Results

G. 19 Prepare and Administer Medications as Directed by Physician

G. 20 Maintain Medication Records

G. 21 Utilize Proper Body Mechanics

G. 22 Apply Basic Math to Medically Related Problems.

G. 25 Use Formulas and Equations to Solve Health-Related Math Problems

G. 26 Transfer and Transport Patients With or Without Assistive Devices Using Proper Body Mechanics

Duty H: Apply Legal, Ethical, and Confidentiality Concepts

H. 01 Document Accurately

H. 02 Determine Needs for Documentation and Reporting

H. 03 Use Appropriate Guidelines When Releasing Records or Information

H. 04 Follow Established Policy in Initiating, Withdrawing, Withholding, or Terminating Medical Treatment

H. 05 Dispose of Controlled Substances in Compliance With Government Regulations

H. 06 Maintain Licenses and Certification

H. 07 Monitor Legislation Related to Current Health Care and Practice

H. 08 Perform Within Ethical Boundaries

Duty I: Manage the Office

I. 01 Maintain the Physical Plant

I. 02 Operate and Maintain Facilities and Equipment Safely

I. 03 Maintain and Operate Medical Equipment

I. 04 Observe Safety Precautions in the Office

I. 05 Inventory Equipment and Supplies

I. 06 Identify Supply Resources

I. 07 Evaluate and Recommend Equipment and Supplies

I. 08 Maintain Liability Coverage

I. 09 Maintain Documentation of Continuing Education

I. 10 Exercise Efficient Time Management

Duty J: Provide Patient Instruction

J. 01 Orient Patients to Office Policies and Procedures

J. 02 Instruct Patients With Special Needs

J. 03 Teach Patients Methods of Health Promotion and Disease Prevention

J. 04 Provide Verbal and Written Information

J. 05 Orient and Train Personnel

Duty K: Manage Practice Finances

K. 01 Use Bookkeeping Systems

K. 02 Implement Current Diagnostic/Procedural Coding Systems (CPT and ICD-9-CM coding)

K. 03 Analyze and Use Current Third-Party Guidelines for Reimbursement

K. 04 Manage Accounts Receivable

K. 05 Manage Accounts Payable

K. 06 Maintain Records for Accounting and Banking Purposes

APPENDIX IV
Prefixes and Suffixes Commonly Used in Medical Terms

a-, an- without, not
ab- from, away
ad-, -ad to, toward
adeno- gland, glandular
aero- air
-aesthesia sensation
-al characterized by
-algia pain
ambi-, amph-, amphi- both, on both sides, around
andr-, andro- man, male
angio- blood vessel
ano- anus
ante- before
antero- in front of
anti- against, opposing
arterio- artery
arthro- joint
-ase enzyme
-asthenia weakness
auto- self
bi- twice, double
bili- bile
bio- life
blasto-, -blast developing stage, bud
brachy- short
brady- slow
broncho- bronchial (windpipe)
cardio- heart
cata- down, lower, under
-cele swelling, tumor
-centesis puncture, tapping
centi- hundred
cephal-, cephalo- head
cerebr-, cerebro- brain
chol-, chole-, cholo- gall
chondro- cartilage
chromo- color
-cidal killing
-cide causing death
circum- around
-cise cut
co-, com-, con- together, with
-coele cavity
colo- colon
colp-, colpo- vagina
contra- against
cost-, costo- rib

crani-, cranio- skull
cryo- cold
cysto-, -cyst bladder, bag
-cyte, cyto- cell, cellular
dacry-, dacryo- tears, lacrimal apparatus
dactyl-, dactylo- finger, toe
de- down, from
deca- ten
deci- tenth
demi- half
dent-, denti-, dento- teeth
derma-, dermat-, dermato-, -derm skin
dextro- to the right
di- double, twice
dia- through, apart, between
dipla-, diplo- double, twin
dis- apart, away from
dorsi-, dorso- back
dynia- pain
dys- difficult, painful, bad, abnormal
e-, ec-, ecto- away, from, without, outside
-ectomy cutting out, surgical removal
em-, en- in, into, inside
-emesis vomiting
-emia blood
encephalo- brain
endo- within, inside
entero- intestine
ento- within, inner
epi- on, above
erythro- red
esthesio-, -esthesia sensation
eu- good, true, normal
ex-, exo- outside of, beyond, without
extra- outside of, beyond, in addition
fibro- connective tissue
fore- before, in front of
-form shape
-fuge driving away
galact-, galacto- milk
gastr-, gastro- stomach
-gene, -genic, -genetic, -genous arising from, origin, formation
glosso- tongue
gluco-, glyco- sugar, sweet
-gram recorded information
-graph instrument for recording

-graphy the process of recording
-gravida pregnant female
gyn-, gyno-, gyne-, gyneco- woman, female
haemo-, hemato-, hem-, hemo- blood
hemi- half
hepa-, hepar-, hepato- liver
herni- rupture
hetero- other, unlike
histo- tissue
homeo, homo- same, like
hydra-, hydro- water
hyper- above, over, increased, excessive
hypo- below, under, decreased
hyster-, hystero- uterus
-ia condition
-iasis condition of
-ic, -ical pertaining to
ictero- jaundice
idio- personal, self-produced
ileo- ileum
im-, in-, ir- not
in- in, into
infra- beneath
inter- between, among
intra-, intro- into, within, during
-ism condition, process, theory
-itis inflammation of
-ium membrane
-ize to cause to be, to become, to treat by special method
juxta- near, nearby
karyo- nucleus, nut
kata-, kath- down, lower, under
kera-, kerato- horn, hardness, cornea
kineto-, -kinesis, -kinetic motion
lact- milk
laparo- abdomen
latero- side
-lepsis, -lepsy seizure, convulsion
leuco-, leuko- white
levo- to the left
lipo- fat
lith-, -lith stone
-logy science of, study of
-lysis setting free, disintegration, decomposition

macro-   large, long
mal-   bad
-malacia   abnormal softening
-mania   insanity, abnormal desire
mast-, masto-   breast
med-, medi-   middle
mega-, megalo-   large, great
meio-   contraction
melan-, melano-   black
meno-   month
mes-, meso-   middle
meta-   beyond
-meter   measure
metro-, metra-   uterus
-metry   process of measuring
micro-   small
mio-   smaller, less
mono-   single, one
multi-   many
my-, myo-   muscle
myel-, myelo-   marrow
narco-   sleep
nas-, naso-   nose
necro-   dead
neo-   new
nephr-, nephro-   kidney
neu-, neuro-   nerve
niter-, nitro-   nitrogen
non-, not-   no
nucleo-   nucleus
-nuli   none
ob-   against
oculo-   eye
odont-   tooth
-odynia   pain
-oid   resembling
-ole   small, little
olig-, oligo-   few, less than normal
-oma   tumor
onco-   tumor
oo-   ovum, egg
oophor-   ovary
ophthalmo-   eye
-opia   vision
-opsy   to view
orchid-   testicle
ortho-   straight
os-   mouth, bone
-osis   disease, condition of
oste-, osteo-   bone
-ostomy   to make a mouth, opening
oto-   ear

-otomy   incision, surgical cutting
-ous   having
oxy-   sharp, acid
pachy-   thick
paedo, pedo-   child
pan-   all, every
par; para-   alongside of, with; woman who has given birth
path-, patho-, -pathy   disease, suffering
ped-, pedi-, pedo-   foot
-penia   too few, lack, decreased
per-   through, excessive
peri-   around
pes-   foot
-pexy   surgical fixation
phag-, phagia, phago-, -phage   eating, consuming, swallowing
pharyng-   throat, pharynx
phlebo-   vein
-phobia   fear, abnormal fear
-phylaxis   protection
-plasia   formation or development
-plastic   molded
-plasty   operation to reconstruct, surgical repair
-plegia   paralysis
pleuro-   side, rib
pluri-   more, several
pneo-, -pnea   breathing
pneumo-   air, lungs
-pod   foot
poly-   many, much
post-   after, behind
pre-, pro-   before, in front of
presby-, presbyo-   old age
primi-   first
procto-   rectum
proto-   first
pseudo-   false
psych-   the mind
pulmon-, pulmono-   lung
pyelo-   pelvis (renal)
pyo-   pus
pyro-   fever, heat
quadri-   four
re-   back, again
reni-, reno-   kidney
retro-   backward, behind
rhino-   nose
-rrhage, -rrhagia   abnormal or excessive discharge, hemorrhage, flow
-rrhaphy   suture of

-rrhea   flow, discharge
sacchar-   sugar
sacro-   sacrum
salpingo-   tube, fallopian tube
sarco-   flesh
sclero-   hard, sclera
-sclerosis   hardening
-scopy   examining
semi-   half
septi-, septic-, septico-   poison, infection
-spasm   cramp or twitching
-stasis   stoppage
steno-   contracted, narrow
stereo-   firm, solid, three-dimensional
stomato-   mouth
-stomy   opening
sub-   under
super-, supra-   above, upon, excess
sym-, syn-   with, together
tachy-   fast
tele-   distant, far
teno-, tenoto-   tendon
tetra-   four
-therapy   treatment
thermo-, -thermy   heat
thio-   sulfur
thoraco-   chest
thrombo-   blood clot
thyro-   thyroid gland
-tome   cutting instrument
tomo-, -tomy   incision, section
trans-   across
tri-   three
-tripsy   surgical crushing
tropho-, -trophy   nutrition, growth
-tropy   turning, tendency
ultra-   beyond, excess
uni-   one
-uria   urine
urino-, uro-   urine, urinary organs
utero-   uterus, uterine
vaso-   vessel
ventri-, ventro-   abdomen
xanth-   yellow

APPENDIX V
Latin and Greek Equivalents Commonly Used in Medical Terms

abdomen venter
adhesion adhaesio
and et
arm brachium; brachion (Gr)
artery arteria
back dorsum
backbone spina
backward retro; opistho (Gr)
bend flexus
bile bilis; chole (Gr)
bladder vesica, cystus
blister vesicula
blood sanguis; haima (Gr)
body corpus; soma (Gr)
bone os, ossis; osteon (Gr)
brain encephalon
break ruptura
breast mamma; mastos (Gr)
buttock gloutos (Gr)
cartilage cartilago; chondros (Gr)
cavity cavum
chest pectoris, pectus; thorax (Gr)
child puer, puerilis
choke strangulo
corn clavus
cornea kerat (Gr)
cough tussis
deadly lethalis
death mors
dental dentalis
digestive pepticos
disease morbus
dislocation luxatio
doctor medicus
dose dosis (Gr)
ear auris; ous (Gr)
egg ovum
erotic erotikos (Gr)
exhalation exhalatio, expiro
external externus
extract extractum
eye oculus; ophthalmos (Gr)
eyelid palpebra
face facies
fat adeps; lipos (Gr)
female femella

fever febris
finger (or toe) digitus
flesh carnis, caro
foot pes
forehead frons
gum gingiva
hair capillus, pilus; thrix (Gr)
hand manus; cheir (Gr)
harelip labrum fissum;
   cheiloschisis (Gr)
head caput; kephale (Gr)
health sanitas
hear audire
heart cor; kardia (Gr)
heat calor; therme (Gr)
heel calx, talus
hysterics hysteria
infant infans
infectious contagiosus
injection injectio
intellect intellectus
internal internus
intestine intestinum; enteron (Gr)
itching pruritis
jawbone maxilla
joint vertebra; arthron (Gr)
kidney ren, renis; nephros (Gr)
knee genu
kneecap patella
lacerate lacerare
larynx guttur
lateral lateralis
limb membrum
lip labium, labrum; cheilos (Gr)
listen auscultare
liver jecur; hepar (Gr)
loin lapara
looseness laxativus
lung pulmo; pneumon (Gr)
male masculinus
malignant malignons
milk lac
moisture humiditas
month mensis
monthly menstruus
mouth oris, os; stoma, stomato (Gr)

nail unguis; onyx (Gr)
navel umbilicus; omphalos (Gr)
neck cervix; trachelos (Gr)
nerve nervus; neuron (Gr)
nipple papilla; thele (Gr)
no, none nullus
nose nasus; rhis (Gr)
nostril naris
nourishment alimentum
ointment unguentum
pain dolor; algia
patient patiens
pectoral pectoralis
pimple pustula
poison venenum
powder pulvis
pregnant praegnans, gravida
pubic bone os pubis
pupil pupilla
rash exanthema (Gr)
recover convalescere
redness rubor
rib costa
ringing tinnitus
scaly squamosus
sciatica sciaticus; ischiadikos (Gr)
seed semen
senile senilis
sheath vagina; theke (Gr)
short brevis; brachys (Gr)
shoulder omos (Gr)
shoulder blade scapula
side latus
skin cutis; derma (Gr)
skull cranium; kranion (Gr)
sleep somnus
solution solutio
spinal spinalis
stomach stomachus; gaster (Gr)
stone calculus
sugar saccharum
swallow glutio
tail cauda
taste gustatio
tear lacrima
testicle testis; orchis (Gr)

*Parenthetical "Gr" means the preceding term is Greek. Other terms in the column are Latin.

thigh   femur
throat   fauces; pharynx (Gr)
tongue   lingua; glossa (Gr)
tooth   dens; odontos (Gr)
touch   tactus
tremor   tremere
twin   gemellus

ulcer   ulcus
urine   urina; ouran (Gr)
uterus   hystera (Gr)
vagina   vagina; kolpos (Gr)
vein   vena; phlebos, phleps (Gr)
vertebra   spondylos (Gr)
vessel   vas

wash   diluere
water   aqua
wax   cera
weak   debilis
windpipe   arteria aspera
wrist   carpus; karpos (Gr)

APPENDIX VI
Abbreviations Commonly Used in Medical Notations

a   before

a.c.   before meals

ADD   attention deficit disorder

ADL   activities of daily living

ad lib   as desired

ADT   admission, discharge, transfer

AIDS   acquired immunodeficiency syndrome

a.m.a.   against medical advice

AMA   American Medical Association

amp.   ampule

amt   amount

aq., AQ   water; aqueous

ausc.   auscultation

ax   axis

Bib, bib   drink

b.i.d., bid, BID   twice a day

BM   bowel movement

BP, B/P   blood pressure

BPC   blood pressure check

BPH   benign prostatic hypertrophy

BSA   body surface area

c̄., c̄   with

Ca   calcium; cancer

cap, caps   capsules

CBC   complete blood (cell) count

C.C., CC   chief complaint

CDC   Centers for Disease Control and Prevention

CHF   congestive heart failure

chr   chronic

CNS   central nervous system

Comp, comp   compound

COPD   chronic obstructive pulmonary disease

CP   chest pain

CPE   complete physical examination

CPR   cardiopulmonary resuscitation

CSF   cerebrospinal fluid

CT   computed tomography

CV   cardiovascular

d   day

D&C   dilation and curettage

DEA   Drug Enforcement Administration

Dil, dil   dilute

DM   diabetes mellitus

DOB   date of birth

DTP   diptheria-tetanus-pertussis vaccine

Dr.   doctor

DTs   delirium tremens

D/W   dextrose in water

Dx, dx   diagnosis

ECG, EKG   electrocardiogram

ED   emergency department

EEG   electroencephalogram

EENT   eyes, ears, nose, and throat

EP   established patient

ER   emergency room

ESR   erythrocyte sedimentation rate

FBS   fasting blood sugar

FDA   Food and Drug Administration

FH   family history

Fl, fl, fld   fluid

F/u   follow-up

Fx   fracture

GBS   gallbladder series

GI   gastrointestinal

Gm   gram

gr   grain

gt, gtt   drops

GTT   glucose tolerance test

GU   genitourinary

GYN   gynecology

HB, Hgb   hemoglobin

HEENT   head, ears, eyes, nose, throat

HIV   human immunodeficiency virus

HO   history of

h.s., hs, HS   hour of sleep/at bedtime

Hx   history

ICU   intensive care unit

I&D   incision and drainage

I&O   intake and output

IM   intramuscular

inf.   infusion; inferior

inj   injection

IT   inhalation therapy

IUD   intrauterine device

IV   intravenous

KUB   kidneys, ureters, bladder

L1, L2, etc.   lumbar vertebrae

lab   laboratory

liq   liquid

LLL   left lower lobe

LLQ   left lower quadrant

LMP   last menstrual period

LUQ   left upper quadrant

MI   myocardial infarction

mL   millileter

MM   mucous membrane

MRI   magnetic resonance imaging

MS   multiple sclerosis

NB   newborn

NED   no evidence of disease

no.   number

noc, noct   night

npo, NPO   nothing by mouth

NPT   new patient

NS   normal saline

NSAID   nonsteroidal anti-inflammatory drug

NTP   normal temperature and pressure

N&V   nausea and vomiting

NYD   not yet diagnosed

OB   obstetrics

OC   oral contraceptive

OD   overdose

O.D., OD   right eye

oint   ointment

OOB   out of bed

OPD   outpatient department

OPS   outpatient services

OR   operating room

O.S., OS   left eye

OTC   over-the-counter

O.U., OU   both eyes

P&P   Pap smear (Papanicolaou smear) and pelvic examination

PA   posteroanterior

Pap   Pap smear

Path   pathology

p.c., pc   after meals

PE   physical examination

per   by, with

PH   past history

PID   pelvic inflammatory disease

p/o   postoperative

POMR   problem-oriented medical record

PMFSH   past medical, family, social history

PMS   premenstrual syndrome

p.r.n., prn, PRN   whenever necessary

Pt   patient

PT   physical therapy

PTA   prior to admission

PVC   premature ventricular contraction

pulv   powder

q.   every

q2, q2h   every 2 hours

q.a.m., qam   every morning

q.h., qh   every hour

qhs   every night, at bedtime

q.i.d., QID   four times a day

qns, QNS   quantity not sufficient

qs, QS   quantity sufficient

RA   rheumatoid arthritis; right atrium

RBC   red blood cells; red blood (cell) count

RDA   recommended dietary allowance, recommended daily allowance

REM   rapid eye movement

RF   rheumatoid factor

RLL   right lower lobe

RLQ   right lower quadrant

R/O   rule out

ROM   range of motion

ROS/SR   review of systems/systems review

RUQ   right upper quadrant

RV   right ventricle

Rx   prescription, take

SAD   seasonal affective disorder

SIDS   sudden infant death syndrome

Sig   directions

sig   sigmoidoscopy

SOAP   subjective, objective, assessment, plan

SOB   shortness of breath

sol   solution

S/R   suture removal

$\overline{ss}$, $\overline{ss}$ one-half

Staph   staphylococcus

stat, STAT   immediately

STD   sexually transmitted disease

Strep   streptococcus

subling, SL   sublingual

subq, SubQ   subcutaneously

surg   surgery

S/W   saline in water

SX   symptoms

T1, T2, etc.   thoracic vertebrae

T & A   tonsillectomy and adenoidectomy

tab   tablet

TB   tuberculosis

TBS, tbs.   tablespoon

TIA   transient ischemic attack

t.i.d., tid, TID   three times a day

tinc, tinct, tr   tincture

TMJ   temporomandibular joint

top   topically

TPR   temperature, pulse, and respiration

TSH   thyroid stimulating hormone

tsp   teaspoon

Tx   treatment

UA   urinalysis

UCHD   usual childhood diseases

UGI   upper gastrointestinal

ung, ungt   ointment

URI   upper respiratory infection

US   ultrasound

UTI   urinary tract infection

VA   visual acuity

VD   venereal disease

Vf   visual field

VS   vital signs

WBC   white blood cells; white blood (cell) count

WNL   within normal limits

wt   weight

y/o   year old

APPENDIX VII
Symbols Commonly Used in Medical Notations

Apothecaries' Weights and Measures

ʒ dram
℥ ounce
fʒ fluidounce
O pint
lb pound

Other Weights and Measures

pounds
° degrees
′ foot; minute
″ inch; second
μm micrometer
μ micron (former term for micrometer)
mμ millimicron; nanometer
mEq milliequivalent
mL milliliter
dL deciliter
mg% milligrams percent; milligrams per 100 mL

Abbreviations

a̅a̅, A̅A̅ of each
c̅ with
M mix (Latin *misce*)
m- meta-
o- ortho-

p- para-
p̅ after
s̅ without
ss, s̅s̅ one-half (Latin *semis*)

Mathematical Functions and Terms

number
+ plus; positive; acid reaction
− minus; negative; alkaline reaction
± plus or minus; either positive or negative; indefinite
× multiply; magnification; crossed with, hybrid
÷ , / divided by
= equal to
≈ approximately equal to
> greater than; from which is derived
< less than; derived from
≮ not less than
≯ not greater than
≤ equal to or less than
≥ equal to or greater than
≠ not equal to
√ square root
₃√ cube root
∞ infinity
: ratio; "is to"
∴ therefore

% percent
π pi (3.14159)—the ratio of circumference of a circle to its diameter

Chemical Notations

Δ change; heat
⇌ reversible reaction
↑ increase
↓ decrease

Warnings

Ⓒ Schedule I controlled substance
Ⓒ Schedule II controlled substance
Ⓒ Schedule III controlled substance
Ⓒ Schedule IV controlled substance
Ⓒ Schedule V controlled substance
☠ poison
☢ radiation
☣ biohazard

Others

℞ prescription; take
□, ♂ male
○, ♀ female
† one
†† two
††† three

APPENDIX VIII
Professional Organizations and Agencies

American Academy of Dental Practice Administrators
1063 Whippoorwill Lane
Palatine, IL 60067
(847) 934-4404

American Academy of Medical Administrators
30555 Southfield Road, Suite 150
Southfield, MI 48076
(313) 540-4310

American Academy of Ophthalmology
655 Beach Street
San Francisco, CA 94109
(415) 561-8500

American Academy of Pediatrics
141 Northwest Point Blvd.
Elk Grove, IL 60007-1098
(847) 434-4000

American Academy of Professional Coders (AAPC)
2480 South 3850 West, Suite B
Salt Lake City, UT. 84120
(800) 626-CODE (2633)

American Association for Medical Transcription
PO Box 576187
Modesto, CA 95355
(209) 527-9620

American Association for Respiratory Care
9425 McArthur Blvd, Suite 100
Irving, TX 75063
(972) 243-2272

American Association of Medical Assistants
20 N. Wacker Drive
Suite 1575
Chicago, IL 60606
(312) 899-1500

American Cancer Society
777 Third Avenue
New York, NY 10017
(212) 586-8700

American Collectors Association International
ACA International
P.O. Box 390106
Minneapolis, MN 55439
(952) 926–6547

American College of Cardiology
9111 Old Georgetown Road
Bethesda, MD 20814
(301) 897-5400

American College of Physicians
2011 Pennsylvania Avenue NW
Washington, DC 20006
(202) 261-4500

American Diabetes Association
1701 North Beauregard Street
Alexandria, VA 22311
(800) 342-2383

American Dietetic Association
120 South Riverside Plaza, Suite 2000
Chicago, Illinois 60606-6995
(800) 877-1600

American Health Information Management Association (formerly the American Medical Record Association)
233 N. Michigan Avenue, 21st Floor
Chicago, IL 60601-5800
(312) 233-1100

American Heart Association
National Center
7272 Greenville Avenue
Dallas, TX 75231-4596
(800) 242-8721, or call your local center

American Hospital Association
One North Franklin
Suite 2706
Chicago, IL 60606-3421
(312) 422-3000

American Lung Association
61 Broadway, 6th Floor
New York, NY 10006
(212) 315-8700 or 1-800-LUNGUSA

American Medical Association Division of Allied Health Education and Accreditation
515 North State Street
Chicago, IL 60610
(800) 621-8335

American Medical Technologists
10700 West Higgins Road
Suite 150
Rosemont, IL 60018
(847) 823-5169

American Occupational Therapy Association
4720 Montgomery Lane
PO Box 31220
Bethesda, MD 20824-1220
(301) 652-2682
TDD: (800) 377-8555

American Pharmacists Association
2215 Constitution Avenue NW
Washington, DC 20037-2985
(202) 628-4410

American Physical Therapy Association/Foundation for Physical Therapy
1111 North Fairfax Street
Alexandria, VA 22314
(703) 684-2782

American Red Cross
2025 E Street, NW
Washington, DC 20006
(202) 303-4498, or call your local chapter

American Red Cross
HIV/AIDS Education, Health and Safety
  Services
8111 Gatehouse Road
6th Floor
Falls Church, VA 22042
(703) 206-7180

American Society for Cardiovascular Professionals
120 Falcon Drive, Unit 3
Fredericksburg, VA 22408
(540) 891-0079

American Society for Clinical Laboratory Science
7910 Woodmont Avenue
Suite 1301
Bethesda, MD 20814
(301) 657-2768

American Society of Clinical Pathologists
33 West Monroe, Suite 1600
Chicago, IL 60603
(312) 541-4999

American Society of Hand Therapists
401 North Michigan Avenue
Chicago, IL 60611-4267
(312) 321-6866

American Society of Phlebotomy Technicians
PO Box 1831
Hickory, NC 28603
(704) 322-1334

American Society of Radiologic Technologists
15000 Central Avenue SE
Albuquerque, NM 87123
(505) 298-4500

Anorexia Nervosa and Related Eating Disorders
Box 7
Highland Park, IL 60035
(847) 831-3438

The Arthritis Foundation
1314 Spring Street, NW
Atlanta, GA 30309
(404) 872-7100

Association of Surgical Technologists
6 West Dry Creek Circle
Littleton, CO 80120
(303) 694-9130

Association of Technical Personnel in Ophthalmology
50 Lee Road
Chestnut Hill, MA 02167
(617) 232-4433

Asthma and Allergy Foundation of America
1717 Massachusetts Avenue
Suite 305
Washington, DC 20036
(202) 265-0265

International Society for Clinical Laboratory Technology
818 Olive Street
Suite 918
St. Louis, MO 63101
(314) 241-1445

Joint Commission on Allied Health Personnel in Ophthalmology
2025 Woodlane Drive
St. Paul, MN 55125-2995
(800) 284-3937

Medical Collection Agency
517 S. Livingston Ave.
Livingston, NJ 07039
Toll Free: 1-877-77-Collect
Phone: 1-973-740-0044

Medical Group Management Association
104 Inverness Terrace East
Englewood Cliffs, CA 80112
(313) 799-1111

National Accrediting Agency for Clinical Laboratory Services
8410 West Bryn Mawr Avenue
Suite 670
Chicago, IL 60631
(773) 714-8880

National AIDS Hotline
215 Park Avenue South, Suite 714
New York, NY 10003
(800) 342-AIDS
(800) 344-SIDA (Spanish)

National Association of Anorexia Nervosa and Associated Disorders
Box 7
Highland Park, IL 60035
(847) 831-3438

National Association of Medical Staff Services
PO Box 23590
Knoxville, TN 37933-1590
(615) 531-3571

National Cancer Institute
9000 Rockville Pike Building 31
Room 10A18
Bethesda, MD 20205
(800) 4-CANCER

National Clearinghouse for Alcohol and Drug Information
PO Box 2345
Rockville, MD 20852
(301) 468-2600

National Eating Disorders Association
603 Stewart Street
Suite 803
Seattle, WA 98101
(206) 382-3587

National Healthcare Association
134 Evergreen Place, 9th Floor
East Orange, NJ 07018
(800) 499-9092

National Health Council
1730 Street NW
Suite 500
Washington, DC 20036
(202) 785-3910

National Health Information Center
PO Box 1133
Washington, DC 20013-1133
(800) 336-4797

National Institute of Mental Health Office of Communications
6001 Executive Boulevard
Room 8184, MSC 9663
Bethesda, MD 20892-9663
(301) 443-4513

National Institute on Aging
Building 31, Room 5C27
31 Center Drive, MSC 2292
Bethesda, MD 20892
(301) 496-1752

National Kidney Foundation
30 East 33rd Street
New York, NY 10016
(212) 889-2210

National Mental Health Association
2001 N. Beauregard Street, 12th Floor
Alexandria, VA 22311
(703) 684-7722

National Organization for Rare Disorders
100 Route 37
PO Box 8923
New Fairfield, CT 06812
(800) 999-NORD

National Phlebotomy Association
1901 Brightseat Road
Landover, MD 20785
(866) 329-9108

National Rehabilitation Association
633 South Washington Street
Alexandria, VA 22314
(703) 836-0850

National Society for Histotechnology
4201 Northview Drive
Suite 502
Bowie, MD 20716-1073
(301) 262-6221

Overeaters Anonymous (OA)
P. O. Box 44020
Rio Rancho, NM 87174
(505) 891-2664

President's Council on Physical Fitness and Sports
Department of Health and Human
    Services
Washington, DC 20001
(202) 272-3421

Society of Diagnostic Medical Sonographers
2745 Dallas Pkwy, Suite 350
Plano, TX 75093-8730
(214) 473-8057 or (800) 229-9506

GLOSSARY

Note: (†) Pronunciation from *Stedman's Medical Dictionary*, 26th edition; all others from *American Heritage*, 4th edition, in case you need to consult.

10× lens (tĕn) A magnifying lens in the ocular of a microscope that magnifies an image ten times.

24-hour urine specimen (twĕnt̄ē fôr our yŏŏr´ in spĕs´ ə-mən) A urine specimen collected over a 24-hour period and used to complete a quantitative and qualitative analysis of one or more substances, such as sodium, chloride, and calcium.

abandonment (ə-băn´dən-mənt) A situation in which a health-care professional stops caring for a patient without arranging for care by an equally qualified substitute.

ABA number (nŭm´ber) A fraction appearing in the upper right corner of all printed checks that identifies the geographic area and specific bank on which the check is drawn.

abduction (ab-dŭk´shuň)(†) Movement away from the body.

abscess (ăb´sĕs´) A collection of pus (white blood cells, bacteria, and dead skin cells) that forms as a result of infection.

absorption (əb-sôrp´shən) The process by which one substance is absorbed, or taken in and incorporated, into another, as when the body converts food or drugs into a form it can use.

abuse (ə-byŏŏz´) A practice or behavior that is not indicative of or in line with sound medical or fiscal activity.

access (ăk´sĕs) The way patients enter and exit a medical office.

accessibility (ăk-sĕs´ə-bĭl´ĭ-tē) The ease with which people can move into and out of a space.

accommodation (ă-kom´ə-dā-shən) The ability of the lens to change shape, allowing the eye to focus images of objects that are near or far away.

accounts payable (ə-kounts´ pā´-ă-bəl) Money owed by a business; the practice's expenses.

accounts receivable (ə-kounts´ rĭ-sē´ və-bəl) Income or money owed to a business.

accreditation (ə-krĕd´ĭ-tā´shən) The documentation of official authorization or approval of a program.

acetabulum (as´ətab´yələm) The hip socket.

acetylcholine (as-e-til-kō´lēn)(†) A neurotransmitter released by the parasympathetic nerves onto organs and glands for resting and digesting.

acetylcholinesterase (as´e-til-kō-lin-es´ter-ās) An enzyme within the nervous system that hydrolyzes acetylcholine to acetate and choline.

acid-fast stain (ăs´ĭd făst stān) A staining procedure for identifying bacteria that have a waxy cell wall.

acids (ăs´ĭds) Electrolytes that release hydrogen ions in water.

acinar cells (as´i-nar sĕlz)(†) Cells in the pancreas that produce pancreatic juice.

acquired immunodeficiency syndrome (AIDS) (ə-kwīrd im´yū-nō-dē-fĭsh´en-sē sĭn´drōm´)(†) The most advanced stage of HIV infection; it severely weakens the body's immune system.

acromegaly (ak-rō-meg´ă-lē)(†) A disorder in which too much growth hormone is produced in adults.

acrosome (ak´rō-sōm)(†) An enzyme-filled sac covering the head of a sperm that aids in the penetration of the egg during fertilization.

action potential (ăk´shən pə-tĕn´shəl) The flow of electrical current along the axon membrane.

active file (ăk´tĭv fĭl) A file used on a consistent basis.

active listening (ăk´tĭv lĭs´ənĭng) Part of two-way communication, such as offering feedback or asking questions; contrast with **passive listening.**

active transport (ak´-tiv trans-pórt) The movement of a substance across a cell membrane from an area of low concentration to an area of high concentration.

acupressure (ak-you-presh-er) Pressure applied by hands to various areas of the body to restore balance in the body's energy flow.

acupuncture (ak-you-punk-chūr) The practice of inserting needles into various areas of the body to restore balance in the body's energy flow.

acupuncturist (ăk´yŏŏ-pŭngk´chər-ĭst) A practitioner of acupuncture. The acupuncturist uses hollow needles inserted into the patient's skin to treat pain, discomfort, or systemic imbalances.

acute (ə-kyŏŏt´) Having a rapid onset and progress, as acute appendicitis.

addiction (ă-dĭk′shun)(†) A physical or psychological dependence on a substance, usually involving a pattern of behavior that includes obsessive or compulsive preoccupation with the substance and the security of its supply, as well as a high rate of relapse after withdrawal.

Addison's disease (ă-dĭsuns dĭzēz) A condition in which the adrenal glands fail to produce enough corticosteroids.

add-on code (ăd′on′ kōd) A code indicating procedures that are usually carried out in addition to another procedure. Add-on codes are used together with the primary code.

adduction (ă-dŭk′shŭn)(†) Movement toward the body.

adenoids (ăd′n-oidz′) See **pharyngeal tonsils.**

adjustment (ə-jŭst′-ment) Manual treatments given by a chiropractor that move the joints of the spine and other joints into proper alignment.

administer (ăd-mĭn′ĭ-stər) To give a drug directly by injection, by mouth, or by any other route that introduces the drug into the body.

adrenocorticotropic hormone (ACTH) (ă-drē′nō-kōr′ti-kō-trō′pik hor′mōn) Hormone that stimulates the adrenal cortex to release its hormones.

advance scheduling (ăd-văns skĕj′ōōl-ĭng) Booking an appointment several weeks or even months in advance.

aerobes (ăr′ōbs′) Bacteria that grow best in the presence of oxygen.

aerobic respiration (â-rō′bĭk rĕs′pə-rā′shən) A process that requires large amounts of oxygen and uses glucose to make ATP.

afebrile (ā-feb′ril)(†) Having a body temperature within one's normal range.

afferent arterioles (ăf′ər-ənt ar-tēr′ē-ōlz)(†) Structures that deliver blood to the glomeruli of the kidneys.

afferent nerves (ăf′ər-ənt nûrvs) A type of sensory nerves are responsible for detecting sensory information from the environment or even from inside the body and bringing it to the CNS for interpretation.

affiliation agreement (ə-fĭl′ē-ā′shən ə-grē′mənt) An agreement that externship participants must sign that states the expectations of the facility and the expectations of the student.

agar (ā′gär′) A gelatin-like substance derived from seaweed that gives a culture medium its semisolid consistency.

age analysis (āj ə-năl′ĭ-sĭs) The process of clarifying and reviewing past due accounts by age from the first date of billing.

agenda (ə-jĕn′də) The list of topics discussed or presented at a meeting, in order of presentation.

agent (ā′jənt) (legal) A person who acts on a physician's behalf while performing professional tasks; (clinical) an active principal or entity that produces a certain effect, for example, an infectious agent.

agglutination (ă-glū-ti-nā′shŭn)(†) The clumping of red blood cells following a blood transfusion.

aggressive (ə-grĕs′ĭv) Imposing one's position on others or trying to manipulate them.

agonist (ăg′ənist) See **antagonist.**

agranular leukocyte (ă-gran′-yulər lū′kō-sīt)(†) A type of leukocyte (white blood cell) with a solid nucleus and clear cytoplasm; includes lymphocytes and monocytes.

agranulocyte (ă-gran′yū-lō-sīt)(†) See **agranular leukocyte.**

albumins (ăl-byōō′mĭns) The smallest of the plasma proteins. Albumins are important for pulling water into the bloodstream to help maintain blood pressure.

aldosterone (al-dos′ter-ōn)(†) A hormone produced in the adrenal glands that acts on the kidney. It causes the body to retain sodium and excrete potassium. Its role is to maintain blood volume and pressure.

alimentary canal (ăl′ə-mĕn′tə-rē kə-năl′) The organs of the digestive system that extend from the mouth to the anus.

allele (ə-lēl′) Any one of a pair or series of **genes** that occupy a specific position on a specific **chromosome.**

allergen (ăl′ər-jən) An antigen that induces an allergic reaction.

allergic rhinitis (al′ərjik rīni′tis) A hypersensitivity reaction to various airborne allergens.

allergist (ăl′ər-jĭst) A specialist who diagnoses and treats physical reactions to substances including mold, dust, fur, pollen, foods, drugs, and chemicals.

allopathy (ə-lō-păth-ē) The usual medical practice of physicians and other health professionals; also known as conventional medicine.

allowed charge (ə-loud′ chärj) The amount that is the most the payer will pay any provider for each procedure or service.

alopecia (ăl′ə-pē′shə) The clinical term for baldness.

alphabetic filing system (ăl′fə-bĕt′ĭk fī′lĭng sis′təm) A filing system in which the files are arranged in alphabetic order, with the patient's last name first, followed by the first name and middle initial.

Alphabetic Index (ăl′fə-bĕt′ĭk ĭn′dĕks′) One of two ways diagnoses are listed in the ICD-9-CM. They appear in alphabetic order with their corresponding diagnosis codes.

alternative medicine (ôl-tûr′-nə-tĭv mĕd′-ĭ-sĭn) The type of medicine used in place of conventional medicine to promote health and treat disease.

alveolar glands (al-vē´ō-lăr glăndz)(†) Glands that make milk under the influence of the hormone **prolactin.**

alveoli (ăl-vē´ə-lī´) Clusters of air sacs in which the exchange of gases between air and blood takes place; located in the lungs.

American Association of Medical Assistants (AAMA) (ə-měr´ĭkən ə-sō´sē-ā´shən měd´ĭ-kəl ə-sĭs´tənts) The professional organization that certifies medical assistants and works to maintain professional standards in the medical assisting profession.

Americans With Disabilities Act (ADA) (ə-měr´ĭ-kəns dĭs´ə-bĭl´ĭ-tēs ăkt) A U.S. civil rights act forbidding discrimination against people because of a physical or mental handicap.

amblyopia (am-blē-ō´pē-ă)(†) Poor vision in one eye without a detectable cause.

amino acids (ə-mē´nō ăs´ĭds) Natural organic compounds found in plant and animal foods and used by the body to create protein.

amnion (ăm´nē-ən) The innermost membrane enveloping the embryo and containing amniotic fluid.

anabolism (ənab´əlĭz´əm) The stage of metabolism in which substances such as nutrients are changed into more complex substances and used to build body tissues.

anaerobe (ăn´ə-rōb´) A bacterium that grows best in the absence of oxygen.

anal canal (ā´nəl kə-năl´) The last few centimeters of the rectum.

anaphase (an´əfāz) The period of mitosis when the centromeres divide and pull the chromosomes (formerly chromatids) toward the centrioles at opposite sides of the cell.

anaphylaxis (an´ă-fī-lak´sis) A severe allergic reaction with symptoms that include respiratory distress, difficulty in swallowing, pallor, and a drastic drop in blood pressure that can lead to circulatory collapse.

anatomical position (ăn´ə-tŏm´ĭ-kəl pə-zĭsh´ən) When the body is standing upright and facing forward with the arms at the side and the palms of the hands facing forward.

anatomy (ə-năt´ə-mē) The scientific term for the study of body structure.

anemia (ə-nē´mē-ə) A condition characterized by low red blood cell count. This condition decreases the ability to transport oxygen throughout the body.

anergic reaction (an-er´jik rē-ăk´shən) A lack of response to skin testing that indicates the body's inability to mount a normal response to invasion by a pathogen.

anesthesia (ăn´ĭs-thē´zhə) A loss of sensation, particularly the feeling of pain.

anesthetic (ăn´ĭs-thĕt´ik) A medication that causes anesthesia.

anesthetist (ă-nes´thĕ-tist)(†) A specialist who uses medications to cause patients to lose sensation or feeling during surgery.

aneurysm (ăn´yə-rĭz´əm) A serious and potentially life-threatening bulge in the wall of a blood vessel.

angiography (an-jē-og´ră-fē)(†) An x-ray examination of a blood vessel, performed after the injection of a contrast medium, that evaluates the function and structure of one or more arteries or veins.

annotate (ăn´ō-tāt´) To underline or highlight key points of a document or to write reminders, make comments, and suggest actions in the margins.

anorexia nervosa (ăn´ə-rĕk´sē-ə nûr-vō´sə) An eating disorder in which people starve themselves because they fear that if they lose control of eating they will become grossly overweight.

antagonist (ăn-tăg´ə-nĭst) A muscle that produces the opposite movement of the **prime mover.**

antecubital space (an-te-kyū´bi-tăl spās) The inner side or bend of the elbow; the site at which the brachial artery is felt or heard when a pulse or blood pressure is taken.

anterior (ăn-tîr´ē-ər) Anatomical term meaning toward the front of the body; also called ventral.

anthracosis (an´thrə kō´sis) Chronic lung disease caused by the inhalation of coal deposits; also known as Black Lung Disease.

antibodies (ăn´tĭ-bod´ēs) Highly specific proteins that attach themselves to foreign substances in an initial step in destroying such substances, as part of the body's defenses.

antidiuretic hormone (ADH) (an´tē-dī-yū-ret´ik hôr´mōn´)(†) A hormone that increases water reabsorption, which decreases urine production and helps to maintain blood pressure.

antigen (an´tĭ-jən) A foreign substance that stimulates white blood cells to create antibodies when it enters the body.

antihistamines (ăn´tē-hĭs´tə-mēnz) Medications used to treat allergies.

antimicrobial (an´tē-mī-krō´bē-ăl)(†) An agent that kills microorganisms or suppresses their growth.

antioxidants (ăn´tē-ŏk´sĭ-dənt) Chemical agents that fight cell-destroying chemical substances called free radicals.

antiseptic (ăn´tĭ-sĕp´tĭk) A cleaning product used on human tissue as an anti-infection agent.

anuria (an-yū´rē-ă)(†) The absence of urine production.

aortic semilunar valve (ā ôr´tĭk sem´ē loonər valv) Heart valve that is a semilunar valve and that is situated between the left ventricle and the aorta.

apex (ā′pĕks) The left lower corner of the heart, where the strongest heart sounds can be heard.

apical (ap′i-kăl)(†) Located at the **apex** of the heart.

apnea (an′nēə) The absence of respiration.

apocrine gland (ap′ō-krin glănd)(†) A type of sweat gland. It produces a thicker type of sweat than other sweat glands and contains more proteins.

aponeurosis (ap′ō-nū-rō′sis)(†) A tough, sheet-like structure that is made of fibrous connective tissue. It typically attaches muscles to other muscles.

appendicitis (ə-pĕn′dĭ-sī′t ĭs) Inflammation of the appendix.

appendicular (ap′en-dik′yū-lăr) The division of the skeletal system that consists of the bones of the arms, legs, pectoral girdle, and pelvic girdle.

approximate (a-prŏk′s i măt) To bring the edges of a wound together so the tissue surfaces are close in order to protect the area from further contamination and to minimize scar and scab formation.

aqueous humor (a′kwē-əs hyo͞o′mər) A liquid produced by the eye's ciliary body that fills the space between the cornea and the lens.

arbitration (är′bĭ-trā′shən) A process in which opposing sides choose a person or persons outside the court system, often someone with special knowledge in the field, to hear and decide a dispute.

areflexia (ā-rē-flek′sē-ă)(†) The absence of reflexes.

areola (ă-rē′ō-lă)(†) The pigmented area that surrounds the nipple.

aromatherapy (a-rō′-mə-thēr′-ə-pē) The use of essential oil extracts or essences from flowers, herbs, and trees to promote health and well-being.

arrector pili (ă-rek′tōr pī′lī)(†) Muscles attached to most hair follicles and found in the dermis.

arrhythmia (ə-rĭth′mē-ə) Irregularity in heart rhythm.

arterial blood gases (är-tîr′ē-əl blŭd găs′ses) A test that measures the amount of gases, such as oxygen and carbon dioxide, dissolved in arterial blood.

arthritis (arth rīt′is) A general term meaning joint inflammation.

arthrography (ar-throg′ră-fē)(†) A radiologic procedure performed by a radiologist, who uses a contrast medium and fluoroscopy to help diagnose abnormalities or injuries in the cartilage, tendons, or ligaments of the joints— usually the knee or shoulder.

arthroscopy (är-thŏs′kə-pē) A procedure in which an orthopedist examines a joint, usually the knee or shoulder, with a tubular instrument called an arthroscope; also used to guide surgical procedures.

articular cartilage (ar-tik′yu-lăr kär′tl-ĭj) (†) The cartilage that covers the **epiphysis** of long bones.

articulations (ärtik′yəla′shəns) The area where bones are joined together; joints.

artifact (är′tə-făkt′) Any irrelevant object or mark observed when examining specimens or graphic records that is not related to the object being examined; for example, a foreign object visible through a microscope or an erroneous mark on an ECG strip.

asbestosis (asbestō′sis) Chronic lung disease caused by the inhalation of asbestos fibers.

ascending colon (ə-sĕnd′ing ko′lən) The segment of the large intestine that runs up the right side of the abdominal cavity.

ascending tracts (ə-sĕnd′ing trăkts) The tracts of the spinal cord that carry sensory information to the brain.

asepsis (ă-sep′sis)(†) The condition in which pathogens are absent or controlled.

assault (ə-sôlt′) The open threat of bodily harm to another.

assertive (ə-sûrt′tĭv) Being firm and standing up for oneself while showing respect for others.

asset (ăs′ĕt′) An item owned by the practice that has a dollar value, such as the medical practice building, office equipment, or accounts receivable.

assignment of benefits (ə-sīn′mənt bĕn′ə-fĭts) An authorization for an insurance carrier to pay a physician or practice directly.

asthma (az′mə) A condition in which the tubes of the bronchial tree become obstructed due to inflammation.

astigmatism (ə-stĭg′mə-tĭz′əm) A condition in which the cornea has an abnormal shape, which causes blurred images during near or distant vision.

astrocytes (ăs′-trō-sīts) Star-shaped cells within the nervous system that anchor blood vessels to the nerve cells.

atelectasis (at′ilek′təsis) The collapse of a lung because of fluid, air, pus, or blood.

atherosclerosis (ăth′ə-rō-sklə-rō′sĭs) The accumulation of fatty deposits along the inner walls of arteries.

atlas (ăt′ləs) The first cervical vertebra.

atoms (ăt′əmz) The simplest units of all matter.

atria (ā′trē-ă)(†) [*Singular:* **atrium**] Chambers of the heart that receive blood from the veins and circulate it to the ventricles.

atrial natriuretic peptide (ā′trē-ăl nā′trēyū-ret′ik pep′tīd)(†) A hormone secreted by the heart that regulates blood pressure.

atrioventricular bundle (ā′trē-ō-ventrik′yū-lar bŭn′dl)(†) A structure that is located between the ventricles of the heart and that sends the electrical impulse to the Purkinje fibers.

atrioventricular node (ā´trē-ō-ventrik´yū-lar nōd) A node that is located between the atria of the heart. After the electrical impulse reaches the atrioventricular node, the atria contract and the impulse is sent to the ventricles.

atrioventricular septum (a´treo-ventrik´yu-lar səp´təm) The wall separating the upper atrial chambers from the lower ventricular chambers of the heart.

audiologist (aw-dē-ol´ōjist)(†) A health-care specialist who focuses on evaluating and correcting hearing problems.

audiometer (aw-dē-om´ĕ-ter) An electronic device that measures hearing acuity by producing sounds in specific frequencies and intensities.

auricle (ôr´ĭ-kəl) The outside part of the ear, made of cartilage and covered with skin.

auscultated blood pressure (ô´skəl-tāt-ĕd blŭd prĕsh´ər) Blood pressure as measured by listening with a stethoscope.

auscultation (ô´skəl-tā´shən) The process of listening to body sounds.

authorization (ô´thər-ĭ-zā´shən) A form that explains in detail the standards for the use and disclosure of patient information for purposes other than treatment, payment, or health-care operations.

autoclave (aw´tō-klāv)(†) A device that uses pressurized steam to sterilize instruments and equipment.

autoimmune disease (aw´tō-ĭmyoŏn di-zēz´) Any condition in which the body attacks its own antigens, causing illness to the patient.

automated external defibrillator (AED) (ô´tə-mā´tĭd ĭk-stûr´nəl dē-fib´ri-lā-ter) A computerized defibrillator programmed to recognize lethal heart rhythms and deliver an electrical shock to restore a normal rhythm.

autonomic (ô´tə-nŏm´ĭk) A division of the peripheral nervous system that connects the central nervous system to viscera such as the heart, stomach, intestines, glands, blood vessels, and bladder.

autonomic nervous system (ANS) (ô´tə-nŏm´ĭk nūr´vəs sĭs´təm) A system that is in charge of the body's automatic functions, such as the respiratory and gastrointestinal systems.

autopsy (ô-top´-sē) The examination of a cadaver to determine or confirm the cause of death.

autosome (ô´tə-sōm´) A chromosome that is not a sex chromosome.

axial (ăk´sē-əl) The division of the skeletal system that consists of the skull, vertebral column, and rib cage.

axilla (ăk-sĭl´ə) Armpit; one of the four locations for temperature readings.

axis (ak´-səs) The second vertebra of the neck on which the head turns.

axon (ăk´sŏn´) A type of nerve fiber that is typically long and branches far from the cell body. Its function is to send information away from the cell body.

Ayurveda (eye-yer-vay-duh) A form of medicine, originated in India, that uses herbal preparations, dietary changes, exercises, and meditation to restore health and promote well-being.

bacillus (ba-sil´ŭs)(†) A rod-shaped bacterium.

bacterial spore (băk-tîr´ēăl spôr) A primitive, thick-walled reproductive body capable of developing into a new individual; resistant to killing through disinfection.

balance billing (băl´əns bĭl´ĭng) Billing a patient for the difference between a higher usual fee and a lower allowed charge.

balloon angioplasty (buh-loon an´je-o-plas´te-) A procedure using a slender, hollow tube passed through a coronary artery to compress a blockage in the artery.

bandwidth (bānd´wĭdth´) A measurement, calculated in bits or bytes, of how much information can be sent or processed with one single instruction.

barium enema (bâr´ē-əm ĕn´ə-mə) A radiologic procedure performed by a radiologist who administers barium sulfate through the anus, into the rectum, and then into the colon to help diagnose and evaluate obstructions, ulcers, polyps, diverticulosis, tumors, or motility problems of the colon or rectum; also called a lower GI (gastrointestinal) series.

barium swallow (bâr´ē-əm swŏl´ō) A radiologic procedure that involves oral administration of a barium sulfate drink to help diagnose and evaluate obstructions, ulcers, polyps, diverticulosis, tumors, or motility problems of the esophagus, stomach, duodenum, and small intestine; also called an upper GI (gastrointestinal) series.

baroreceptors (bar´ō-rē-sep´ters)(†) Structures, located in the aorta and carotid arteries, that help regulate blood pressure.

Bartholin's glands (bär´ tə linz glăndz) Glands lateral to the vagina that produce mucus for lubrication of the vagina.

bases (bā´sēz´) Electrolytes that release hydroxyl ions in water.

basophil (bā-sō-fil)(†) A type of granular leukocyte that produces the chemical histamine, which aids the body in controlling allergic reactions and other exaggerated immunologic responses.

battery (băt´ə-rē) An action that causes bodily harm to another.

behavior modification (bĭ-hāv´yər mŏd´ə-fī-kā-shən) The altering of personal habits to promote a healthier lifestyle.

benefits (bĕn´ə-fĭts) Payments for medical services.

benign (bē-nīn´) A noncancerous or nonmalignant growth or condition.

benign prostatic hypertrophy (bē nīn´ pros-tat´ik hī pur´trə fē) A noncancerous enlargement of the prostate gland.

bicarbonate ions (bī-kar´bon-āt ī´onz) Elements formed when carbon dioxide gets into the bloodstream and reacts with water. In the alimentary canal, these ions neutralize acidic chyme arriving from the stomach.

bicuspids (bī-kŭs´pĭds) Teeth with two cusps. There are two in front of each set of molars.

bicuspid valve (bī-kŭs´pĭd vălv) Heart valve that has two cusps and that is located between the left atrium and the left ventricle. Also known as the mitral valve.

bile (bīl) A substance created in the liver and stored in the gallbladder. Bile is a bitter yellow-green fluid that is used in the digestion of fats.

bilirubin (bili-rū´bin)(†) A bile pigment formed by the breakdown of hemoglobin in the liver.

bilirubinuria (bil´i-rū-bi-nū´rē-ă)(†) The presence of bilirubin in the urine; one of the first signs of liver disease or conditions that involve the liver.

biliverdin (bil-i-ver´din)(†) A pigment released when a red blood cell is destroyed.

biochemistry (bī´ō-kĕm´ĭ-strē) The study of matter and chemical reactions in the body.

bioelectromagnetic-based therapies (bī´ō-ī-lĕk´trĭk basĕd thĕr´-ə-pēs) The use of measurable energy fields in such things as magnetic therapy, millimeter wave therapy, sound energy therapy, and light therapy.

bioethics (bī-ō-ĕth´ĭks) Principles of right and wrong in issues that arise from medical advances.

biofeedback (bī-ō-fēd´-bāk) A type of therapy in which an individual learns how to control involuntary body responses in order to promote health and treat disease.

biofield therapies (bī-ō-field thĕr´-ə-pēs) Treatments that affect the energy fields that surround and penetrate the human body in order to promote health and well-being.

biohazard symbol (bī-ō-hăz´ərd sĭm´bəl) A symbol that must appear on all containers used to store waste products, blood, blood products, or other specimens that may be infectious.

biohazardous materials (bī-ō-hăz´ərd-əs mə-tîr´ə-əls) Biological agents that can spread disease to living things.

biohazardous waste container (bī-ō-hăz´ərd-əs wāst kən-tā´nər) A leakproof, puncture-resistant container, color-coded red or labeled with a special biohazard symbol, that is used to store and dispose of contaminated supplies and equipment.

biopsy (bī-op´-sē) The removal and examination of a sample of tissue from a living body for diagnostic purposes.

biopsy specimen (bī´ŏp´sē spĕs´ə-mən) A small amount of tissue removed from the body for examination under a microscope to diagnose an illness.

bioterrorism (bī-ō´tĕr´ə-rĭz´əm) The intentional release of a biologic agent with the intent to harm individuals.

birthday rule (bûrth´dā´rool) A rule that states that the insurance policy of a policyholder whose birthday comes first in the year is the primary payer for all dependents.

blastocyst (blas´tō-sist) A morula that travels down the uterine tube to the uterus and is invaded with fluid. It then implants into the wall of the uterus.

blood-borne pathogen (blŭd-bôrn păth´ə-jən) A disease-causing microorganism carried in a host's blood and transmitted through contact with infected blood, tissue, or body fluids.

blood-brain barrier (blŭd brān băr´ē-ər) A structure that is formed from tight capillaries to protect the tissues of the central nervous system from certain substances.

B lymphocyte (bē lĭm´fə-sīt´) A type of nongranular leukocyte that produces antibodies to combat specific pathogens.

body (bod-ee) Single-spaced lines of text that are the content of a business letter.

body language (bŏd´ē lăng´gwĭj) Nonverbal communication, including facial expressions, eye contact, posture, touch, and attention to personal space.

bolus (bō´ləs) The mass created when food is combined with saliva and mucus.

bone conduction (bōnkən-dŭk´shən) The process by which sound waves pass through the bones of the skull directly to the inner ear, bypassing the outer and middle ears.

bookkeeping (book´kē´pĭng) The systematic recording of business transactions.

botulism (bŏch´ə-lĭz´əm) A life-threatening type of food poisoning that results from eating improperly canned or preserved foods that have been contaminated with the bacterium *Clostridium botulinum*.

Bowman's capsule (bō´mənz kap´səl) A capsule that surrounds the **glomerulus** of the kidney.

brachial artery (brāke´əl är´tə-rē) An artery that provides a palpable pulse and audible vascular sounds in the antecubital space (the bend of the elbow).

brachytherapy (brak-ē-thār´ə-pē´)(†) A radiation therapy technique in which a radiologist places temporary radioactive implants close to or directly into cancerous tissue; used for treating localized cancers.

bradycardia (braid uh card e uh) A slow heart rate; usually less than 60 beats per minute.

brain stem (brān stēm) A structure that connects the cerebrum to the spinal cord.

breach of contract (brēch kŏn′trăkt′) The violation of or failure to live up to a contract's terms.

bronchi (brŏn-kī) The two branches of the trachea that enter the lungs.

bronchial tree (brŏng′kē-al trē) A series of tubes that begins where the distal end of the trachea branches.

bronchioles (brŏng′kē-ōlz) A part of the respiratory tract that branches from the tertiary bronchi.

buccal (bŭk′ăl)(†) Between the cheek and gum.

buffy coat (buf′ē kōt) The layer between the packed red blood cells and plasma in a centrifuged blood sample; this layer contains the white blood cells and platelets.

bulbourethral glands (bŭl′bō-yū-rē′thrăl glăndz)(†) Glands that lie beneath the prostate and empty their fluid into the urethra. Their fluid aids in sperm movement.

bulimia (boo-lē′mē-ə) An eating disorder in which people eat a large quantity of food in a short period of time (bingeing) and then attempt to counter the effects of bingeing by self-induced vomiting, use of laxatives or diuretics, and/or excessive exercise.

bundle of His (bēn′ dl ov hiss) Also known as the AV bundle, this is the node located between the ventricles of the heart that carries the electrical impulse from the AV node to the bundle branches.

burnout (′bər-naửt) The end result of prolonged periods of stress without relief. Burnout is an energy-depleting condition that can affect one's health and career. It can be common for those who work in health care.

bursitis (bər-sī′tĭs) Inflammation of a bursa.

calcaneus (kal-kā′nē-ŭs)(†) The largest tarsal bone; also called the heel bone.

calcitonin (kal-si-tō′nin) A hormone produced by the thyroid gland that lowers blood calcium levels by activating osteoblasts.

calibrate (kīal′-brat) To **determine the caliber of;** to standardize a measuring instrument.

calibration syringe (kăl′ə-brā′shənsə-rĭnj) A standardized measuring instrument used to check and adjust the volume indicator on a spirometer.

calorie (kăl′ə-rē) A unit used to measure the amount of energy food produces; the amount of energy needed to raise the temperature of 1 kg of water by 1°C.

calyces (kă′lĭ-sēz′) Small cavities of the renal pelvis of the kidney.

CAM (kăm) The acronym for complementary and alternative medicine. Complementary medicine is used with conventional medicine. Alternative medicine is used in place of conventional medicine.

canaliculi (kan-ă-lik′yū-lī) Tiny canals that connect lacunae to each other.

cancellous (kan′siləs) Bone also known as spongy bone. It contains spaces within it containing the red bone marrow.

capillary (kăp′ə-lĕr′ē) Branches of arterioles and the smallest type of blood vessel.

capillary puncture (kăp′ə-lĕr′ē pŭngk′chər) A blood-drawing technique that requires a superficial puncture of the skin with a sharp point.

capitation (kăp′ĭ-tā′shən) A payment structure in which a health maintenance organization prepays an annual set fee per patient to a physician.

carboxyhemoglobin (kärbok′sēhē′məglō′bin) The term used when the hemoglobin of red blood cells is carrying carbon dioxide.

carboxypeptidase (kar-bok-sē-pep′ti-dās) (†) A pancreatic enzyme that digests proteins.

carcinogen (kär-sĭn′ə-jən) A factor that is known to cause the formation of cancer.

cardiac catheterization (kär′dē-ăk′ kath′ě-ter-ī-zā′shun) (†) A diagnostic method in which a catheter is inserted into a vein or artery in the arm or leg and passed through blood vessels into the heart.

cardiac cycle (kär′dē-ăk′ sī′kəl) The sequence of contraction and relaxation that makes up a complete heartbeat.

cardiac sphincter (kär′dē-ăk sfingk′tər) The valve-like structure composed of a circular band of muscle at juncture of the esophagus and stomach. Also known as the esophageal sphincter.

cardiologist (kär′dē-ŏl′ə-jĭst) A specialist who diagnoses and treats diseases of the heart and blood vessels (cardiovascular diseases).

carditis (kar-dĭ′tis)(†) Inflammation of the heart.

carpal (kär′pəl) Bones of the wrist.

carpal tunnel syndrome (kär′pəl tŭn′əl sĭn′drōm′) A painful disorder caused by compression of the median nerve in the carpal tunnel of the wrist.

carrier (kär′ē-ər) A reservoir host who is unaware of the presence of a pathogen and so spreads the disease while exhibiting no symptoms of infection.

cast (kăst) A rigid, external dressing, usually made of plaster or fiberglass, that is molded to the contours of the body part to which it is applied; used to immobilize a fractured or dislocated bone. Cylinder-shaped elements with flat or rounded ends, differing in composition and size, that form when protein from the breakdown of cells accumulates and precipitates in the kidney tubules and is washed into the urine.

catabolism (kə tab′əliz′am) The stage of metabolism in which complex substances, including nutrients and body tissues, are broken down into simpler substances and converted into energy.

cataracts (kăt′ə-răkts′) Cloudy areas that form in the lens of the eye that prevent light from reaching visual receptors.

cash flow statement (kăsh flō stā′mənt) A statement that shows the cash on hand at the beginning of a period, the income and disbursements made during the period, and the new amount of cash on hand at the end of the period.

cashier's check (kă-shîrz′ che′k) A bank check issued by a bank on bank paper and signed by a bank representative; usually purchased by individuals who do not have checking accounts.

catheterization (kath′ē-ter-ī-zăshun)(†) The procedure during which a catheter is inserted into a vessel, an organ, or a body cavity.

caudal (kôd′l) See **inferior**.

CD-ROM (sē′dē′rŏm′) A compact disc that contains software programs; an abbreviation for "compact disc—read-only memory."

cecum (sē′kəm) The first section of the large intestine.

cell body (sĕl bŏd′ē) The portion of the neuron that contains the nucleus and organelles.

cell membrane (sĕl mĕm′brăn′) The outer limit of a cell that is thin and selectively permeable. It controls the movement of substances into and out of the cell.

cells (sĕlz) The smallest living units of structure and function.

cellulitis (sel-yū-lī′tis) Inflammation of cellular or connective tissue.

cellulose (sĕl′yə-lōs′) A type of carbohydrate that is found in vegetables and cannot be digested by humans; commonly called fiber.

Celsius (centigrade) (sē l′sē-əs) One of two common scales for measuring temperature; measured in degrees Celsius, or °C.

Centers for Medicare and Medicaid Services (CMS) (sĕn′tərs mĕd′ĭ-kâr′ mĕd′ĭ-kād′ sûr′vĭs-əz) A congressional agency designed to handle Medicare and Medicaid insurance claims. It was formerly known as the Health Care Financing Administration.

central nervous system (CNS) (sĕn′trəl nûr′vəs sĭs′təm) A system that consists of the brain and the spinal cord.

central processing unit (CPU) (sĕn′trəl prŏs′es′ĭng yōō′nĭt) A microprocessor, the primary computer chip responsible for interpreting and executing programs.

centrifuge (sĕn′trə-fyōōj′) A device used to spin a specimen at high speed until it separates into its component parts.

centrioles (sen′trē ōz) Two cylinder-shaped organs near the cell nucleus that are essential for cell division, by equally dividing chromosomes to the daughter cells.

cerebellum (sĕr′ə-bĕl′əm) An area of the brain inferior to the cerebrum that coordinates complex skeletal muscle coordination.

cerebrospinal fluid (CSF) (ser′ē-brō-spĭ-năl flōō′ĭd) The fluid in the subarachnoid space of the meninges and the central canal of the spinal cord.

cerebrovascular accident (ser′əbrovas′kyələr ak′sidənt) A stroke. Caused by a hemorrhage in the brain or more often by a clot lodged in a cerebral artery.

cerebrum (sĕr′ə-brəm) The largest part of the brain; it mainly includes the cerebral hemispheres.

Certificate of Waiver tests (sər-tĭf′ĭ-kĭt wā′vər tĕsts) Laboratory tests that pose an insignificant risk to the patient if they are performed or interpreted incorrectly, are simple and accurate to such a degree that the risk of obtaining incorrect results is minimal, and have been approved by the Food and Drug Administration for use by patients at home; laboratories performing only Certificate of Waiver tests must meet less stringent standards than laboratories that perform tests in other categories.

certified check (sûr′tə-fīd′ chĕk) A payer's check written and signed by the payer, which is stamped "certified" by the bank. The bank has already drawn money from the payer's account to guarantee that the check will be paid.

Certified Medical Assistant (CMA) (sûr′tə-fīd′ mĕd′ĭ-kəl ə-sĭs′tənt) A medical assistant whose knowledge about the skills of medical assistants, as summarized by the 2003 AAMA Role Delineation Study areas of competence, has been certified by the Certifying Board of the American Association of Medical Assistants (AAMA).

cerumen (sə-rōō′mən) A wax-like substance produced by glands in the ear canal; also called earwax.

cervical enlargement (sûr′vĭ-kəl in-lär′j-mənt) The thickening of the spinal cord in the neck region.

cervical orifice (sûr′vĭ-kəl ôr′ə-fĭs) The opening of the uterus through the cervix into the vagina.

cervicitis (ser-vi-sī′tis) Inflammation of the cervix.

cervix (sûr′vĭks) The lowest portion of the uterus that extends into the vagina.

cesarean section (si zer´ē ən sək´ shən)   A surgical incision of the abdomen and uterus to deliver a baby transabdominally.

chain of custody (chān kŭs´tə-dē)   A procedure for ensuring that a specimen is obtained from a specified individual, is correctly identified, is under the uninterrupted control of authorized personnel, and has not been altered or replaced.

CHAMPVA (Civilian Health and Medical Program of the Veterans Administration)(sĭ-vĭl´yən hĕlth mĕd´ĭ-kəl prō´ğram vĕtər-enz ăd-mĭn´ĭ-strä´shən)   A type of health insurance that covers the expenses of families (dependent spouses and children) of veterans with total, permanent, and service-connected disabilities. It also covers the surviving families of veterans who die in the line of duty or as a result of service-connected disabilities.

chancre (shang´ker)(†)   A painless ulcer that may appear on the tongue, the lips, the genitalia, the rectum, or elsewhere.

charge slip (chärj slĭp)   The original record of services performed for a patient and the charges for those services.

check (chĕk)   A bank draft or order written by a payer that directs the bank to pay a sum of money on demand to the payee.

chemistry (kĕm´ĭ-strē)   The study of the composition of matter and how matter changes.

chemoreceptor (kē´mo-rĭ-sĕp´tôr)   Any cell that is activated by a change in chemical concentration and results in a nerve impulse. The olfactory or smell receptors in the nose are an example of a chemoreceptor.

Cheyne-Stokes respirations (chain stokes RES per ra shuns)   A pattern of breathing that gradually alternates between deep and shallow breaths with a period of apnea or no breathing that can last from 5 to 40 seconds.

chief cells (chēf sĕlz)   Cells in the lining of the stomach that secrete **pepsinogen.**

chief complaint (chēf kəm-plān´t)   The patient's main issue of pain or ailment.

chiropractor (kī´rə-prăk´tôr)   A physician who uses a system of therapy, including manipulation of the spine, to treat illness or pain. This treatment is done without drugs or surgery.

chlamydia (klə mid´ē ah)   A common bacterial STD caused by bacterium *Chlamydia trachomatis* that can lead to PID in women.

cholangiography (kō-lan-jē-og´rä-fē)(†)   A test that evaluates the function of the bile ducts by injection of a contrast medium directly into the common bile duct (during gallbladder surgery) or through a T-tube (after gallbladder surgery or during radiologic testing) and taking an x-ray.

cholecystography (kō-lē-sis-tog´rä-fē)(†)   A gallbladder function test performed by x-ray after the patient ingests an oral contrast agent; used to detect gallstones and bile duct obstruction.

cholesterol (kə-lĕs´tə-rôl)   A fat-related substance that the body produces in the liver and obtains from dietary sources; needed in small amounts to carry out several vital functions. High levels of cholesterol in the blood increase the risk of heart and artery disease.

chordae tendineae (kōr´dĕ ten-din´ā)(†)   Cord-like structures that attach the cusps of the heart valves to the papillary muscles in the ventricles.

choroid (kôr´oid´)   The middle layer of the eye, which contains the iris, the ciliary body, and most of the eye's blood vessels.

chromosome (krō´mə-sōm´)   Thread-like structures composed of DNA.

chronic (krŏn´ĭk)   Lasting a long time or recurring frequently, as in chronic osteoarthritis.

chronic obstructive pulmonary disease (COPD) (krŏn´ĭk ob-strŭk´tiv poōolmə-nĕr´ē dĭ-zēz´)   A disease characterized by the presence of airflow obstruction as a result of chronic bronchitis or emphysema. It is typically progressive. Cigarette smoking is the leading cause.

chronological résumé (krŏn´ə-lŏj´ĭ-kəl rĕzoŏo-mā´)   The type of résumé used by individuals who have job experience. Jobs are listed according to date, with the most recent being listed first.

chylomicron (kī-lō-mi´kron)   The least dense of the lipoproteins; it functions in lipid transportation.

chyme (kīm)(†)   The mixture of food and gastric juice.

chymotrypsin (kī-mō-trip´sin)(†)   A pancreatic enzyme that digests proteins.

cilia (sil´ēa)   Hair-like projections from the outside of the cell membrane on some cell types.

ciliary body (sĭl´ē-ĕr´ē bŏd´ē)   A wedge-shaped thickening in the middle layer of the eyeball that contains the muscles that control the shape of the lens.

circumduction (ser-kŭm-dŭk´shŭn)   Moving a body part in a circle; for example, tracing a circle with your arm.

cirrhosis (sĭ-rō´sĭs)   A long-lasting liver disease in which normal liver tissue is replaced with nonfunctioning scar tissue.

civil law (sĭv´əl lô)   Involves crimes against persons. A person can sue another person, business, or the government. Judgments often require a payment of money.

clarity (klăr´i-tē)   Clearness in writing or stating a message.

class action lawsuit (klăs-ăk´shən lô´soōt)   A lawsuit in which one or more people sue a company or other legal entity that allegedly wronged all of them in the same way.

clavicle (klăv´ĭ-kəl) A slender, curved long bone that connects the sternum and the scapula; also called the collar bone.

clean-catch midstream urine specimen (klēn-kăch mĭd´strēm yōōr´ĭn spĕs´əmən) A type of urine specimen that requires special cleansing of the external genitalia to avoid contamination by organisms residing near the external opening of the urethra and is used to identify the number and types of pathogens present in urine; sometimes referred to as midvoid.

clearinghouse (klîr´ĭng-hous´) A group that takes nonstandard medical billing software formats and translates them into the standard EDI formats.

cleavage (klē´vĭj) The rapid rate of mitosis of a zygote immediately following fertilization.

clinical coordinator (klĭn´ĭ-kəlkō-ôr´dn-ā´tor) The person associated with the medical assisting school that procures externship sites and qualifies them to ensure that they provide a thorough educational experience.

clinical diagnosis (klĭn´ĭ-kəl dī´əg-nō´sĭs) A diagnosis based on the signs and symptoms of a disease or condition.

clinical drug trial (klĭn´ĭ-kəl drŭg trī´əl) An internationally recognized research protocol designed to evaluate the efficacy or safety of drugs and to produce scientifically valid results.

Clinical Laboratory Improvement Amendments of 1988 (CLIA '88) (klē´ə) A law enacted by Congress in 1988 that placed all laboratory facilities that conduct tests for diagnosing, preventing, or treating human disease or for assessing human health under federal regulations administered by the Health Care Financing Administration (HCFA) and the Centers for Disease Control and Prevention (CDC).

clitoris (klĭt´ər-ĭs) Located anterior to the urethral opening in females. It contains erectile tissue and is rich in sensory nerves.

clock speed (klŏk spēd) A measurement of how many instructions per second that a CPU can process. Clock speed is measured in megahertz (MHz) or gigahertz (GHz).

closed file (klōzd fīl) A file for a patient who has died, moved away, or for some other reason no longer consults the office for medical expertise.

closed posture (klōzd pŏs´chər) A position that conveys the feeling of not being totally receptive to what is being said; arms are often rigid or folded across the chest.

cluster scheduling (klŭs´tər skĕj´ōōl-ĭng) The scheduling of similar appointments together at a certain time of the day or week.

coagulation (kō-ăg´yə-lā´shən) The process by which a clot forms in blood.

coccus (kŏk´əs) A spherical, round, or ovoid bacterium.

coccyx (kŏk´sĭks) A small, triangular-shaped bone consisting of three to five fused vertebrae.

cochlea (kŏk´lē-ă) A spiral-shaped canal in the inner ear that contains the hearing receptors.

code linkage (kōd lĭng´kĭj) Analysis of the connection between diagnostic and procedural information in order to evaluate the medical necessity of the reported charges. This analysis is performed by insurance company representatives.

coinsurance (kō-ĭn-shōōr´əns) A fixed percentage of covered charges paid by the insured person after a deductible has been met.

colitis (kə-lī´tĭs) Inflammation of the colon.

colonoscopy (kō-lon-os´ kŏ-pē)(†) A procedure used to determine the cause of diarrhea, constipation, bleeding, or lower abdominal pain by inserting a scope through the anus to provide direct visualization of the large intestine.

colony (kōl´ə-nē) A distinct group of microorganisms, visible with the naked eye, on the surface of a culture medium.

color family (kūl´ər făm´ə-lē) A group of colors that share certain characteristics, such as warmth or coolness, allowing them to blend well together.

colposcopy (kol-pos´kŏ-pē)(†) The examination of the vagina and cervix with an instrument called a colposcope to identify abnormal tissue, such as cancerous or precancerous cells.

common bile duct (kŏm´ən bīl dŭkt) Duct that carries bile to the duodenum. It is formed from the merger of the cystic and hepatic ducts.

compactible file (kəm-păkt´-əbəl fīl) Files kept on rolling shelves that slide along permanent tracks in the floor and are stored close together or stacked when not in use.

complement (kŏm´plə-mənt) A protein present in serum that is involved in specific defenses.

complementary medicine (kŏm´-plə-mĕn-tə-rē mĕd´-ĭ-sĭn) A type of medicine that is used with conventional medicine.

complete proteins (kəm-plēt´ prō´ten´) Proteins that contain all nine essential amino acids.

complex carbohydrates (kəm-plĕks´ kär´bō-hī´drāt´s) Long chains of sugar units; also known as polysaccharides.

complex inheritance (kəm-plĕks´ ĭn-hĕr´ĭ-təns) The inheritance of traits determined by multiple genes.

compliance plan (kəm-plī´əns plăn) A process for finding, correcting, and preventing illegal medical office practices.

complimentary closing (kom-pluh-men-tuh-ree kloh-zing) The closing remark of a business letter found two spaces below the last line of the body of the letter.

compound (kŏm´pound´) A substance that is formed when

two or more atoms of more than one element are chemically combined.

compound microscope (kŏm′pound′ mī′krə-skōp′) A microscope that uses two lenses to magnify the image created by condensed light focused through the object being examined.

computed tomography (kəm-pyōōt′ĕd tō-mogra-fē)(†) A radiographic examination that produces a three-dimensional, cross-sectional view of an area of the body; may be performed with or without a contrast medium.

concise (k n-sīs′) Brevity; the use of no unnecessary words.

concussion (kən-kŭsh′ən) A jarring injury to the brain; the most common type of head injury.

conductive hearing loss (kon-dŭk-tiv′hēr′ing lôs)(†) A type of hearing loss that occurs when sound waves cannot be conducted through the ear. Most types are temporary.

condyle (kon′dīl)(†) Rounded articular surface on a bone.

cones (kōnz) Light-sensing nerve cells in the eye, at the posterior of the retina, that are sensitive to color, provide sharp images, and function only in bright light.

conflict (kŏn′flīkt′) An opposition of opinions or ideas.

conjunctiva (kŏn′jŭngk-tī′və) The protective membrane that lines the eyelid and covers the anterior of the sclera, or the white of the eye.

conjunctivitis (kən-jŭngk′tə-vī′tĭs) A contagious infection of the conjunctiva caused by bacteria, viruses, and allergies. The symptoms may include discharge, red eyes, itching, and swollen eyelids; also commonly called pinkeye.

connective tissue (kə-nĕk′tĭv) A tissue type that is the framework of the body.

consent (kən-′sēnt) A voluntary agreement that a patient gives to

allow a medically trained person the permission to touch, examine, and perform a treatment.

constructive criticism (kən-stre′k-tiv kr′i-tə-si-zəm) A type of critique that is aimed at giving an individual feedback about his or her performance in order to improve that performance.

consumable (kən-sōō′mə-bəl) Able to be emptied or used up, as with supplies.

consumer education (kən-sōō′mər ĕj′ə-ka′shən) The process by which the average person learns to make informed decisions about goods and services, including health care.

contagious (kən-tā′jəs) Having a disease that can easily be transmitted to others.

contaminated (kən-tăm′ə-nāt′ĕd) Soiled or stained, particularly through contact with potentially infectious substances; no longer clean or sterile.

contract (kŏn′trăct′) A voluntary agreement between two parties in which specific promises are made.

contraindication (kŏn′trə-ĭn′dĭ-kā′-shən) A symptom that renders use of a remedy or procedure inadvisable, usually because of risk.

contrast medium (kŏn′trast′ mē′dē-əm) A substance that makes internal organs denser and blocks the passage of x-rays to photographic film. Introducing a contrast medium into certain structures or areas of the body can provide a clear image of organs and tissues and highlight indications of how well they are functioning.

controlled substance (kən-trōld′ sūb′stəns) A drug or drug product that is categorized as potentially dangerous and addictive and is strictly regulated by federal laws.

control sample (kən-trōl′ săm′pəl) A specimen that has a known value; used as a comparison

for test results on a patient sample.

contusion (kon-tŭ′shŭn) (†) A closed wound, or bruise.

conventional medicine (kən-vĕn′-shən-əl mĕd′-ĭ-sĭn) The usual practice of physicians and other allied health professionals, such as physical therapists, psychologists, medical assistants, and registered nurses. Also known as allopathy.

conventions (kən-vĕn′shənz) A list of abbreviations, punctuation, symbols, typefaces, and instructional notes appearing in the beginning of the ICD-9. The items provide guidelines for using the code set.

convolutions (kŏn′və-lōō′shənz) The ridges of brain matter between the sulci; also called gyri.

coordination of benefits (kō-ôr′dn-ā′shən bĕn′ə-fĭts) A legal principle that limits payment by insurance companies to 100% of the cost of covered expenses.

co-payment (kō-pā′mənt) A small fee paid by the insured at the time of a medical service rather than by the insurance company.

cornea (kôr′nē-ə) A transparent area on the front of the outer layer of the eye that acts as a window to let light into the eye.

coronary artery bypass graft (CABG) (kor′-uh-ner-ee, ahr′-tuh-ree, bahy′-pas, grahft) A surgery performed to bypass a blockage within a coronary artery with a vessel taken from another area.

coronary sinus (kôr′ə-nĕr′ē sī′nəs) The large vein that receives oxygen-poor blood from the cardiac veins and empties it into the right atrium of the heart.

corporation (kôr-pə-′rā-shən) A type of business group, such as a medical practice, that is established by law and managed by a board of directors.

corpus callosum (kôr′pəs ka-l′ō-səm) A thick bundle of nerve fibers that connects the cerebral hemispheres.

corpus luteum (kôr´pŭs lū-tē´ŭm)(†) A ruptured follicle cell in the ovary following ovulation.

cortex (kôr´tăks´) The outermost layer of the cerebrum.

cortisol (kōr´ti-sol) (†) A steroid hormone that is released when a person is stressed. It decreases protein synthesis.

coryza (côrĭ´zə) Another name for an upper respiratory tract infection. The common cold.

costal (kos´tăl)(†) Cartilage that attaches true ribs to the sternum.

counter check (koun´tər chĕk) A special bank check that allows a depositor to draw funds from his own account only, as when he has forgotten his checkbook.

courtesy title (kûr´tĭ-sē tīt´l) A title used before a person's name, such as Dr., Mr., or Ms.

cover sheet (kŭr´ər shēt) A form sent with a fax that provides details about the transmission.

covered entity (kūv´ərd en-tə-tē) Any organization that transmits health information in an electronic form that is related in any way with a HIPAA-covered business.

Cowper's glands (kou´ pərz glāndz) Bulbourethral glands.

coxal (koks-al´)(†) Pertaining to the bones of the pelvic girdle. The coxa is composed of the ilium, ischium, and pubis.

CPT See *Current Procedural Terminology.*

cranial (krā´-nē-ăl)(†) See **superior.**

cranial nerves (krā´nē-ăl nûrvs)(†) Peripheral nerves that originate from the brain.

crash cart (krăsh kärt) A rolling cart of emergency supplies and equipment.

creatine phosphate (krē´ă-tēn fos´fāt)(†) A protein that stores extra phosphate groups.

credit (krĕd´ĭt) An extension of time to pay for services, which are provided on trust.

credit bureau (kre´-dit byür´-o) A company that provides information about the credit worthiness of a person seeking credit.

cricoid cartilage (krī´koyd kär´tl-ĭj)(†) A cartilage of the larynx that forms most of the posterior wall and a small part of the anterior wall.

crime (krīm) An offense against the state committed or omitted in violation of public law.

criminal law (krĭm´ə-nəl lô) Involves crimes against the state. When a state or federal law is violated, the government brings criminal charges against the alleged offender.

cross-reference (krôs´rĕf´ər-əns) The notation within the ICD-9 of the word *see* after a main term in the index. The *see* reference means that the main term first checked is not correct. Another category must then be used.

cross-referenced (krôs´rĕf´ər-ənsd) Filed in two or more places, with each place noted in each file; the exact contents of the file may be duplicated, or a cross-reference form can be created, listing all the places to find the file.

cross-training (krȯs-trā´ning) The acquisition of training in a variety of tasks and skills.

cryosurgery (krī´ō-sûr´jə-rē) The use of extreme cold to destroy unwanted tissue, such as skin lesions.

cryotherapy (krī´ō-thĕr´ə-pē) The application of cold to a patient's body for therapeutic reasons.

cryptorchidism (kriptôr´kidiz´əm) Congenital failure of the testes to descend into the scrotal sac.

crystals (krĭs´təls) Naturally produced solids of definite form; commonly seen in urine specimens, especially those permitted to cool.

culture (kŭl´chər) In the sociologic sense, a pattern of assumptions, beliefs, and practices that shape the way people think and act.

To place a sample of a specimen in or on a substance that allows microorganisms to grow in order to identify the microorganisms present.

culture and sensitivity (C and S) (kŭl´chər sĕn´sĭ-tĭv´ə-tē) A procedure that involves culturing a specimen and then testing the isolated bacteria's susceptibility (sensitivity) to certain antibiotics to determine which antibiotics would be most effective in treating an infection.

culture medium (kŭlchər mē´de-əm) A substance containing all the nutrients a particular type of microorganism needs to grow.

***Current Procedural Terminology* (CPT) (kûr´ənt prə-sē´jər-əl tûr´mə-nŏl´ə-jē)** A book with the most commonly used system of procedure codes. It is the HIPAA-required code set for physicians' procedures.

cursor (kûr´sər) A blinking line or cube on a computer screen that shows where the next character that is keyed will appear.

Cushing's disease (kush´ingz dī-zēz´) A condition in which a person produces too much **cortisol** or has used too many steroid hormones. Some of the signs and symptoms include buffalo hump obesity, a moon face, and abdominal stretch marks; also called hypercortisolism.

cuspids (kūs´pĭdz) The sharpest teeth; they act to tear food.

cyanosis (sī´ə-no´sīs) A bluish color of skin that results when the supply of oxygen is low in the blood.

cycle billing (sī´kəl bĭl´ĭng) A system that sends invoices to groups of patients every few days, spreading the work of billing all patients over the month while billing each patient only once.

cystic duct (sĭs´tĭk dŭkt) The duct from the gallbladder that merges with the hepatic duct to form the common bile duct.

cystitis (sis-tī′tis)(†) Inflammation of the urinary bladder caused by infection.

cytokines (sī′tō-kīnz) A chemical secreted by T lymphocytes in response to an antigen. Cytokines increase T- and B-cell production, kill cells that have antigens, and stimulate red bone marrow to produce more white blood cells.

cytokinesis (sī′tō-ki-nē′sis)(†) Splitting of the cytoplasm during cell division.

cytoplasm (sī′tə-plăz′əm) The watery intracellular substance that consists mostly of water, proteins, ions, and nutrients.

damages (dăm′ĭjz) Money paid as compensation for violating legal rights.

database (dā′tə-bās) A collection of records created and stored on a computer.

dateline (dāt′līn′) The line at the top of a letter that contains the month, day, and year.

debridement (dā-brēd-mont′)(†) The removal of debris or dead tissue from a wound to expose healthy tissue.

decibel (děs′ə-bəl) A unit for measuring the relative intensity of sounds on a scale from 0 to 130.

deductible (dĭ-dŭk′tə-bəl) A fixed dollar amount that must be paid by the insured before additional expenses are covered by an insurer.

deep (dēp) Anatomical term meaning closer to the inside of the body.

defamation (děf′ə-mā′shən) Damaging a person's reputation by making public statements that are both false and malicious.

defecation reflex (def-ĕ-kā′shŭn rē′flěks′) The relaxation of the anal sphincters so that feces can move through the anus in the process of elimination.

deflection (dĭ-flěk′shən) A peak or valley on an electrocardiogram.

dehydration (dē-hī′drā′shən) The condition that results from a lack of adequate water in the body.

dementia (dĭ-měn′shə) The deterioration of mental faculties from organic disease of the brain.

dendrite (děn′drīt′) A type of nerve fiber that is short and branches near the cell body. Its function is to receive information from the neuron.

deoxyhemoblobin (dē-oks-ē-hē-mō-glō′bin)(†) A type of hemoglobin that is not carrying oxygen. It is darker red in color than hemoglobin.

dependent (dĭ-pěn′dənt) A person who depends on another person for financial support.

depolarization (dē-pō′lär-i-za-shŭn)(†) The loss of polarity, or opposite charges inside and outside; the electrical impulse that initiates a chain reaction resulting in contraction.

depolarized (dē-pō′lär-īzd)(†) A state in which sodium ions flow to the inside of the cell membrane, making the outside less positive. Depolarization occurs when a neuron responds to stimuli such as heat, pressure, or chemicals.

depression (di′-pre-shan) The lowering of a body part.

dermatitis (dûr′mə-tī′tĭs) Inflammation of the skin.

dermatologist (der-mă-tol′ō-jist)(†) A specialist who diagnoses and treats diseases of the skin, hair, and nails.

dermatome (dur′mə tōm) An area of skin innervated by a spinal nerve.

dermis (dûr′mĭs) The middle layer of the skin, which contains connective tissue, nerve endings, hair follicles, sweat glands, and oil glands.

descending colon (dĭ-sĕnd′ĭng kō′lən) The segment of the large intestine after the transverse colon that descends the left side of the abdominal cavity.

descending tracts (dĭ-sĕnd′ĭng trăkts) Tracts of the spinal cord that carry motor information from the brain to muscles and glands.

detrusor muscle (dē-trŭs′or mŭs′əl) A smooth muscle that contracts to push urine from the bladder into the urethra.

diabetes insipidus (dī′ə bētis ĭnsĭp′ĭdəs) The condition of excessive thirst and excessive urination related to hyposecretion of ADH so that water is not retained by the kidney.

diabetes mellitus (dī′ə-bē′tĭs mə-lī′təs) Any of several related endocrine disorders characterized by an elevated level of glucose in the blood, caused by a deficiency of insulin or insulin resistance at the cellular level.

diagnosis (Dx) (dī′əg-nō′sĭs) The primary condition for which a patient is receiving care.

diagnosis code (dī′əg-nō′sĭs kōd) The way a diagnosis is communicated to the third-party payer on the health-care claim.

diagnostic radiology (dī′əg-nos′tik rā′dē-ŏl′ə-jē) The use of x-ray technology to determine the cause of a patient's symptoms.

diapedesis (dī′ă-pĕ-dē′sis)(†) The squeezing of a cell through a blood vessel wall.

diaphoresis (dī′əfarē′sis) Excessive sweating as a result of illness or injury.

diaphragm (dī′ə-frăm′) A muscle that separates the thoracic and abdominopelvic cavities.

diaphysis (dī′-af′i-sis) The shaft of a long bone.

diastolic pressure (dī′ə-stŏl′ĭk prěsh′ər) The blood pressure measured when the heart relaxes.

diathermy (dī′ə-thŭr′mē) A type of heat therapy in which a machine produces high-frequency waves that achieve deep heat penetration in muscle tissue.

diencephalon (dī-en-sef´ă-lon)(†) A structure that includes the thalamus and the hypothalamus. It is located between the cerebral hemispheres and is superior to the brain stem.

dietary supplement (dī´-ĭ-tĕr-ē sŭp´-lə-mənt) Vitamins, minerals, herbals, and other substances taken by mouth without a prescription to promote health and well-being.

differential diagnosis (dĭf´ə-rĕn´shəl dī´ăg-nō´sĭs) The process of determining the correct diagnosis when two or more diagnoses are possible.

differently abled (dĭf´ər-ənt-lē ā´bəld) Having a condition that limits or changes a person's abilities and may require special accommodations.

diffusion (di-fyū´zhŭn)(†) The movement of a substance from an area of high concentration to an area of low concentration.

digital examination (dĭj´ĭ-tl ĭg-zam´ə-nā´shən) Part of a physical examination in which the physician inserts one or two fingers of one hand into the opening of a body canal such as the vagina or the rectum; used to palpate canal and related structures.

diluent (dĭl´yōo-ənt) A liquid used to dissolve and dilute another substance, such as a drug.

disability insurance (dĭs´ə-bĭlĭ-tē ĭn-shōor´əns) Insurance that provides a monthly, prearranged payment to an individual who cannot work as the result of an injury or disability.

disaccharide (dī-sak´ă-rīd) (†) A type of carbohydrate that is a simple sugar.

disbursement (dĭs-bûrs´mənt) Any payment of funds made by the physician's office for goods and services.

disclaimer (dĭs-klā´mər) A statement of denial of legal liability or that refutes the authenticity of a claim.

disclosure (dĭ-sklō´zhər) The release of, the transfer of, the provision of access to, or the divulgence in any manner of patient information.

disclosure statement (dĭ-sklō´zhər stāt´mənt) A written description of agreed terms of payment; also called a federal Truth in Lending statement.

discrimination (dĭs-´skrĭm-ə-´nā-shən) Unequal and unfair treatment.

disinfectant (dĭs´ĭn-fĕk´tănt) A cleaning product applied to instruments and equipment to reduce or eliminate infectious organisms; not used on human tissue.

dislocation (dĭs´lō-kā´shən) The displacement of a bone end from a joint.

dispense (dĭ-spĕns´) To distribute a drug, in a properly labeled container, to a patient who is to use it.

distal (dĭs´təl) Anatomic term meaning farther away from a point of attachment or farther away from the trunk of the body.

distal convoluted tubule (dĭs´təl kon´vō-lū-ted tū´byūl) The last twisted section of the renal tubule; it is located after the loop of Henle. Several of these tubules merge together to form collecting ducts.

distribution (dĭs´trĭ-byōo´shən) The biochemical process of transporting a drug from its administration site in the body to its site of action.

diverticulitis (dī´ver-tik-yū-li´tis)(†) Inflammation of the diverticuli, which are abnormal dilations in the intestine.

diverticulosis (dī´ver-tik-yū-lō-sis) Abnormal outpouchings or dilations of the intestine.

DNA (dē´ĕn-ā´) A nucleic acid that contains the genetic information of cells.

doctor of osteopathy (dok´tər ŏs´tē-ŏp´ə-thē) A doctor who focuses special attention on the musculo-skeletal system and uses hands and eyes to identify and adjust structural problems, supporting the body's natural tendency toward health and self-healing.

doctrine of informed consent (dōk-´trĭn of ĭn-fôrmd´ kən-´sēnt) The legal basis for informed consent, usually outlined in a state's medical practice act.

doctrine of professional discretion (dōk-´trĭn of prə-fĕsh´ə-nəl dĭ-skĕsh´ən) A principle under which a physician can exercise judgment as to whether to show patients who are being treated for mental or emotional conditions their records.

documentation (dōk´yə-mən-tā´shən) The recording of information in a patient's medical record; includes detailed notes about each contact with the patient and about the treatment plan, patient progress, and treatment outcomes.

dorsal (dôr´səl) See **posterior.**

dorsal root (dôr´səl rōot) A portion of a spinal nerve that contains axons of sensory neurons only.

dorsiflexion (dōr-si-flek´shŭn)(†) Pointing the toes upward.

dosage (dōs´āj) The size, frequency, and number of doses.

dose (dōs) The amount of a drug given or taken at one time.

dot matrix printer (dŏt mā´trĭks prĭn´tər) An impact printer that creates characters by placing a series of tiny dots next to one another.

double-booking system (dŭb´əl bōok´ing sĭs´təm) A system of scheduling in which two or more patients are booked for the same appointment slot, with the assumption that both patients will be seen by the doctor within the scheduled period.

douche (dōosh) Vaginal irrigation, which can be used to administer vaginal medication in liquid form.

drainage catheter (drā'nĭj kăth'ĭ-tər) A type of catheter used to withdraw fluids.

dressing (drĕs'ĭng) A sterile material used to cover a surgical or other wound.

DSL (digital subscriber line) (dĭj'ĭ-tl səb-skrīb'lĭn) A type of modem that operates over telephone lines but uses a different frequency than a telephone, allowing a computer to access the Internet at the same time that a telephone is being used.

ductus arteriosus (dŭk'tŭs ar-tēr'ē-ō'sus)(†) The connection in the fetus between the pulmonary trunk and the aorta.

ductus venosus (duk'tŭs ven-ō'sus)(†) A blood vessel that allows most of the blood to bypass the liver in the fetus.

duodenum (dōō'ə-dē'nəm) The first section of the small intestine.

durable item (dŏŏr'ə-bəl ī'təm) A piece of equipment that is used repeatedly, such as a telephone, computer, or examination table; contrast with **expendable item.**

durable power of attorney (dŏŏr'ə-bəl poúər ə-tûr'nē)(†) A document naming the person who will make decisions regarding medical care on behalf of another person if that person becomes unable to do so.

dwarfism (dwôrf'ĭzm) A condition in which too little growth hormone is produced, resulting in an abnormally small stature.

dysmenorrhea (dis-men-ōr-ē'ă)(†) Severe menstrual cramps that limit daily activity.

dyspnea (disp-nē'ă)(†) Difficult or painful breathing.

ear ossicles (îr os'i-kl)(†) Three tiny bones called the malleus, the incus, and the stapes located in the middle ear cavity. They are the smallest bones of the body.

eccrine gland (ek'rin glănd)(†) The most numerous type of sweat gland. Eccrine sweat glands produce a watery type of sweat and are activated primarily by heat.

echocardiography (ek'ō-kar-dē-og'rǎ-fē)(†) A procedure that tests the structure and function of the heart through the use of reflected sound waves, or echoes.

E code (ē kŏd) A type of code in the ICD-9. E-codes identify the external causes of injuries and poisoning.

ectoderm (ek'tō-derm)(†) The primary germ layer that gives rise to nervous tissue and some epithelial tissue.

ectropian (ek-trō'pē-ŭn) Eversion of the lower eyelid.

eczema (ĕk'sə-mə) Inflammatory condition of the skin.

edema (ĭ-dē'mə) An excessive buildup of fluid in body tissue.

editing (ĕd'ĭt-ĭng) The process of ensuring that a document is accurate, clear, and complete; free of grammatical errors; organized logically; and written in the appropriate style.

effacement (i fās'mənt) Thinning of the cervix in preparation for childbirth.

effectors (ĭ-fĕk'tərs) Muscles and glands that are stimulated by motor neurons in the peripheral nervous system.

efferent arterioles (ĕf'ər-ənt ar-tēr'ē-ōlz)(†) Structures that deliver blood to peritubular capillaries that are wrapped around the renal tubules of the nephron in the kidneys.

efferent nerves (ĕf'ər-ənt nûrvs) Motor nerves that bring information or impulses from the Central nervous System to the Peripheral nervous System to allow for the movement or action of a muscle or gland.

efficacy (ĕf'ĭ-kə-sē) The therapeutic value of a procedure or therapy, such as a drug.

efficiency (ĭ-fĭsh'ən-sē) The ability to produce a desired result with the least effort, expense, and waste.

elective procedure (ĭ-lĕk'tĭv prə-sē'jər) A medical procedure that is not required to sustain life but is requested for payment to the third-party payer by the patient or physician. Some elective procedures are paid for by third-party payers, whereas others are not.

electrocardiogram (ECG or EKG) (ĭ-lĕk'trō-kär'dē-ə-grăm') The tracing made by an **electrocardiograph.**

electrocardiograph (ĭ-lĕk'trō-kär'dē-ə-grăf') An instrument that measures and displays the waves of electrical impulses responsible for the cardiac cycle.

electrocardiography (ĭ-lĕk'trō-kär'dē-ŏg'rə-fē) The process by which a graphic pattern is created to reflect the electrical impulses generated by the heart as it pumps.

electrocauterization (ĭ-lĕk'trō-kô'tər-ĭ-zā'shən) The use of a needle, probe, or loop heated by electric current to remove growths such as warts, to stop bleeding, and to control nosebleeds that either will not subside or continually recur.

electrodes (ĭ-lĕk'trōds') Sensors that detect electrical activity.

electroencephalography (ĭ-lĕk'trō-ĕn-sĕf'ə-lŏ'grə-fē) A procedure that records the electrical activity of the brain as a tracing called an electroencephalogram, or EEG, on a strip of graph paper.

electrolytes (ĭ-lĕk'trə-līts) Substances that carry electrical current through the movement of ions.

electromyography (ĭ-lĕk'trō-mī-og'rə-fē) A procedure in which needle electrodes are inserted into some of the skeletal muscles and a monitor records the nerve impulses and measures conduction time; used to detect neuromuscular disorders or nerve damage.

electronic data interchange (EDI) (ĭ-lĕk-trŏn´ĭk dā´tə ĭn´tər-chānj´) Transmitting electronic medical insurance claims from providers to payers using the necessary information systems.

electronic mail (ĭ-lĕk´trŏn´ĭks) A method of sending and receiving messages through a computer network; commonly known as e-mail.

electronic media (i-lek-tron´-ik mee´-dee-uh) Any transmissions that are physically moved from one location to another through the use of magnetic tape, disk, compact disk media, or any other form of digital or electronic technology.

electronic transaction record (ĭ-lĕk´trŏn´ĭk trăn-săk´shən rĭ-kôrd) The standardized codes and formats used for the exchange of medical data.

elevation (e-lə-v´ā-shən) The raising of a body part.

embolism (ĕm´bə-lĭz´əm) An obstruction in a blood vessel.

embolus (ĕm´bə-ləs) A portion of a thrombus that breaks off and moves through the bloodstream.

embryonic period (em-brē-on´ik pîr´ē-əd)(†) The second through eighth weeks of pregnancy.

E/M code (ē/ĕm kōd) Evaluation and management codes that are often considered the most important of all CPT codes. The E/M section guidelines explain how to code different levels of services.

empathy (ĕm´pə-thē) Identification with or sensitivity to another person's feelings and problems.

emphysema (em´fəsēmə) A chronic lung condition consisting of damage to the alveoli of the lungs. It is heavily associated with smoking, which causes stretching of the spaces between the alveoli and paralyzes the cilia of the respiratory system.

employment contract (ĕm-ploi´mənt kŏn´trăkt´) A written agreement of employment terms between employer and employee that describes the employee's duties and the considerations (money, benefits, and so on) to be given by the employer in exchange.

empyema (em´pīē´mə) A collection of pus in the pleural cavity.

enclosure (ĕn-klō´zhərz) Materials that are included in the same envelope as the primary letter.

encounter form (en-´kaun-tər form) A form that combines the charges for services rendered, an invoice for payment or insurance copayment, and all the information for submitting an insurance claim; also known as a superbill.

endocardium (en-dō-kar´dē-ŭm)(†) The innermost layer of the heart.

endochondral (en-dō-kon´drăl)(†) A type of ossification in which bones start out as cartilage models.

endocrine gland (ĕn´də-kra-n glănd) A gland that secretes its products directly into tissue, fluid, or blood.

endocrinologist (ĕn´də-kra-nŏl´ə-jĭst) A specialist who diagnoses and treats disorders of the endocrine system, which regulates many body functions by circulating hormones that are secreted by glands throughout the body.

endoderm (ĕn´dō-derm)(†) The primary germ layer that gives rise to epithelial tissues only.

endogenous infection (ĕn´-dŏj´ə-nəs ĭn-fĕk´shən) An infection in which an abnormality or malfunction in routine body processes causes normally beneficial or harmless microorganisms to become pathogenic.

endolymph (ĕn´dō-limf)(†) A fluid in the inner ear. When this fluid moves, it activates hearing and equilibrium receptors.

endometriosis (en´dō-mē-trē-ō´sis)(†) A condition in which tissues that make up the lining of the uterus grow outside the uterus.

endometrium (en´dō-mē´trē-ŭm)(†) The innermost layer of the uterus. It undergoes significant changes during the menstrual cycle.

endomysium (en´dō-miz´e-ŭm)(†) A connective tissue covering that surrounds individual muscle cells.

endoplasmic reticulum (en´doplaz´mik ritik´yəlum) The organelles of the endoplasmic reticulum is composed of both smooth and rough types. The rough type contains ribosomes on its surface. The smooth type has no ribosomes. Both types create a network of passageways throughout the cytoplasm.

endorse (ĕn-dôrs´) To sign or stamp the back of a check with the proper identification of the person or organization to whom the check is made out, to prevent the check from being cashed if it is stolen or lost.

endoscopy (ĕn-dôs´kə-pē) Any procedure in which a scope is used to visually inspect a canal or cavity within the body.

endosteum (en-dos´tē-ŭm)(†) A membrane that lines the medullary cavity and the holes of spongy bone.

entropion (en-trō´pē-ūn) Inversion of the lower eyelid.

enunciation (ĭ-nŭn´sē-ā´shən) Clear and distinct speaking.

enzyme immunoassay (EIA) (ĕn´zīm im´yū-nō-as´ā)(†) The detection of substances by immunologic methods. This method involves an antigen, an antibody specific for the antigen, and a second antibody conjugated to an enzyme.

enzyme-linked immunosorbent assay (ELISA) test (ĕn´zīm-lĭngkt im´yū-nō-sōr´bent ăs´ā tĕst)(†) A blood test that confirms the presence of antibodies developed by the body's immune system in response to an initial HIV infection.

eosinophil (ē-ō-sin´ō-fil)(†) A type of granular leukocyte that captures invading bacteria and antigen-antibody complexes through phagocytosis.

epicardium (ep-i-kar´dē-ŭm)(†) The outermost layer of the wall of the heart. Also known as the **visceral pericardium.**

epidermis (ĕp´ĭ-dûr´mĭs) The most superficial layer of the skin.

epididymis (ep-i-diď´i-mis) (†) An elongated structure attached to the back of the testes and in which sperm cells mature.

epididymitis (ep-i-did-i-mī´tis)(†) Inflammation of an **epididymis.** Most cases result from infection.

epiglottic cartilage (ep-i-glot´ik kär´tl-ĭj)(†) A cartilage of the larynx that forms the framework of the epiglottis.

epiglottis (ep-i-glot-ī´tis)(†) The flap-like structure that closes off the larynx during swallowing.

epilepsy (ĕp´ə-lĕp´sē) A condition that occurs when parts of the brain receive a burst of electrical signals that disrupt normal brain function; also called **seizures.**

epimysium (ep-i-mis´-ē-ŭm)(†) A thin covering that is just deep to the fascia of a muscle. It surrounds the entire muscle.

epinephrine (ĕp´ə-nĕf´rĭn) An injectable medication used to treat anaphylaxis by causing vasoconstriction to increase blood pressure. A hormone secreted from the adrenal glands. It increases heart rate, breathing rate, and blood pressure.

epiphyseal disk (ep-i-fiz´ē-ăl dĭsk)(†) A plate of cartilage between the **epiphysis** and the **diaphysis.**

epiphysis (e-pif´i-sis)(†) The expanded end of a long bone.

episiotomy (epē´zēot´əmē) A surgical incision of the female perineum to enlarge the vaginal opening for delivery.

epistaxis (ĕp´i-stak´sis) Nosebleed.

epithelial tissue (ep-i-thē´lē-ĕl tĭsh´oo)(†) A tissue type that lines the tubes, hollow organs, and cavities of the body.

erectile tissue (ĭ-rĕk´tĕl tĭsh´oo) A highly specialized tissue located in the shaft of the penis. It fills with blood to achieve an erection.

erythema (er-i-thē´mă) Redness of the skin.

erythroblastosis fetalis (ĕ-rith´rō-blas-tō´sis fe´tăl-is)(†) A serious anemia that develops in a fetus with Rh-positive blood as a result of antibodies in an Rh-negative mother's body.

erythrocytes (ĭ-rĭth´rə-sīt´s) Red blood cells.

erythrocyte sedimentation rate (ESR) (ĭ-rĭth´rə-sīt´ sĕd´ə-mən-tā´shən rāt) The rate at which red blood cells, the heaviest blood component, settle to the bottom of a blood sample.

erythropoietin (ĕ-rith-rō-poy´ē-tin)(†) A hormone secreted by the kidney and is responsible for regulating the production of red blood cells.

esophageal hiatus (ĭ-sŏf´ə-jē´əl) Hole in the diaphragm through which the esophagus passes.

established patient (ĭ-stăb´lĭsht pā´shənt) A patient who has seen the physician within the past 3 years. This determination is important when using E/M codes.

estrogen (ĕs´trə-jən) A female sex hormone; when produced during ovulation, estrogen causes a buildup of the lining of the uterus (womb) to prepare it for a possible pregnancy.

ethics (ĕth´ĭks) General principles of right and wrong, as opposed to requirements of law.

ethmoid (ĕth´moyd)(†) Bones located between the sphenoid and nasal bone that form part of the floor of the cranium.

etiologic agent (ē´tē-ə-lŏj´ĭkā´jənt) A living microorganism or its toxin that may cause human disease.

etiquette (ĕt´ĭ-ket´) Good manners.

eustachian tube (yoo-stā´shən toob) An opening in the middle ear, leading to the back of the throat, that helps equalize air pressure on both sides of the eardrum.

eversion (ē-ver´zhŭn)(†) Turning the sole of the foot laterally.

exclusion (ĭk-skloozh´ən) An expense that is not covered by a particular insurance policy, such as an eye examination or dental care.

excretion (ĭk-skrē´shən) The elimination of waste by a discharge; in drug metabolism, the manner in which a drug is eliminated from the body.

exocrine gland (ĕk´sə-krĭn glănd) A gland that secretes its product into a duct.

exogenous infection (ĕk-sŏj´ə-nəs ĭn-fĕk´shən) An infection that is caused by the introduction of a pathogen from outside the body.

exophthalmos (k´s f´th lm s) Bulging of the eyeballs, often related to hyperthyroidism.

expendable item (ĭk-spĕn´dəbəl ī´təm) An item that is used and must then be restocked; also known collectively as supplies. Contrast with **durable item.**

expiration (ĕk´spə-rā´shən) The process of breathing out; also called exhalation.

explanation of benefits (EOB) (ĕk´splə-nā´shən ŭv bĕn´ə-fits) Information that explains the medical claim in detail; also called **remittance advice (RA).**

expressed contract (ĭk-sprĕst´ kŏn´trăct) A contract clearly stated in written or spoken words.

extension (ĭk-stĕn´shən) An unbending or straightening movement of the two elements of a jointed body part.

external auditory canal (ĭk-stûr´nəl ô´dĭ-tôr´ē kə-năl´)   Canal that carries sound waves to the tympanic membrane; commonly called the ear canal.

externship (ĭk-stûrn´shĭp)   A period of practical work experience performed by a medical assisting student in a physician's office, hospital, or other health-care facility.

extrinsic eye muscles (ĭk-strĭn´ sĭk ĭmūs´əlz)   The skeletal muscles that move the eyeball.

facsimile machine (făk-sĭm´ə-lē mə-shēn´)   A piece of office equipment used to send a facsimile, or fax, over telephone lines from one modem to another; more commonly called a fax machine.

facultative (fak-ŭl-tā´tĭv)(†)   Able to adapt to different conditions; in microbiology, able to grow in environments either with or without oxygen.

Fahrenheit (făr´ən-hīt)   One of two common scales used for measuring temperature; measured in degrees Fahrenheit, or °F.

fallopian tubes (fə-lō-pē-ən tübz)   Tubes that extend from the uterus on each side and that open near an ovary.

family practitioner (făm´ə-lē prăk-tĭsh´ə-nər)(†)   A physician who does not specialize in a branch of medicine but treats all types and ages of patients; also called a general practitioner.

fascia (fash´e-ă)(†)   A structure that covers entire skeletal muscles and separates them from each other.

fascicle (făs´ĭ-kəl)   Sections of a muscle divided by connective tissue called perimysium.

febrile (fĕb´rəl)   Having a body temperature above one's normal range.

feces (fē´sēz)   Material found in the large intestine and made from leftover chyme. Faces are eventually eliminated through the anus.

Federal Unemployment Tax Act (FUTA)   This act requires employers to pay a percentage of each employee's income up to a certain dollar amount.

feedback (fēd´băk´)   Verbal and nonverbal evidence that a message was received and understood.

feedback loop (fēd´băk lōōp)   A mechanism to control hormone levels. The two types are positive and negative feedback loops.

fee-for-service (fēfôr sûr´vĭs)   A major type of health plan. It repays policyholders for the costs of health care that are due to illness and accidents.

fee schedule (fē skĕj´ōol)   A list of the costs of common services and procedures performed by a physician.

felony (fĕl´ə-nē)   A serious crime, such as murder or rape, that is punishable by imprisonment. In certain crimes, a felony is punishable by death.

femoral (fem´ŏ-răl)(†)   Relating to the femur or thigh.

femur (fē´mər)   The bone in the upper leg; commonly called the thigh bone.

fenestrated drape (fĕn´ĭ-strāt´ĕd drāp)   A drape that has a round or slit-like opening that provides access to the surgical site.

fertilization (fer´til-i-zā´shŭn)   The process in which an egg unites with a sperm.

fetal period (fĕt´l pîr´e-əd)   A period that begins at week nine of pregnancy and continues through delivery of the offspring.

fiber (fī´bər)   The tough, stringy part of vegetables and grains, which is not absorbed by the body but aids in a variety of bodily functions.

fibrinogen (fī-brin´ō-jen)(†)   A protein found in plasma that is important for blood clotting.

fibroid (fī´broid)   A benign tumor in the uterus composed of fibrous tissue.

fibromyalgia (fī-brō-mī-al´jē-ă)(†)   A condition that exhibits chronic pain primarily in joints, muscles, and tendons.

fibula (fĭb´yə-lə)   The lateral bone of the lower leg.

file guide (fīlgīd)   A heavy cardboard or plastic insert used to identify a group of file folders in a file drawer.

filtration (fĭl-trā´shən)   A process that separates substances into solutions by forcing them across a membrane.

fimbriae (fĭm-brē-ə)   Fringe-like structures that border the entrances of the **fallopian tubes.**

first morning urine specimen (fûrst môr´nĭng yōōr´ĭn spĕs´ə-mən)   A urine specimen that is collected after a night's sleep; contains greater concentrations of substances that collect over time than specimens taken during the day.

fixative (fĭk´sə-tĭv)   A solution sprayed on a slide immediately after the specimen is applied. It is used to preserve and hold the cells in place until a microscopic examination is performed.

flaccid (flak´sid)   Weak, soft; not erect.

flagellum (flajel´əm)   The "tail-like" structure on some cell membranes that provides cell movement.

flexion (flek´shŭn)(†)   A bending movement of the two elements of a jointed body part.

floater (flō´tər)   A nonsterile assistant who is free to move about the room during surgery and attend to unsterile needs.

fluidotherapy (flōō´ĭd-ōthĕr´ə-pē)   A technique for stimulating healing, particularly in the hands and feet, by placing the affected body part in a container of glass beads that are heated and agitated with hot air.

follicle (fŏl´ĭ-kəl)   An accessory organ of the skin that is found in the dermis and the sites at which hairs emerge.

follicle-stimulating hormone (FSH) (fŏl´ĭ-kəl stim´yū-lā-ting hôr´mōn) A hormone that in females stimulates the production of estrogen by the ovaries; in males, it stimulates sperm production.

follicular cells (fə-li´-kyə-lər selz) Small cells contained in the primordial follicle along with a large cell called a primary **oocyte.**

folliculitis (fŏ-lik-yū-lī´tis)(†) Inflammation of the hair follicle.

fomite (fō´mĭt)(†) An inanimate object, such as clothing, body fluids, water, or food, that may be contaminated with infectious organisms and thus serve to transmit disease.

fontanel (fän-tə-n´el) The soft spot in an infant's skull that consists of tough membranes that connect to incompletely developed bone.

food exchange (fōod ĭks-chānj´) A unit of food in a particular food category that provides the same amounts of protein, fat, and carbohydrates as all other units of food in that category.

foramen magnum (fə-rā´-mən mag-nəm) The large hole in the occipital bone that allows the brain to connect to the spinal cord.

foramen ovale (fō-rā´men ō-va´lē)(†) A hole in the fetal heart between the right atrium and the left atrium.

forced vital capacity (FVC) (fôrst vīt´l kə-păs´ĭ-tē) The greatest volume of air that a person is able to expel when performing rapid, forced expiration.

formalin (fōr-mă-lin)(†) A dilute solution of formaldehyde used to preserve biological specimens.

formed elements (fôrmd ĕl´ə-mənts) Red blood cells, white blood cells, and platelets; compose 45% of blood volume.

formulary (fōr´myū-lā-rē)(†) An insurance plan's list of approved prescription medications.

fracture (frăk´chər) Any break in a bone.

fraud (frôd) An act of deception that is used to take advantage of another person or entity.

frequency (frē´kwən-sē) The number of complete fluctuations of energy per second in the form of waves.

frontal (frŭn´tl) Anatomic term that refers to the plane that divides the body into anterior and posterior portions. Also called coronal.

fulgurated (ful´gy ə rā təd) The ise of heat or laser to burn or destroy tissue.

full-block letter style (fōol blŏk lĕt´ər stīl) A letter format in which all lines begin flush left; also called block style.

functional résumé (fŭngk´shə-nəl rĕz´ōo-mā´) A résumé that highlights specialty areas of a person's accomplishments and strengths.

fundus (fun´dus) The upper domed portion of an organ.

fungus (fŭng´gəs) A eukaryotic organism that has a rigid cell wall at some stage in the life cycle.

gait (gāt) The way a person walks, consisting of two phases: stance and swing.

ganglia (găng´glē-ə) Collections of neuron cell bodies outside the central nervous system.

gastic juice (găs´trĭk jüs) Secretions from the stomach lining that begin the process of digesting protein.

gastritis (gă-strī´tĭs) Inflammation of the stomach lining.

gastroenterologist (găs´trō-ĕn-ter-ol´ō-jist)(†) A specialist who diagnoses and treats disorders of the entire gastrointestinal tract, including the stomach, intestines, and associated digestive organs.

gastroesophageal reflux disease (GERD) (gas´trō-ē-sof´ă-jē´ăl rē´flĕks dĭ-zēz´) A condition that occurs when stomach acids are pushed into the esophagus and cause heartburn.

gene (jēn) A segment of DNA that determines a body trait.

general physical examination (jĕn´ər-əl fĭz´ĭ-kəl ĭg-zăm´ə-nā´shən) An examination performed by a physician to confirm a patient's health or to diagnose a medical problem.

generic name (jə-nĕr´ĭk nām) A drug's official name.

gerontologist (jĕr´ən-tŏl´ə-jist) A specialist who studies the aging process.

giantism (jī´an-tizm)(†) A condition in which too much growth hormone is produced in childhood, resulting in an abnormally increased stature.

glans penis (glanz pē´nĭs) A cone-shaped structure at the end of the penis.

glaucoma (glou-kō´mə) A condition in which too much pressure is created in the eye by excessive aqueous humor. This excess pressure can lead to permanent damage of the optic nerves, resulting in blindness.

global period (glō´bəl pîr´ē-əd) The period of time that is covered for follow-up care of a procedure or surgical service.

globulins (glob´yū-lin)(†) Plasma proteins that transport lipids and some vitamins.

glomerular filtrate (glō-măr´yū-lăr fĭl´trāt´)(†) The fluid remaining in the **glomerular capsule** after **glomerular filtration.**

glomerular filtration (glō-măr´yū-lăr fĭl-trā´shən)(†) The process by which urine forms in the kidneys as blood moves through a tight ball of capillaries called the glomerulus.

glomerulonephritis (glō-măr´yū-lō-nef-rī´tis)(†) An inflammation of the glomeruli of the kidney.

glomerulus (glō-mār′yū-lŭs)(†)   A group of capillaries in the renal corpuscle.

glottis (glot′is)(†)   The opening between the vocal cords.

glucagon (glōō′kə-gŏn′)   A hormone that increases glucose concentrations in the bloodstream and slows down protein synthesis.

glycogen (glī′kə-jən)   An excess of glucose that is stored in the liver and in skeletal muscle.

glycosuria (glī-kō-sū′rē-ă)(†)   The presence of significant levels of glucose in the urine.

goiter (goi′tər)   Enlargement of the thyroid gland, which causes swelling of the neck, often related to iodine insufficiency in the diet.

Golgi apparatus (gôl′jē ap′ərat′es)   The cell's Golgi apparatus synthesizes carbohydrates and also appears to prepare and store secretions for discharge from the cell.

gonadotropin-releasing hormone (GnRH) (gō′na-dō-trō′pinr ĭ-lēs′ing hôr′mōn′)   Hormone that stimulates the anterior pituitary gland to release **follicle-stimulating hormone (FSH).**

gonads (gō′nădz)   The reproductive organs; namely, in women, the ovaries, and in men, the testes.

goniometer (gō-ne-ä′-me-tər)   A protractor device that measures range of motion.

gout (gowt)(†)   A medical condition characterized by an elevated uric acid level and recurrent acute arthritis.

G-protein (jē-prō′tēn)(†)   A substance that causes enzymes in the cell to activate following the activation of the hormone-receptor complex in the cell membrane.

gram-negative (grăm′nĕg′ə-tĭv)   Referring to bacteria that lose their purple color when a decolorizer has been added during a Gram's stain.

gram-positive (grăm′pŏz′ĭ-tĭv)   Referring to bacteria that retain their purple color after a decolorizer has been added during a Gram's stain.

Gram's stain (grămz stăn)   A method of staining that differentiates bacteria according to the chemical composition of their cell walls.

granular leukocyte (grăn′yə-lər lōō′kəsīt′)   A type of leukocyte (white blood cell) with a segmented nucleus and granulated cytoplasm; also known as a polymorphonuclear leukocyte.

granulocyte (grăn′yū-lō-sīt)(†)   See **granular leukocyte.**

Grave's disease (grāvz dĭ-zēz′)   A disorder in which a person develops antibodies that attack the thyroid gland.

gray matter (grā măt′ər)   The inner tissue of the brain and the spinal cord that is darker in color than **white matter.** It contains all the bodies and dendrites of nerve cells.

gross earnings (grōs ûr′nĭngz)   The total amount an employee earns before deductions.

group practice (grōōp prăk′ tĭs)   A medical management system in which a group of three of more licensed physicians share their collective income, expenses, facilities, equipment, records, and personnel. (3)

growth hormone (GH) (grōth hôr′mōn′)   A hormone that stimulates an increase in the size of the muscles and bones of the body.

gustatory receptors (gə′s-tə-tör-ē ri-se′p-tər)   Taste receptors that are found on taste buds.

gynecologist (gī′nĭ-kŏi′ə-jĭst)   A specialist who performs routine physical care and examinations of the female reproductive system.

gyri (jī′rī)(†)   The ridges of brain matter between the sulci; also called **convolutions.**

hairy leukoplakia (hâr′ē lū-kō-plā′kē-ă)(†)   A white lesion on the tongue associated with AIDS.

hapten (hap′tĕn)(†)   Foreign substances in the body too small to start an immune response by themselves.

hard copy (härd′ kŏp′ē)   A readable paper copy or printout of information.

hardware (härd′wâr′)   The physical components of a computer system, including the monitor, keyboard, and printer.

hazard label (hăz′ərd lā′bəl)   A shortened version of the Material Safety Data Sheet; permanently affixed to a hazardous substance container.

HCPCS Level II codes (āch sē pē sē ĕs lĕv′əl tōō kōdz)   Codes that cover many supplies such as sterile trays, drugs, and durable medical equipment; also referred to as national codes. They also cover services and procedures not included in the CPT.

Health Care Common Procedure Coding System (HCPCS) (hĕlth kâr kŏm′ən prə-sē′jər kōd′ĭng sĭs′təm)   A coding system developed by the Centers for Medicare and Medicaid Services that is used in coding services for Medicare patients.

health fraud (hĕlth frôd)   A deception or trickery related to health prevention or care for profit.

health maintenance organization (HMO) (hĕlth mān′tə-nəns ôr′gə-nĭ-zā′shən)   A health-care organization that provides specific services to individuals and their dependents who are enrolled in the plan. Doctors who enroll in an HMO agree to provide certain services in exchange for a prepaid fee.

helper T-cells (hĕl′pər tē′ sĕlz)   White blood cells that are a key component of the body's immune system and that work in coordination with other white blood cells to combat infection.

hematemesis (hē′-mă-tem′ĕ-sis)   The vomiting of blood.

hematocrit (hē′mă-tō-krit)(†) The percentage of the volume of a sample made up of red blood cells after the sample has been spun in a centrifuge.

hematology (hē′mə-tŏl′ə-jē) The study of blood.

hematoma (hē′mə-tō′me) A swelling caused by blood under the skin.

hematopoiesis (hēmətōpōē′sis) The process of new blood cell formation in the red bone marrow of cancellous bone.

hematuria (hē-mă-tu′rē-ă)(†) The presence of blood in the urine.

hemocytoblast (hē′mă-sī′tō-blast)(†) Cells of the red bone marrow that produce most red blood cells.

hemoglobin (hē′mə-glō′bĭn) A protein that contains iron and bonds with and carries oxygen to cells; the main component of erythrocytes.

hemoglobinuria ((hē′mō-glō-bi-nū′rē-ă) (†) The presence of free **hemoglobin** in the urine; a rare condition caused by transfusion reactions, malaria, drug reactions, snake bites, or severe burns.

hemolysis (hē-mol′ĭ-sis)(†) The rupturing of red blood cells, which releases hemoglobin.

hemolytic anemias (hē mō lit′ ik ənē′mēə) Types of anemia that cause red blood cells to be destroyed faster than they can be made.

hemoptysis (hi mop′ ti sis) The spitting up of blood from the respiratory tract.

hemorrhoids (hĕm′ə-roidz′) Varicose veins of the rectum or anus.

hemostasis (hē′mō-stā-sis)(†) The stoppage of bleeding.

hemothorax (hē′ mō thôr′ aks) Blood collection in the pleural cavity causing collapse of the lung.

hepatic duct (hĭ-păt′ĭk dŭkt) A duct that leaves the liver carrying bile and merges with the cystic duct to form the common bile duct.

hepatic lobule (he-păt′ĭk lob′yūl)(†) Smaller divisions within the lobes of the liver.

hepatic portal system (he-pat′ik pôr′tl sĭs′təm)(†) The collection of veins carrying blood to the liver.

hepatic portal vein (hĭ-păt′ĭk pôr′tl vān) A blood vessel that carries blood from the other digestive organs to the **hepatic lobules.**

hepatitis (hĕp′ə-tī′tĭss) Inflammation of the liver usually caused by viruses or toxins.

hepatocytes (hep′ă-tō-sītz)(†) The cells within the lobules of the liver. Hepatocytes process nutrients in the blood and make bile.

hernia (hûr′nē-ə) The protrusion of an organ through the wall that usually contains it, such as a hiatal or inguinal hernia.

herpes simplex (her′pēz sĭm′plĕks)(†) A medical condition characterized by an eruption of one or more groups of vesicles on the lips or genitalia.

herpes zoster (her′pēz zos′ter)(†) A medical condition characterized by an eruption of a group of vesicles on one side of the body following a nerve root.

hierarchy (hī′ə-rär′kē) A term that pertains to Abraham Maslow's hierarchy of needs. This hierarchy states that human beings are motivated by unsatisfied needs and that certain lower needs must be satisfied before higher needs can be met.

hilum (hī′lŭm)(†) The indented side of a lymph node. The entrance of the renal sinus that contains the renal artery, renal vein, and ureter.

HIPAA (Health Insurance Portability and Accountability Act) (hĭp′ə) A set of regulations whose goals include the following: (1) improving the portability and continuity of health-care coverage in group and individual markets; (2) combating waste, fraud, and abuse in health-care insurance and health-care delivery; (3) promoting the use of a medical savings account; (4) improving access to long-term care services and coverage; and (5) simplifying the administration of health insurance.

Holter monitor (hol′tər mŏn′ĭ-tər) An electrocardiography device that includes a small portable cassette recorder worn around a patient's waist or on a shoulder strap to record the heart's electrical activity.

homeopathic medicine (hō-mē-ō-păth′-ĭk mĕd′-ĭ-sĭn) A system of medicine that uses remedies in an attempt to stimulate the body to recover itself.

homeostasis (hō′mē-ō-stā′sĭs) A balanced, stable state within the body.

homologous chromosome (hŏ-mŏl′ō-gŭs krō′mə-sōm′)(†) Members in each pair of chromosomes.

hormone (hôr′mōn′) A chemical secreted by a cell that affects the functions of other cells.

hospice (hŏs′pĭs) Volunteers who work with terminally ill patients and their families.

human chorionic gonadotropin (HCG) (hyōō′mən kō-rē-on′ik gō′nad-ōtrō′pin) A hormone secreted by cells of the embryo after implantation. It maintains the corpus luteum in the ovary so it will continue to secrete estrogen and progesterone.

human immunodeficiency virus (HIV) (hyōō′mən im′yū-nō-dē-fish′en-sē vī′rəs) A retrovirus that gradually destroys the body's immune system and causes AIDS.

humerus (hyü′-mə-rəs) The bone of the upper arm.

humors (hyōō′mərz) Fluids of the body.

hydrotherapy (hī′drə-thĕr′ə-pē) The therapeutic use of water to treat physical problems.

hydrothorax (hī' drō thôr' aks) Fluid collection in the pleural cavity causing collapse of the lung.

hyoid (hī'-öid) The bone that anchors the tongue.

hyperextension (hī'per-eks-ten'shŭn)(†) Extension of a body part past the normal anatomic position.

hyperglycemia (hī'pər-glī-sē'mē-ə) High blood sugar.

hyperopia (hī-per-ō'pē-ă) A condition that occurs when light entering the eye is focused behind the retina; commonly called farsightedness.

hyperpnea (hī-per-nē'ă)(†) Abnormally deep, rapid breathing.

hyperpyrexia (hy per py rex' e a) An exceptionally high fever.

hyperreflexia (hī'per-rē-flek'sē-ă) Reflexes that are stronger than normal reflexes.

hypertension (hī'pər-tĕn'shən) High blood pressure.

hyperventilation (hī'pər-vĕn'tl-ā'shən) The condition of breathing rapidly and deeply. Hyperventilating decreases the amount of carbon dioxide in the blood.

hypnosis (hĭp-nō'-sĭs) A trance-like state usually induced by another person to access the subconscious mind and promote healing.

hypodermis (hī'pə-dûr'mĭs) The subcutaneous layer of the skin that is largely made of adipose tissue.

hypoglycemia (hī'pō-glī-sē'mē-ə) Low blood sugar.

hyporeflexia (hī'pō-rē-flek'sē-ă)(†) A condition of decreased reflexes.

hypotension (hi'pō-tĕn'shən) Low blood pressure.

hypothalamus (hī'pō-thăl'ə-məs) A region of the **diencephalon.** It maintains homeostasis by regulating many vital activities such as heart rate, blood pressure, and breathing rate.

hypovolemic shock (hī'per-vō-lē'mē-ă shŏk)(†) A state of shock resulting from insufficient blood volume in the circulatory system.

hypoxia (hī pôk' sē ə) Inadequate oxygenation of the cells of the body.

hysterectomy (hĭs'tə-rĕk'tə-mē) Surgical removal of the uterus.

ICD-9 See *International Classification of Diseases, Ninth Revision, Clinical Modification.*

icon (ī'kŏn') A pictorial image; on a computer screen, a graphic symbol that identifies a menu choice.

identification line (ī-dĕn'tə-fĭ-kā'shən līn) A line at the bottom of a letter containing the letter writer's initials and the typist's initials.

idiopathic (ĭd-ē-ō-path'ik) A disease or condition of unknown cause.

ileocecal sphincter (ĭl'ē ō sē'kəl sfĭngk'ter) A structure that controls the movement of **chime** from the ileum to the **cecum.**

ileum (ĭl'ē-əm) The last portion of the small intestine. It is directly attached to the large intestine.

ilium (i'-lē-əm) The most superior part of the hip bone. It is broad and flaring.

immunity (ĭ-myoōn'ĭ-tē) The condition of being resistant or not susceptible to pathogens and the diseases they cause.

immunization (im'yū-nī-zā-shən) The administration of a vaccine or toxoid to protect susceptible individuals from communicable diseases.

immunocompromised (im'yū-nōkom'pro-mīzd)(†) Having an impaired or weakened immune system.

immunofluorescent antibody (IFFA) test(im'yū-nō-flūr-es'ent ăn'tĭ-bŏd-ē tĕst)(†) A blood test used to confirm enzyme-linked immunosorbent assay (ELISA) test results for HIV infection.

immunoglobulins (im'yū-nō-glob'yū-linz)(†) A class of structurally related proteins that include IgG, IgA, IgM, and IgE; also called **antibodies.**

impetigo (im'pĭ-tī'gō) A contagious skin infection usually caused by germs commonly called staph and strep.

implied contract (ĭm-plīd kŏn'trăct') A contract that is created by the acceptance or conduct of the parties rather than the written word.

impotence (ĭm'pŏ-tens)(†) A disorder in which a male cannot maintain an erect penis to complete sexual intercourse; also called erectile dysfunction.

inactive file (ĭn-ăk'tĭv fīl) A file used infrequently.

incision (ĭn-sĭzh'ən) A surgical wound made by cutting into body tissue.

incisors (ĭn-sī'zərz) The most medial teeth. They act as chisels to bite off food.

incomplete proteins (ĭn'kəm-plēt' prō'tēnz') Proteins that lack one or more of the essential amino acids.

incontinence (in-kon'ti-nens)(†) The involuntary leakage of urine.

incus (ĭng'kəs) A small bone in the middle ear, located between the malleus and the stapes; also called the anvil.

indexing (n'dēks' ing) The naming of a file.

indexing rules (n'dēks' ing roōls) Rules used as guidelines for the sequencing of files based on current business practice.

indication (ĭn'dĭ-kā'shən) The purpose or reason for using a drug, as approved by the FDA.

individual identifiable health information (IIHI) (in-duh-vij-oo-uh ahy-den-tuh-fahy-able hĕlth ĭn'fər-mā'shən) Any part of an individual's health information, including demographic information, collected from an individual that is received by a covered entity (e.g., a health-care provider).

induration (in-də-´rā-shən) The process of hardening or of beccomming hard.

infection (ĭn-fĕk´shən) The presence of a pathogen in or on the body.

infectious waste (ĭn-fĕk´shəs wāst) Waste that can be dangerous to those who handle it or to the environment; includes human waste, human tissue, and body fluids as well as potentially hazardous waste, such as used needles, scalpels, and dressings, and cultures of human cells.

inferior (ĭn-fîr´ē-ər) Anatomic term meaning below or closer to the feet; also called caudal.

inflammation (ĭn´flə-mā´shən) The body's reaction when tissue becomes injured or infected. The four cardinal signs are redness, heat, pain, and swelling.

inflammatory phase (in-flam´-a-tor-ee fāz) The initial phase of wound healing in which bleeding is reduced as blood vessels in the affected area constrict.

informed consent (ĭn-fôrmd´ kən-sĕnt) The patient's right to receive all information relative to his or her condition and then make a decision regarding treatment based upon that knowledge.

informed consent form (ĭn-fôrmd´ kən-sĕnt fôrm) A form that verifies that a patient understands the offered treatment and its possible outcomes or side effects.

infundibulum (in-fŭn-dib´yū-lŭm)(†) The funnel-like end of the uterine tube near an ovary. It catches the secondary oocyte as it leaves the ovary.

infusion (in-fyū´zhŭn)(†) A slow drip, as of an intravenous solution into a vein.

ink-jet printer (ĭngk´jĕt´ prĭn´tər) A nonimpact printer that forms characters by using a series of dots created by tiny drops of ink.

innate immunity (ĭn āt ĭmyoōn´ītē) The body's mechanisms to protect itself against pathogens in general; also called nonspecific defenses.

inner cell mass (ĭn´ər sĕl măs) A group of cells in a blastocyte that gives rise to an embryo.

inorganic (ĭn´ôr-găn´ĭk) Matter that generally does not contain carbon and hydrogen.

insertion (ĭn-sûr´shən) An attachment site of a skeletal muscle that moves when a muscle contracts.

inside address (ĭn-sĭd´ ə-drĕs´) The name and address of the person to whom the letter is being sent. It appears on a business letter two to four spaces down from the date. It should be two, three, or four lines in length.

inspection (ĭn-spĕk´shən) The visual examination of the patient's entire body and overall appearance.

inspiration (in-spə-rā´-shən)(†) The act of breathing in; also called inhalation.

instruction set (ĭn-strŭk´shən set) Includes the groups of instructions from installed programming that a CPU can implement.

insulin (ĭn´sə-lĭn) A hormone that regulates the amount of sugar in the blood by facilitating its entry into the cells.

integrative medicine (ĭn´-tĭ-grāt´-tĭv mĕd´-ĭ-sĭn) The combination of components of conventional medicine with complementary and alternative medicine modalities.

interactive pager (ĭn´tər-ăk´tĭv pāj´ər) A pager designed for two-way communication. The pager screen displays a printed message and allows the physician to respond by way of a mini keyboard.

interatrial septum (in´tər ā´trē əl səp´təm) The wall separating the right and left atria from each other.

intercalated disc (in-ter´kă-lā-ted disk)(†) A disk that connects groups of cardiac muscles. This disc allows the fibers in that group to contract and relax together.

interferon (in-ter-fēr´on)(†) A protein that blocks viruses from infecting cells.

interim room (ĭn´tər-ĭm rōōm) A room off the patient reception area and away from the examination rooms for occasions when patients require privacy.

***International Classification of Diseases, Ninth Revision, Clinical Modification*(ICD-9) (ĭn´tər-năsh´ə-nəl klăs´ə-fīkā´ shən dĭ-zēz´əz nīnth rĭ-vĭzh´ən klĭn´ĭ-kəl mŏd´ə-fī-kā´shən)** Code set that is based on a system maintained by the World Health Organization of the United Nations. The use of the ICD-9 codes in the health-care industry is mandated by **HIPAA** for reporting patients' diseases, conditions, and signs and symptoms.

Internet (ĭn´tər-nĕt´) A global network of computers.

interneuron (ĭn´ter-nū´ron)(†) A structure found only in the central nervous system that functions to link sensory and motor neurons together.

internist (ĭn-tûr´nĭst) A doctor who specializes in diagnosing and treating problems related to the internal organs.

interpersonal skills (ĭn´tər-pûr´sə-nəl skĭlz) Attitudes, qualities, and abilities that influence the level of success and satisfaction achieved in interacting with other people.

interphalangeal (intərfəlan´jeal) Pertaining to the joints between the phalangeal bones.

interphase (in´ter-fāz)(†) The state of a cell carrying out its normal daily functions and not dividing.

interstitial cell (in-ter-stish´ăl sĕl)
A cell located between the seminiferous tubules that is responsible for making testosterone.

interstitial fluid (in-ter-stish´ăl flōō´ĭd) Fluid found between tissue cells that is absorbed by lymph capillaries to become lymph.

interventricular septum (in´tər ventrik´yələr səp´təm) The wall separating the right and left ventricles from each other.

intestinal lipase (ĭn-tĕs´tĭ-n lip´ās) An enzyme that digests fat.

intradermal (ID) (in´tră-der´măl) Within the upper layers of the skin.

intradermal test (in´tră-der´măl tĕst) An allergy test in which dilute solutions of allergens are introduced into the skin of the inner forearm or upper back with a fine-gauge needle.

intramembranous (in-tra-mē´m-brə-nəs) A type of ossification in which bones begin as tough fibrous membranes.

intramuscular (IM) (in´tră-mŭs´kyū-lăr) Within muscle; an IM injection allows administration of a larger amount of a drug than a subcutaneous injection allows.

intraoperative (in´tră-ŏp´ər-ə-tĭv) Taking place during surgery.

intravenous IV (in´tră-vē´năs) Injected directly into a vein.

intravenous pyelography (IVP) (in´tra-vē´nəs pī´ĕ-log´ră-fē)(†) A radiologic procedure in which the doctor injects a contrast medium into a vein and takes a series of x-rays of the kidneys, ureters, and bladder to evaluate urinary system abnormalities or trauma to the urinary system; also known as excretory urography.

intrinsic factor (ĭn-trĭn´zĭk făk´tər) A substance secreted by **parietal cells** in the lining of the stomach. It is necessary for vitamin B$_{12}$ absorption.

invasive (ĭn-vā´sĭv) Referring to a procedure in which a catheter, wire, or other foreign object is introduced into a blood vessel or organ through the skin or a body orifice. Surgical asepsis is required during all invasive tests.

inventory (ĭn´vən-tôrē) A list of supplies used regularly and the quantities in stock.

inversion (ĭn-vûr´zhən) Turning the sole of the foot medially.

invoice (ĭn´vois´) A bill for materials or services received by or services performed by the practice.

ions (ī´ənz) Positively or negatively charged particles.

iris (ī´rĭs) The colored part of the eye, made of muscular tissue that contracts and relaxes, altering the size of the pupil.

ischium (is´-kē-əm) A structure that forms the lower part of the hip bone.

islets of Langerhans (ī´lĭt lan´gerhans) Structures in the pancreas that secrete insulin and glucagon into the bloodstream.

itinerary (ī-tĭn´ə-rĕr´ē) A detailed travel plan listing dates and times for specific transportation arrangements and events, the location of meetings and lodgings, and phone numbers.

jaundice (jôn´dĭs) A condition characterized by yellowness of the skin, eyes, mucous membranes, and excretions; occurs during the second stage of hepatitis infection.

jejunum (jə-jōō´nəm) The midportion and the majority of the small intestine.

journalizing (jûr´nə-lĭz´ĭng) The process of logging charges and receipts in a chronological list each day; used in the single-entry system of bookkeeping.

juxtaglomerular apparatus (jŭks´tă-glŏmĕr´yū-lăr ăp´ə-răt´əs)(†) A structure contained in the nephron and made up of the macula densa and **juxtaglomerular cells.**

juxtaglomerular cells (jŭks´tă-glŏmer´yū-lăr sĕlz) Enlarged smooth muscle cells in the walls of either the afferent or efferent arterioles.

Kaposi's sarcoma (kap´ō-sēz sar-kō´mă) Abnormal tissue occurring in the skin, and sometimes in the lymph nodes and organs, manifested by reddish-purple to dark blue patches or spots on the skin.

keratin (kĕr´ə-tĭn) A tough, hard protein contained in skin, hair, and nails.

keratinocyte (kĕ-rat´i-nō-sīt)(†) The most common cell type in the epidermis of the skin.

key (kē) The act of inputting or entering information into a computer.

KOH mount (kā´ō-āch mount) A type of mount used when a physician suspects a patient has a fungal infection of the skin, nails, or hair and to which potassium hydroxide is added to dissolve the keratin in cell walls.

Krebs cycle (krēbz sī´kəl) Also called the citric acid cycle. This cycle generates ATP for muscle cells.

KUB radiography (kā´yōō-bē rā´dēog´ră-fē)(†) The process of x-raying the abdomen to help assess the size, shape, and position of the urinary organs; evaluate urinary system diseases or disorders; or determine the presence of kidney stones. It can also be helpful in determining the position of an intrauterine device (IUD) or in locating foreign bodies in the digestive tract; also called a flat plate of the abdomen.

kyphosis (kī-fō´sis) A deformity of the spine characterized by a bent-over position; more commonly called humpback.

labeling (lā´bəl-ĭng) Information provided with a drug, including FDA-approved indications and the form of the drug.

labia majora (lā´bē-ă mă´jôr-ă) The rounded folds of adipose tissue and skin that serve to protect the other female reproductive organs.

labia minora (lā´bē-ă mĭ´nôr-ă) The folds of skin between the labia majora.

labyrinth (lăb´ə-rĭnth´) The inner ear.

laceration (lăs´ə-rā´shən) A jagged, open wound in the skin that can extend down into the underlying tissue.

lacrimal apparatus (lăk´rə-məl ăp´ə-răt´əs) A structure that consists of the lacrimal glands and nasolacrimal ducts.

lacrimal gland (lăk´rə-məl glănd) A gland in the eye that produces tears.

lactase (lăk´tās)(†) An enzyme that digests sugars.

lactic acid (lăk´tĭk ăs´ĭd) A waste product that must be released from the cell. It is produced when a cell is low on oxygen and converts pyruvic acid.

lactiferous (lak-tif´ə rus) Pertaining to producing milk.

lactogen (lak´tō-jen) Substance secreted by the placenta that stimulates the enlargement of the mammary glands.

lacunae (l-kü-na) Holes in the matrix of bone that hold osteocytes.

lamella (lə-me´-lə) Layers of bone surrounding the canals of osteons.

LAN (lān) Abbreviation for Local Area Network.

lancet (lăn´sĭt) A small, disposable instrument with a sharp point used to puncture the skin and make a shallow incision; used for capillary puncture.

laryngopharynx (lă-ring´gō-far-ingks) (†) The portion of the pharynx behind the **larynx.**

larynx (lăr´ingks) The part of the respiratory tract between the pharynx and the trachea that is responsible for voice production; also called the voice box.

laser printer (lā´zər prĭn´tər) A high-resolution printer that uses a technology similar to that of a photocopier. It is the fastest type of computer printer and produces the highest-quality output.

lateral (lăt´ər-əl) A directional term that means farther away from the midline of the body.

lateral file (lăt´ər-əl fĭl) A horizontal filing cabinet that features doors that flip up and a pull-ut drawer, where files are arranged with sides facing out.

law (lô) A rule of conduct established and enforced by an authority or governing body, such as the federal government.

law of agency (lô ā´jən-sē) A law stating that an employee is considered to be acting on the physician's behalf while performing professional duties.

lead (lēd) A view of a specific area of the heart on an electrocardiogram.

lease (lēs)) To rent an item or piece of equipment.

legal custody (lēgəl kŭs´tə-dē) The court-decreed right to have control over a child's upbringing and to take responsibility for the child's care, including health care.

lens (lēnz) A clear, circular disc located in the eye, just posterior to the iris, that can change shape to help the eye focus images of objects that are near or far away.

letterhead (lĕt´ər-hĕd´) Formal business stationery, with the doctor's (or office's) name and address printed at the top, used for correspondence with patients, colleagues, and vendors.

leukemia (loo-kē´mē-ə) A medical condition in which bone marrow produces a large number of white blood cells that are not normal.

leukocyte (loo-kə-sīt) White blood cells.

leukocytosis (lū´kō-sī-tō´sis)(†) A white blood cell count that is above normal.

leukopenia (lū´kō-pē´nē-ă)(†) A white blood cell count that is below normal.

liability insurance (lī´ə-bĭl´ĭ-tē ĭn-shoor´əns) A type of insurance that covers injuries caused by the insured or injuries that occurred on the insured's property.

liable (lī´ə-bəl) Legally responsible.

libel (lī´bəl) A false publication, as in writing, print, signs, or pictures, that damages a person's reputation.

lifetime maximum benefit (līf´tīm´ măk´sə-məm bĕn´ə-fĭt) The total sum that a health plan will pay out over the patient's life.

ligament (lĭg´ə-mənt) A tough, fibrous band of tissue that connects bone to bone.

ligature (lĭg´ə-choor´) Suture material.

limbus (lĭm bŭs) The corneal-scleral junction, which is the area where the sclera (the white of the eye) gives way to the clear covering of the iris (cornea).

limited check (lĭm´ĭ-tĭd chĕk) A check that is void after a certain time limit; commonly used for payroll.

lingual frenulum (ling´gwăl fren´yūlŭm)(†) A flap of mucosa that holds the body of the tongue to the floor of the oral cavity.

lingual tonsils (ling´gwăl ton´silz)(†) Two lumps of lymphatic tissue on the back of the tongue that act to destroy bacteria and viruses.

linoleic acid (lin-ō-lē´ik as´id)(†) An essential fatty acid found in corn and sunflower oils.

lipoproteins (lip-ō-prō´tēnz) Large molecules that are fat-soluble on the inside and water-soluble on the outside and carry lipids such as cholesterol and triglycerides through the bloodstream.

living will (lĭv´ĭng wĭl) A legal document addressed to a patient's family and health-care providers stating what type of treatment the patient wishes or does not wish to receive if he becomes terminally ill, unconscious, or permanently comatose; sometimes called an advance directive.

lobe (lōb) The frontal, parietal, temporal, or occipital regions of the cerebral hemisphere.

locum tenens (lō´kum těn´ens)(†) A substitute physician hired to see patients while the regular physician is away from the office.

loop of Henle (lōōp hen´lē) The portion of the renal tubule that curves back toward the renal corpuscle and twists again to become the distal convoluted tubule.

lubricant (loo-bri-kuh nt) A water-soluble gel used during examination of the rectum or vaginal cavity.

lumbar enlargement (lŭm´bär ěnlärj´mənt) The thickening of the spinal cord in the low back region.

lunula (lū´nū-lă) The white half-moon–shaped area at the base of a nail.

luteinizing hormone (LH) (lū´tē-in-izing hôr´mōn´)(†) Hormone that in females stimulates ovulation and the production of estrogen; in males, it stimulates the production of testosterone.

lymphedema (limf´e-dē´mă) The blockage of lymphatic vessels that results in the swelling of tissue from the accumulation of lymphatic fluid.

lymphocyte (lĭm´fō-sīt)(†) An agranular leukocyte formed in lymphatic tissue. Lymphocytes are generally small. See **T lymphocyte** and **B lymphocyte.**

lymphokines (lĭmf´ō kĭnz) A type of cytokine secreted by T cells that increases T-cell production and directly kill cells with antigens.

lysosomes (lī´səsōmz) Structures that are known to perform the digestive function of the cells.

lysozyme (lī´sō-zīm)(†) An enzyme in tears that destroys pathogens on the surface of the eye.

macrophage (măk´rə-făj´) A type of phagocytic cell found in the liver, spleen, lungs, bone marrow, and connective tissue. Macrophages play several roles in humoral and cell-mediated immunity, including presenting the antigens to the lymphocytes involved in these defenses; also known as monocytes while in the bloodstream.

macula densa (mak´yū-lă den´sa)(†) An area of the distal convoluted tubule that touches afferent and efferent arterioles.

macular degeneration (mak´yū-lăr dējen-er-ā´shŭn)(†) A progressive disease that usually affects people older-than the age of 50. It occurs when the retina no longer receives an adequate blood supply.

magnetic resonance imaging (MRI) (măgnět´ĭk rěz´ə-nəns ĭ-măj´ing) A viewing technique that uses a powerful magnetic field to produce an image of internal body structures.

magnetic therapy (māg-nět´-ĭk thěr´-ə-pē) A type of therapy in which magnets are placed on the body to penetrate and correct the body's energy fields.

maintenance contract (mān´tə-nəns kŏn´trăkt´) A contract that specifies when a piece of equipment will be cleaned, checked for worn parts, and repaired.

major histocompatibility complex (MHC) (mā´jər his´tō-kom-pat-ĭ-bil´i-tē kəm-plěks) A large protein complex that plays a role in T-cell activation.

malignant (mə-lĭg´nənt) A type of tumor or neoplasm that is invasive and destructive and that tends to metastasize; it is commonly known as cancerous.

malleus (măl´ē-əs) A small bone in the middle ear that is attached to the eardrum; also called the hammer.

malpractice claim (măl-prăk´tĭs klām) A lawsuit brought by a patient against a physician for errors in diagnosis or treatment.

maltase (mawl-tās) An enzyme that digests sugars.

mammary glands (mam´ă-rē glăndz) Accessory organs of the female reproductive system that secrete milk after pregnancy.

mammography (mă-mŏg´rə-fē) X-ray examination of the breasts.

managed care organization (MCO) (măn´ĭjd kâr ôr´gə-nĭ-zā´shən) A health-care business that, through mergers and buyouts, can deliver health care more cost-effectively.

mandible (man´-də-bəl) A bone that forms the lower portion of the jaw.

manipulation (mə-nĭp´yə-la´shən) The systematic movement of a patient's body parts.

margin (mahr-jin) The space or measurement around the edges of a form or letter that is left blank.

marrow (mer´-ō) A substance that is contained in the medullary cavity. In adults, it consists primarily of fat.

massage (mə-sāzh) The use of pressure, kneading, stroking, and the human touch to alleviate pain and promote healing through relaxation.

massage therapist (mə-säzh´thěr´ə-pĭst) An individual who is trained to use pressure, kneading, and stroking to promote muscle and full-body relaxation.

mastoid process (mas´-to´id pr´ä-ses) A large bump on each temporal bone just behind each ear. It resembles a nipple, hence the name mastoid.

Material Safety Data Sheet (MSDS) (mə-tîr´e-əl sāf´tē dā´tə shēt) A form that is required for all hazardous chemicals or other substances used in the laboratory and that contains information about the product's name, ingredients, chemical characteristics, physical and health hazards, guidelines for safe handling, and procedures to be followed in the event of exposure.

matrix (mā′trĭks) The basic format of an appointment book, established by blocking off times on the schedule during which the doctor is able to see patients. The material between the cells of connective tissue.

matter (mătˊer) Anything that takes up space and has weight. Liquids, solids, and gases are matter.

maturation phase (măchˊə-rāˊshən fāz) The third phase of wound healing, in which scar tissue forms.

maxillae (mak-siˊ-lə) A bone that forms the upper portion of the jaw.

Mayo stand (māˊō stănd) A movable stainless steel instrument tray on a stand.

medial (mēˊdē-əl) A directional term that describes areas closer to the midline of the body.

Medicaid (mĕdˊĭ-kādˊ) A federally funded health cost assistance program for low-income, blind, and disabled patients; families receiving aid to dependent children; foster children; and children with birth defects.

medical asepsis (mĕdˊĭ-kəl ə-sĕpˊsĭs) Measures taken to reduce the number of microorganisms, such as hand washing and wearing examination gloves, that do not necessarily eliminate microorganisms; also called clean technique.

medical practice act (mĕdˊĭ-kəl prăkˊtĭs ăkt) A law that defines the exact duties that physicians and other health-care personnel may perform.

Medicare (mĕdˊĭ-kârˊ) A national health insurance program for Americans aged 65 and older.

Medicare + Choice Plan (mĕdˊĭ-kârˊ chois plăn) Medicare benefit in which beneficiaries can choose to enroll in one of three major types of plans instead of the **Original Medicare Plan.**

Medigap (mĕdˊĭ-găpˊ) Private insurance that Medicare recipients can purchase to reduce the gap in coverage—the amount they would have to pay from their own pockets after receiving Medicare benefits.

meditation (mĕdˊ-ĭ-tā-shən) A state in which the body is consciously relaxed and the mind becomes calm and focused.

medullary cavity (meˊ-de-ler-ē kaˊ-və-tē) The canal that runs through the center of the **diaphysis.**

megakaryocytes (meg-ă-karˊē-ō-sīts)(†) Cells within red blood marrow that give rise to platelets.

meiosis (mī-ōˊsis)(†) A type of cell division in which each new cell contains only one member of each chromosome pair.

melanin (mĕlˊə-nĭn) A pigment that is deposited throughout the layers of the epidermis.

melanocyte (mĕlˊă-nō-sīt)(†) A cell type within the epidermis that makes the pigment **melanin.**

melanocyte-stimulating hormone (MSH) (məlˊən ō sīt stimˊ yū lāting hôr mōnˊ) A hormone released from the anterior pituitary to stimulate melanin production in the skin's epidermal cells.

melatonin (mĕlˊə-tōˊnĭn) A hormone that helps to regulate circadian rhythms.

membrane potential (mĕmˊbrānˊ pə-tĕnˊshəl) The potential inside a cell relative to the fluid outside the cell.

menarche (me-narˊke) The first menstrual period.

Meniere's disease (Mənˊerz dĭzēz) An inner ear disease characterized by attacks of vertigo, tinnitus, and nausea. Permanent hearing loss may result.

meninges (mĕ-ninˊjēz)(†) Membranes that protect the brain and spinal cord.

meningitis (mĕnˊĭn-jīˊtĭs) An inflammation of the **meninges.**

meniscus (mə-nĭsˊkəs) The curve in the air-to-liquid surface of a liquid specimen in a container.

menopause (mĕnˊə-pôzˊ) The termination of the menstrual cycle due to the normal aging of the ovaries.

menses (mĕnˊsēz) The clinical term for menstrual flow.

menstrual cycle (mĕnˊstroo-əl sīˊkəl) The female reproductive cycle. It consists of regular changes in the uterine lining that lead to monthly bleeding.

mensuration (mĕnˊsə-rāˊ-shən) The process of measuring.

meridian (mə-rĭdˊ-ē-ən) Pathways of energetic flow that are distributed symmetrically throughout the body. These pathways are used in acupuncture, traditional Chinese medicine, and Ayurveda.

mesentery (meˊsenˊtərē) The fan-like tissue that attaches the jejunum and ileum to the posterior abdominal wall.

mesoderm (mezˊō-derm)(†) The primary germ layer that gives rise to connective tissue and some epithelial tissue.

metabolism (mĭ-tăbˊə-lĭzˊəm) The overall chemical functioning of the body, including all body processes that build small molecules into large ones (anabolism) and break down large molecules into small ones (catabolism).

metacarpals (me-tə-kˊär-pəl) The bones that form the palms of the hand.

metacarpophalangeal (metˊəkarˊ pōfəlanˊjēəl) Pertaining to the joints that join the phalanges to the metacarpals.

metaphase (met´əfāz) Period of mitosis when the chromosomes line up on the spindle fibers created by the centrioles during prophase.

metastasis (mə-tăs´tə-sĭs) The transfer of abnormal cells to body sites far removed from the original tumor; the spread of tumor cells.

metatarsals (mĕt´ə-tär´salz) The bones that form the front of the foot.

metatarsophalangeal (met´ətar´sōfəlan´jēəl) Pertaining to the joints that join the phalanges to the metatarsals.

microbiology (mī´krō-bī-ŏl´ə-jē) The study of microorganisms.

microfiche (mī´krō-fēsh´) Microfilm in rectangular sheets.

microfilm (mī´krə-fĭlm´) A roll of film stored on a reel and imprinted with information on a reduced scale to minimize storage space requirements.

microglia (mī-krŏg´lĕa) Small cells within the nervous system that act as phagocytes, watching for and engulfing invaders.

microorganism (mī´krō-ôr´gə-nĭz´əm) A simple form of life, commonly made up of a single cell and so small that it can be seen only with a microscope.

micropipette (mī´krō-pĭ-pet´) A small pipette that holds a small, precise volume of fluid; used to collect capillary blood.

microvilli (mī´krō-vil´-ī)(†) Structures found in the lining of the small intestine. They greatly increase the surface area of the small intestine so it can absorb many nutrients.

micturition (mik-chū-rish´ŭn)(†) The process of urination.

middle digit (´mi-dəl ´di-jət) A small group of two to three numbers in the middle of a patient number that is used as an identifying unit in a filing system.

midsagittal (mid´saj´i-tăl)(†) Anatomical term that refers to the plane that runs lengthwise down the midline of the body, dividing it into equal left and right halves.

minerals (mĭn´ər-əlz) Natural, inorganic substances the body needs to help build and maintain body tissues and carry on life functions.

minors (mī-nərs) Anyone under the age of majority—18 in most states, 21 in some jurisdictions.

minutes (mi-nətz´) A report of what happened and what was discussed and decided at a meeting.

mirroring (mĭr´ər-ĭng) Restating in your own words what a person is saying.

misdemeanor (mĭs´dĭ-mē´nər) A less serious crime such as theft under a certain dollar amount or disturbing the peace. A misdemeanor is punishable by fines or imprisonment.

mitochondria (mīto´kon´drēə) Structures that provide energy for cells and are the respiratory centers for the cell.

mitosis (mī-tō´sĭs) A type of cell division that produces ordinary body, or somatic, cells; each new cell receives a complete set of paired chromosomes.

mitral valve (mī´trăl vălv)(†) See **bicuspid valve.**

mobility aid (mō´bəl-ə-tē ād) Device that improve one's ability to move from one place to another; also called mobility assistive device.

modeling (mŏd´l-ĭng) The process of teaching the patient a new skill by having the patient observe and imitate it.

modem (mō´dəm) A device used to transfer information from one computer to another through telephone lines.

modified-block letter style (mŏd´ə-fīd blŏk lĕt´ər stīl) A letter format similar to full-block style, except that the dateline, complimentary closing, signature block, and notations are aligned and begin at the center of the page or slightly to the right of center.

modified-wave schedule (mŏd´ə-fīd wāv skĕj´ōol) A scheduling system similar to the wave system, with patients arriving at planned intervals during the hour, allowing time to catch up before the next hour begins.

modifier (mŏd´ə-fī´ər) One or more two-digit codes assigned to the five-digit main code to show that some special circumstance applied to the service or procedure that the physician performed.

molars (mō´lərz) Back teeth that are flat and are designed to grind food.

mold (mōld) Fungi that grow into large, fuzzy, multicelled organisms that produce spores.

molecule (mŏl´ĭ-kyōol´) The smallest unit into which an element can be divided and still retain its properties; it is formed when atoms bond together.

money order (mŭn´ē ôr´dər) A certificate of guaranteed payment, which may be purchased from a bank, a post office, or some convenience stores.

monocyte (mon´-o-s-īt)(†) A type of phagocyte that is formed in bone marrow and circulates throughout the blood for a very short period of time. It then migrates to specific tissues and is called a macrophage.

monokines (mon´ō kīnz) A type of cytokine secreted by lymphocytes and macrophages that assists in regulating the immune response by increasing B-cell production and stimulating red bone marrow to produce more white blood cells.

mononucleosis (mon´ō nōo klē ō´sis) A highly contagious viral infection caused by the Epstein-Barr virus (EBV).

monosaccharide (mon-ō-sak′ă-rīd)(†) A type of carbohydrate that is a simple sugar.

mons pubis (m′änz py′ü-bəs) A fatty area that overlies the public bone.

moral values (môr′əl văl′yōōz) Values or types of behavior that serve as a basis for ethical conduct and are formed through the influence of the family, culture, or society.

mordant (môr′dnt) A substance, such as iodine, that can intensify or deepen the response a specimen has to a stain.

morphology (môr-fŏl′ə-jē) The study of the shape or form of objects.

morula (mōr′ū-lă)(†) A zygote that has undergone cleavage and results in a ball of cells.

motherboard (mŭth′ər-bôrd′) The main circuit board of a computer that controls the other components in the system.

motility (mō′ti li tē) To be capable of movement.

motor (mō′tər) Efferent neurons that carry information from the central nervous system to the effectors.

mouse (mous) A pointing device that can be added to a computer that directs activity on the computer screen by positioning a pointer or cursor on the screen. It can be directly attached to the computer or can be wireless.

moxibustion (mŏk-ĭ-bŭs′-chən) The application of heat at the points where the needles are inserted during acupuncture.

mucocutaneous exposure (myü-kō-kyü′-tā-nē-əs ik-spō′-zhər) Exposure to a pathogen through mucous membranes.

mucosa (myōō-kō′sə) The innermost layer of the wall of the alimentary canal.

mucous cells (myōō′-kəs sĕlz) Cells that are found in the salivary glands and the lining of the stomach and that secrete mucous.

MUGA scan (mŭg′ə skăn) A radiologic procedure that evaluates the condition of the heart's myocardium; it involves injection of radioisotopes that concentrate in the myocardium, followed by the use of a gamma camera to measure ventricular contractions to evaluate the patient's heart wall.

multimedia (mŭl′tē-mē′dē-ə) More than one medium, such as in graphics, sound, and text used to convey information.

multitasking (mŭl′tē-tăs′kĭng) Running two or more computer software programs simultaneously.

multi-unit smooth muscle (mŭl′tə-yōō′nĭt smōōth mŭs′əl) A type of smooth muscle that is found in the iris of the eye and in the walls of blood vessels.

murmur (mûr′mər) An abnormal heart sound heard when the ventricles contract and blood leaks back into the atria.

muscle fatigue (mŭs′əl fa-tēg′) A condition caused by a buildup of lactic acid.

muscle fiber (mŭs′əl fī′bər) Muscle cells that are called fibers because of their long lengths.

muscle tissue (mŭs′əl tĭsh′ōō) A tissue type that is specialized to shorten and elongate.

muscular dystrophy (mŭs′kyə-lər dis′trō-fē)(†) A group of inherited disorders characterized by a loss of muscle tissue and by muscle weakness.

mutation (myōō-ta′shən) An error that sometimes occurs when DNA is duplicated. When it occurs, it is passed to descendent cells and may or may not affect them in harmful ways.

myasthenia gravis (mī-as-thē′nē-ă grav′is) An autoimmune disorder that is characterized by muscle weakness.

myelin (mī′ə-lĭn) A fatty substance that insulates the axon and allows it to send nerve impulses quickly.

myelography (mī′ĕ-log′ră-fē) An x-ray visualization of the spinal cord after the injection of a radioactive contrast medium or air into the spinal subarachnoid space (between the second and innermost of three membranes that cover the spinal cord). This test can reveal tumors, cysts, spinal stenosis, or herniated disks.

myocardial infarction (mī′ō-kär′dē-ăl ĭn-fark′shən) A heart attack that occurs when the blood flow to the heart is reduced as a result of blockage in the coronary arteries or their branches.

myocardium (mī′ō-kär′dē-əm) The middle and thickest layer of the heart. It is made primarily of cardiac muscle.

myocytes (mī′ō sīts) Muscle cells; also called muscle fibers.

myofibrils (mī-ō-fī′brils)(†) Long structures that fill the sarcoplasm of a muscle fiber.

myoglobin (mī-ō-glō′bin)(†) A pigment contained in muscle cells that stores extra oxygen.

myoglobinuria (mī′ō-glō-bi-nūrē-ă) The presence of myoglobin in the urine; can be caused by injured or damaged muscle tissue.

myometrium (mī′ō-mē′trē-ŭm)(†) The middle, thick muscular layer of the uterus.

myopia (mī-ō′pē-ə) A condition that occurs when light entering the eye is focused in front of the retina; commonly called nearsightedness.

myxedema (mik-se-dē′mă)(†) A severe type of hypothyroidism that is most common in women older than the age of 50.

nail bed (nāl bĕd) The layer beneath each nail.

narcotic (när-kŏt′ĭk) A popular term for an opioid and term of choice in government agencies; see **opioid.**

nares (ner′ēz) The openings of the nose or nostrils.

nasal (nā′zəl)   Relating to the nose. The nasal bones fuse to form the bridge of the nose.

nasal conchae (nā′zəl kon′kē)(†)   Structures that extend from the lateral walls of the nasal cavity.

nasal mucosa (nā′zəl myōō-kō′sə)   The lining of the nose.

nasal septum (nā′zəl sĕp′təm)   A structure that divides the nasal cavity into a left and right portion.

nasolacrimal duct (nā-zō-lăk′rə-məl dŭkt)   A structure located on the medial aspect of each eyeball. These ducts drain tears into the nose.

nasopharynx (nā′zō-far′ingks)(†)   The portion of the pharynx behind the nasal cavity.

National Center for Complementary and Alternative Medicine (NCCAM) (năsh′ə-nəl sĕn′tər for kŏm′-plə-mĕn-tə-rē and ôl-tûr′-nə-tĭv mĕd′-ĭ-sĭn)   National organization that conducts and supports CAM research and provides CAM information to healthcare providers and the public.

natural killer (NK) cells (năch′ər-el kĭl′ər selz)   Non-B and non-T lymphocytes. NK cells kill cancer cells and virus-infected cells without previous exposure to the antigen.

naturopathic medicine (nă′-chə-rŏp′-ə-ĭk mĕd′-ĭ-sĭn)   A system of medicine that relies on the healing power of the body and supports that power through various healthcare practices, such as nutritional counseling, lifestyle counseling, and exercise.

needle biopsy (nēd′l bī′ŏp′sē)   A procedure in which a needle and syringe are used to aspirate (withdraw by suction) fluid or tissue cells.

negligence (nĕg′lĭ-jəns)   A medical professional's failure to perform an essential action or performance of an improper action that directly results in the harm of a patient.

negotiable (nĭ-gō′shē-ə-bəl)   Legally transferable from one person to another.

neonatal period (nē-ō-nā′tăl pîr′ē-əd)(†)   The first 4 weeks of the postnatal period of an offspring.

neonate (nē′ə-nāt′)   An infant during the first 4 weeks of life.

nephrologist (ne-frol′ō-jĭst)(†)   A specialist who studies, diagnoses, and manages diseases of the kidney.

nephrons (nef′ronz)(†)   Microscopic structures in the kidneys that filter blood and form urine.

nerve fiber (nûrv fī′bər)   A structure that extends from the cell body. It consists of two types: axons and dendrites.

nerve impulse (nûrv ĭm′pŭls′)   Electrochemical messages transmitted from neurons to other neurons and effectors.

nervous tissue (nûr′vəs tĭsh′ōō)   A tissue type located in the brain, spinal cord, and peripheral nerves.

net earnings (nĕt ûr′nĭngz)   Take-home pay, calculated by subtracting total deductions from gross earnings.

network (nĕt′wûrk′)   A system that links several computers together.

networking (nĕt′wûrk′ĭng)   Making contacts with relatives, friends, and acquaintances that may have information about how to find a job in your field.

neuralgia (nŏō-răl′jə)   A medical condition characterized by severe pain along the distribution of a nerve.

neuroglia (nûr-ŏg′lēə)   Structures that function as support cells for other neurons, including astrocytes, microglia, and oligodendrocytes. See also **neuroglial cells.**

neuroglial cell (nū-rog′lē-ăl sĕl)(†)   Non-neuronal type of nervous tissue that is smaller and more abundant than neurons. Neuroglial cells support neurons.

neurologist (nŏō-rəl′ə-jĕst)   A specialist who diagnoses and treats disorders and diseases of the nervous system, including the brain, spinal cord, and nerves.

neuron (nŏōr′ŏn′)   A nerve cell; it carries nerve impulses between the brain or spinal cord and other parts of the body.

neurotransmitter (nŏōr′ō-trăns′mĭt-ər)   A chemical within the vesicles of the synaptic knob that is released into the postsynaptic structures when a nerve impulse reaches the synaptic knob.

neutrophil (nū′trō-fil)(†)   A type of granular leukocyte that aids in phagocytosis by attacking bacterial invaders; also responsible for the release of pyrogens.

new patient (nōō pā′shənt)   Patient that, for CPT reporting purposes, has not received professional services from the physician within the past 3 years.

nocturia (nok-tū′rē-ă)(†)   Excessive nighttime urination.

noncompliant (nŏn′kəm-plī′ent)   The term used to describe a patient who does not follow the medical advice given.

noninvasive (non-in-vā′siv)(†)   Referring to procedures that do not require inserting devices, breaking the skin, or monitoring to the degree needed with invasive procedures.

nonsteroidal hormone (non-stēr′oyd-al hôr′mōn′)(†)   A type of hormone made of amino acids and proteins.

norepinephrine (nōr′ep-i-nef′rin)(†)   A neurotransmitter released by sympathetic neurons onto organs and glands for fight-or-flight (stressful) situations.

no-show (nō shō)   A patient who does not call to cancel and does not come to an appointment.

nosocomial infection (nos-ō-kō′mē-ăl ĭn-fĕk-shən)   An infection contracted in a hospital.

notations (nō-tā´shən) Information found at the end of a business letter indicating enclosures included with the letter and the names of other people who will be receiving copies of the letter.

Notice of Privacy Practices (NPP) (nō´tĭs prī´və-sē prăk´tis-əs) A document that informs patients of their rights as outlined under **HIPAA.**

nuclear medicine (noo´klē-ər mĕd´ĭ-sĭn) The use of radionuclides, or radioisotopes (radioactive elements or their compounds), to evaluate the bone, brain, lungs, kidneys, liver, pancreas, thyroid, and spleen; also known as radionuclide imaging.

nucleases (nū´klē-ās-ez) Pancreatic enzymes that digest nucleic acids.

nucleus (noo´klē-əs)(†) The control center of a cell; contains the chromosomes that direct cellular processes.

numeric filing system (noo-mĕr´ĭk fīl´ĭng sĭs´təm) A filing system that organizes files by numbers instead of names. Each patient is assigned a number in the order in which she joins the practice.

nystagmus (nis-tag´mŭs) Rapid involuntary eye movements that may be the result of drug or alcohol use, brain injury or lesion, or cerebrovascular accident (CVA).

O&P specimen (ō ənd pē spĕs´ə-mən) An ova and parasites specimen, or a stool sample, that is examined for the presence of certain forms of protozoans or parasites, including their eggs (ova).

objective (əb-jĕk´tĭv) Pertaining to data that is readily apparent and measurable, such as vital signs, test results, or physical examination findings.

objectives (ob-jek´tĭvs) The set of magnifying lenses contained in the nosepiece of a compound microscope.

occipital (ŏk-sĭp´ĭ-tl) Relating to the back of the head. The occipital bone forms the back of the skull.

occult blood (ə-kŭlt blŭd) Blood contained in some other substance, not visible to the naked eye.

ocular (ŏk´yə-lər) An eyepiece of a microscope.

oil-immersion objective (oil ĭ-mûr´zhənəb-jĕk´tĭv) A microscope objective that is designed to be lowered into a drop of immersion oil placed directly above the prepared specimen under examination, eliminating the air space between the microscope slide and the objective and producing a much sharper, brighter image.

ointment (oint´mənt) A form of topical drug; also known as a salve.

Older Americans Act of 1965 (ōl´dər ə-mĕr´ĭ-kəns ăkt) A U.S. law that guarantees certain benefits to elderly citizens, including health care, retirement income, and protection against abuse.

olfactory (ŏl-făk´tə-rē) Relating to the sense of smell.

oligodendrocytes (ŏl´igōden´drəsit) Specialized neuroglial cells that assist in the production of the myelin sheath.

oliguria (ol´i-gu´re-ah) Insufficient production (or volume) of urine.

oncologist (ŏn-kŏl´ə-jĭst) A specialist who identifies tumors and treats patients who have cancer.

onychectomy (ŏn-i-kek´tō-mē) The removal of a fingernail or toenail.

oocyte (ō´ō-sīt)(†) The immature egg.

oogenesis (ō-ō-jen´ĕ-sis)(†) The process of egg cell formation.

open-book account (ō´pən book ə-kount´) An account that is open to charges made occasionally as needed.

open-hours scheduling (ō´pən ourz skĕj´ool-ĭng) A system of scheduling in which patients arrive at the doctor's office at their convenience and are seen on a first-come, first-served basis.

open posture (ōpən pŏs´chər) A position that conveys a feeling of receptiveness and friendliness; facing another person with arms comfortably at the sides or in the lap.

ophthalmologist (ŏf-thəl-mŏl´ə-jĭst) A medical doctor who is an eye specialist.

ophthalmoscope (of-thal´mōskōp)(†) A hand-held instrument with a light; used to view inner eye structures.

opioid (ō´-pē-òid) A natural or synthetic drug that produces opium-like effects.

opportunistic infection (ŏp´ər-toon ĭs´tĭk ĭn-fĕk-shən) Infection by microorganisms that can cause disease only when a host's resistance is low.

optical character reader (OCR) (ōp´tī-kəl kār´ək-tər-rek-tər rēdər) An electronic scanner that can "read" typed letters.

optical character recognition (OCR) (ōp´tĭ-kəl kār´ək-tər rek-uh g-nish-uh n) The process or technology of reading data in printed form by a device that scans and identifies characters.

optical microscope (op´ti-kăl mī´krə-skōp´) A microscope that uses light, concentrated through a condenser and focused through the object being examined, to project an image.

optic chiasm (ŏp´tĭk kī´azm)(†) A structure located at the base of the brain where parts of the optic nerves cross. It carries visual information to the brain.

optician (ŏp-tĭ´shən) An eye professional who fills prescriptions for eyeglasses and contact lenses.

optometrist (ŏp-tŏm´ĭ-trĭst) A trained and licensed vision specialist who is not a physician.

orbicularis oculi (ōr-bĭk´yū-lā´ris ok´yū-lī) The muscle in the eyelid responsible for blinking.

orbit (ôr´bĭt) The eye socket, which forms a protective shell around the eye.

organ (ôr´gan) Structure formed by the organization of two or more different tissue types that carries out specific functions.

organ of Corti (ôr´gən əv kôr´tē) The organ of hearing, located within the cochlea of the inner ear.

organelle (ôr´gə-nəl´) A structure within a cell that performs a specific function.

organic (ôr-găn´ĭk) Pertaining to matter that contains carbon and hydrogen.

organism (ôr´gə-nĭz´əm) A whole living being that is formed from organ systems.

organ system (ôr´gən sĭs´təm) A system that consists of organs that join together to carry out vital functions.

orifice (ôr´i fis) An opening.

origin (ôr´ə-jĭn) An attachment site of a skeletal muscle that does not move when a muscle contracts.

Original Medicare Plan (ə-rĭj´ə-nəl mĕd´ĭ-kâr´ plăn) The Medicare fee-for-service plan that allows the beneficiary to choose any licensed physician certified by Medicare.

oropharynx (ōr´ō-far´ingks)(†) The portion of the pharynx behind the oral cavity.

orthopedist (ôr´thə-pēd ĭst) A specialist who diagnoses and treats diseases and disorders of the muscles and bones.

orthopnea (ôr thop´nē a) Condition of difficulty breathing except while in an upright position.

orthostatic hypotension (ôr´-thə-stăt´-ĭk hĭ/po-tĕn´ shən) A situation in which blood pressure becomes low and the pulse increases when a patient is moved from a lying to standing position; also known as postural hypotension.

OSHA (Occupational Safety and Health Act) (ō´shə) A set of regulations designed to save lives, prevent injuries, and protect the health of workers in the United States.

osmosis (ŏz-mō´sĭs) The diffusion of water across a semipermeable membrane such as a cell membrane.

ossification (ä-sə-fə-kā´-shən) The process of bone growth.

osteoblast (os´tē-ō-blast)(†) Bone-forming cells that turn membrane into bone. They use excess blood calcium to build new bone.

osteoclast (os´tē-ō-klast)(†) Bone-dissolving cells. When bone is dissolved, calcium is released into the bloodstream.

osteocyte (äs´-tē-ə-sīt) A cell of osseous tissue; also called a bone cell.

osteon (äs´-tē-ən) Elongated cylinders that run up and down the long axis of bone.

osteopathic manipulative medicine (OMM) (ŏs´tē-ō-păth´ĭk mə-nĭp´ū-lā´tĭv mĕd´ĭ-sĭn) A system of hands-on techniques that help relieve pain, restore motion, support the body's natural functions, and influence the body's structure. Osteopathic physicians study OMM in addition to medical courses.

osteoporosis (ŏs´tē-ō-pə-rō´sĭs) An endocrine and metabolic disorder of the musculoskeletal system, more common in women than in men, characterized by hunched-over posture.

osteosarcoma (os´tē-ō-sar-kō´mă) A type of bone cancer that originates from osteoblasts, the cells that make bony tissue.

otologist (ō-tol´ŏ-jist)(†) A medical doctor who specializes in the health of the ear.

otorhinolaryngologist (ō-tō-rī´nōlar-ing-gol´ŏ-jist) A specialist who diagnoses and treats diseases of the ear, nose, and throat.

otosclerosis (ō-tō-sklŭ rōsis) Hardening or immobilization of the stapes within the inner ear.

out guide (out gīd) A marker made of stiff material and used as a placeholder when a file is taken out of a filing system.

ova (ō va) Eggs.

oval window (ō´vəl wĭn´dō) The beginning of the inner ear.

overbooking (ō´vər-bŏŏk´ĭng) Scheduling appointments for more patients than can reasonably be seen in the time allowed.

oviduct (ō´ və´ duct) A Fallopian tube.

ovulation (ō´vyə-lā´shən) The process by which the ovaries release one ovum (egg) approximately every 28 days.

ovum (ō vəm) One egg. The female "egg" that unites with the male sperm to begin reproduction.

oxygenated (ok´səjənātəd) Oxygenated blood refers to blood that has been to the lungs and is carrying oxygen in the hemoglobin.

oxygen debt (ok´sĭ-jən) A condition that develops when skeletal muscles are used strenuously for a minute or two.

oxyhemoglobin (oks-ē-hē-mō-glō´bin)(†) Hemoglobin that is bound to oxygen. It is bright red in color.

oxytocin OT (ok-sē-tō´sin)(†) A hormone that causes contraction of the uterus during childbirth and the ejection of milk from mammary glands during breast-feeding.

packed red blood cells (păkt rĕd blud sĕlz) Red blood cells that collect at the bottom of a centrifuged blood sample.

palate (pal´ăt)(†) The roof of the mouth.

palatine (pa´-lə-tīn) Bones that form the anterior potion of the roof of the mouth and the **palate.**

palatine tonsils (pal´ă-tīn tŏn´sils)(†) Two masses of lymphatic tissue located at the back of the throat.

palpation (păl-pā´shən) A type of touch used by health-care providers to determine characteristics such as texture, temperature, shape, and the presence of movement.

palpatory method (pal-pa´tôr´ē mĕth´əd) Systolic blood pressure measured by using the sense of touch. This measurement provides a necessary preliminary approximation of the systolic blood pressure to ensure an adequate level of inflation when the actual auscultatory measurement is made.

palpitations (păl´pĭ-tā´shənz) Unusually rapid, strong, or irregular pulsations of the heart.

pancreatic amylase (pan-krē-at´ik am´il-ās)(†) An enzyme that digests carbohydrates.

pancreatic lipase (pan-krē-at´ik lip´ās)(†) An enzyme that digests lipids.

panel (păn´əl) Tests frequently ordered together that are organ or disease oriented.

papillae (pə-pĭl´ē) The "bumps" of the tongue in which the taste buds are found.

paranasal sinuses (par-ă-nā´zəl sī´nŭs-ĕz) Air-filled spaces within skull bones that open into the nasal cavity.

parasite (păr´ə-sīt´) An organism that lives on or in another organism and relies on it for nourishment or some other advantage to the detriment of the host organism.

parasympathetic (păr´ə-sĭm´pə-thĕt´ĭk)(†) A division of the autonomic nervous system that prepares the body for rest and digestion.

parathyroid glands (para-ă-thī royd glăndz) Four small glands embedded in the posterior thyroid gland that secrete parathyroid hormone (PTH); also known as parathormone.

parathyroid hormone PH (par-ă-thī´royd hôr´mōn´)(†) A hormone that helps regulate calcium levels in the bloodstream. It increases blood calcium by decreasing bone calcium.

parenteral nutrition (pă-ren´ter-ăl nōō-trĭsh´ən) Nutrition obtained when specially prepared nutrients are injected directly into patients' veins rather than taken by mouth.

paresthesias (par-es-thē´zē-ăs)(†) Abnormal sensations ranging from burning to tingling.

parietal (pă-rī´ĕ-tăl) Bones that form most of the top and sides of the skull.

parietal cells (pă-rī´ĕ-tăl sĕlz) Stomach cells that secrete hydrochloric acid, which is necessary to convert **pepsinogen** to **pepsin.** Parietal cells also secrete **intrinsic factor,** which is necessary for vitamin B_{12} absorption.

parietal pericardium (pă-rī´ĕ-tăl per-i-kar´dē-ŭm)(†) The layer on top of the visceral pericardium.

parietal peritoneum (pă-rī´ĕ-tăl per-ə-tŏnē´əm) The lining of the abdominal cavity.

parotid glands (pă-rot´id glăndz)(†) The largest of the salivary glands. The parotid glands are located beneath the skin just in front of the ears.

participating physicians (păr-tĭs´ə-pāt´ĭng fĭ-zĭsh´ənz) Physicians who enroll in managed care plans. They have contracts with MCOs that stipulate their fees.

partnership (pärt´n r shĭp) A form of medical practice management in which two or more parties practice together under a written agreement, specifying the rights, obligations, and responsibilities of each partner.

parturition (pär´ tur ish´ ən) The act of giving birth.

passive listening (păs´ĭv lĭs´ən-ĭng) Hearing what a person has to say without responding in any way; contrast with **active listening.**

patch test (păch tĕst) An allergy test in which a gauze patch soaked with a suspected allergen is taped onto the skin with nonallergenic tape; used to discover the cause of contact dermatitis.

patella (pə-té-lə) The bone commonly referred to as the kneecap.

pathogen (păth´ə-jən) A microorganism capable of causing disease.

pathologist (pă-thŏl´ə-jĭst) A medical doctor who studies the changes a disease produces in the cells, fluids, and processes of the entire body.

patient compliance (pā´shənt kəm-plī´əns) Obedience in terms of following a physician's orders.

patient ledger card (pā´shənt lĕj´ər kärd) A card containing information needed for insurance purposes, including the patient's name, address, telephone number, Social Security number, insurance information, employer's name, and any special billing instructions. It also includes the name of the person who is responsible for charges if this is anyone other than the patient.

patient record/chart (pā´shənt rĕk´ərd/chärt) A compilation of important information about a patient's medical history and present condition.

pay schedule (pā skĭej´ool) A list showing how often an employee is paid, such as weekly, biweekly, or monthly.

payee (pā-ē´) A person who receives a payment.

payer (pā´ər) A person who pays a bill or writes a check.

pectoral girdle (pĕk´tər əl) The structure that attaches the arms to the axial skeleton.

pediatrician (pē´dē-ə-trĭshən) A specialist who diagnoses and treats childhood diseases and teaches parents skills for keeping their children healthy.

pediculosis (pədĭk´yoolō´sis) The medical term for lice.

pegboard system (pĕg´bôrd sĭs´təm) A bookkeeping system that uses a lightweight board with pegs on which forms can be stacked, allowing each transaction to be entered and recorded on four different bookkeeping forms at once; also called the one-write system.

pelvic girdle (pĕl´vik) The structure that attaches the legs to the axial skeleton.

pepsin (pep´sin)(†) An enzyme that allows the body to digest proteins.

pepsinogen (pep-sin´ō-jen)(†) Substance that is secreted by the chief cells in the lining of the stomach and becomes **pepsin** in the presence of acid.

peptidases (pep´ti-dās-ez)(†) Enzymes that digest proteins.

percussion (pər-kŭsh´ən) Tapping or striking the body to hear sounds or feel vibration.

percutaneous exposure (per-kyūtā´nē-ŭs ĭk-spō´zhər)(†) Exposure to a pathogen through a puncture wound or needlestick.

pericardium (per-i-kar´dē-ŭm)(†) A membrane that covers the heart and large blood vessels attached to it.

perilymph (per´i-limf)(†) A fluid in the inner ear. When this fluid moves, it activates hearing and equilibrium receptors.

perimetrium (peri-mē´trĕŭm) The thin layer that covers the myometrium of the uterus.

perimysium (per-i-mis´ē-ŭm)(†) The connective tissue that divides a muscle into sections called fascicles.

perineum (per i nē´üm) In the male, the area between the scrotum and anus; in the female, the area between the vagina and rectum.

periosteum (pĕr´ē ŏs´tē əm) The membrane that surrounds the **diaphysis** of a bone.

peripheral nervous system (PNS) (pə-rĭf´ər-əl nûr´vəs sĭs´təm) A system that consists of nerves that branch off the central nervous system.

peristalsis (pĕr´ĭ-stôl´sĭs) The rhythmic muscular contractions that move a substance through a tract, such as food through the digestive tract and the ovum through the fallopian tube.

personal protective equipment (PPE) (pur-suh-nl pruh-tek-tiv i-kwip-muh nt) Any type of protective gear worn to guard against physical hazards.

personal space (pûr´sə-nəl spās) A certain area that surrounds an individual and within which another person's physical presence is felt as an intrusion.

petty cash fund (pĕt´ē kăsh fŭnd) Cash kept on hand in the office for small purchases.

phagocyte (făg´ə-sīt´) A specialized white blood cell that engulfs and digests pathogens.

phagocytosis (fag´ō-sī-tō´sis)(†) The process by which white blood cells defend the body against infection by engulfing invading pathogens.

phalanges The bones of the fingers.

pharmaceutical (fär´mə-soo͞´tĭ-kəl) Pertaining to medicinal drugs.

pharmacodynamics (far´mă-kō-dīnam´iks)(†) The study of what drugs do to the body: the mechanism of action, or how they work to produce a therapeutic effect.

pharmacognosy (far-mă-kog´nō-sē)(†) The study of characteristics of natural drugs and their sources.

pharmacokinetics (far´mă-kō-kinet´iks) (†) The study of what the body does to drugs: how the body absorbs, metabolizes, distributes, and excretes the drugs.

pharmacology (fär´ma-kŏl´ə-jē)(†) The study of drugs.

pharmacotherapeutics (far´mă-kō-thĕr´ə-pyoo͞´tĭks) The study of how drugs are used to treat disease; also called clinical **pharmacology.**

pharyngeal tonsils (fă-rin´jē-ăl tŏn´səls) (†) Two masses of lymphatic tissue located above the palatine tonsils; also called adenoids.

pharynx (făr´ĭngks) Structure below the mouth and nasal cavities that is an organ of the respiratory system as well as the digestive system.

phenylketonuria (PKU) (fen´il-kē´tō-nū´rē-ă)(†) A genetically inherited disorder in which the body cannot properly metabolize the nutrient phenylalanine, resulting in the buildup of phenylketones in the blood and their presence in the urine. The accumulation of phenylketones results in mental retardation.

philosophy (fĭ-lŏs´ə-fē) The system of values and principles an office has adopted in its everyday practice.

phlebotomy (flĭ-bŏt´ə-mē) The insertion of a needle or cannula (small tube) into a vein for the purpose of withdrawing blood.

photometer (fō-tŏm´ĭ-tər) An instrument that measures light intensity.

physiatrist (fiz-ī´ă-trist)(†) A physical medicine specialist, who diagnoses and treats diseases and disorders with physical therapy.

physical therapy (fĭz´ĭ-kəl thĕr´ə-pē) A medical specialty that uses cold, heat, water, exercise, massage, traction, and other physical means to treat musculoskeletal, nervous, and cardiopulmonary disorders.

physician assistant (PA) (fĭ-zĭsh´ən ə-sĭs´tənt) A health-care provider who practices medicine under the supervision of a physician.

physician's office laboratory (POL) (fĭ-zĭsh´ənz ô´fĭs lăb´rə-tôr´ē) A laboratory contained in a physician's office; processing tests in the POL produces quick turnaround and eliminates the need for patients to travel to other test locations.

physiology (fĭz´ē-ŏl´ə-jē) The science of the study of the body's functions.

pineal body (pĭn´ē-ăl bŏd´ē) A small gland located between the cerebral hemispheres that secretes melatonin.

pitch (pĭch) The high or low quality in the sound of a person's speaking voice.

placebo effect (plə´-sē-bō ĭ-fĕkt´) The belief that a medication or treatment works even though it is not scientifically substantiated. In research, a placebo is an inactive substance or preparation used as a control to determine the effectiveness of a medicinal drug.

placenta (plə-sĕn´tə) An organ located between the mother and the fetus. It permits the absorption of nutrients and oxygen. In some cases, harmful substances such as viruses are absorbed through the placenta.

plantar flexion (plan´tăr flek´shŭn)(†) Pointing the toes downward.

plasma (plăz´mə) The fluid component of blood, in which formed elements are suspended; makes up 55% of blood volume.

plastic surgeon (plăs´tĭk sûr´jən) A specialist who reconstructs, corrects, or improves body structures.

platelets (plāt´lĭts) Fragments of cytoplasm in the blood that are crucial to clot formation; also called thrombocytes.

pleura (plŭr´ă)(†) The membranes that surround the lungs.

pleural effusion (plŏŏr´əl if yōō´zhən) A buildup of fluid within the pleural cavity.

pleurisy (plŏŏr´əsē) Also known as pleuritis; this is an inflammation of the parietal pleura of the lungs.

pleuritis A condition in which the **pleura** become inflamed, which causes them to stick together. It can also cause an excess amount of fluid to form between the membranes.

plexus (plĕk´səs) A structure that is formed when spinal nerves fuse together. It includes the cervical, brachial, and lumbosacral nerves.

pneumoconiosis (nŏŏ mŏ kō´nē ō´sis) This is the name given to lung diseases that result from years of exposure to different environmental or occupational types of dust.

pneumothorax (nū-mō-thōr´aks)(†) The presence of air or gas in the pleural cavity. The lung typically collapses with pneumothorax.

polar body (pō´lər bŏd´ē) A nonfunctional cell that is one of two small cells formed during the division of an oocyte.

polarity (pō-lăr´ĭ-tē) The condition of having two separate poles, one of which is positive and the other, negative.

polarized (pō´lə-rīzd´) The state in which the outside of a cell membrane is positively charged and the inside is negatively charged. Polarization occurs when a neuron is at rest.

polysaccharide (pol-ē-sak´ă-rīd)(†) A type of carbohydrate that is a starch.

POMR (pē´ō-ĕm-är) The problem-oriented medical record system for keeping patients' charts. Information in a POMR includes the database of information about the patient and the patient's condition, the problem list, the diagnostic and treatment plan, and progress notes.

portfolio (pôrt-fō´lē-ō´) A collection of an applicant's résumé, reference letters, and other documents of interest to a potential employer.

positive tilt test (pŏz´-ĭ-tĭv tĭlt tĕst) When the pulse rate increases more than 10 beats per minute (bpm) and the blood pressure drops more than 20 points while taking vital signs in the lying, sitting, and standing positions.

positron emission tomography (PET) (pah´-zih-tron ee-mih´-shun toh-mah´-gruh-fee) A radiologic procedure that entails injecting isotopes combined with other substances involved in metabolic activity, such as glucose. These special isotopes emit positrons, which a computer processes and displays on a screen.

posterior (pŏ-stîr´ē-ar) Anatomic term meaning toward the back of the body. Also called dorsal.

postnatal period (pōst-nā´tăl pîr´ē-əd)(†) The period following childbirth.

postoperative (pōst-ŏp´ər-ə-tĭv) Taking place after a surgical procedure.

postural hypotension (pŏs-chĕr-ăl hī-pō-tĕn-shŭn) A situation in which blood pressure becomes low and the pulse increases increases when a patient is moved from a lying to standing position; also known as ortho-static hypotension.

posture (pŏs´chər) Body position and alignment.

power of attorney (pou´ər ə-tûr´nē) The legal right to act as the attorney or agent of another person, including handling that person's financial matters.

practitioner (prăk-tĭsh´ə-nər) One who practices a profession.

pre-authorization (prē ô´thər-ĭ-zā´shən) Authorization or approval for payment from a third-party payer requested in advance of a specific procedure.

pre-certification (prē sûr´tə-fĭ-kā´shən) A determination of the amount of money that will be paid by a third-party payer for a specific procedure before the procedure is conducted.

preferred provider organization (PPO) (prĭ-fûrd′ prə-vīd′ər or′ gə-nĭ-zā′shən) A managed care plan that establishes a network of providers to perform services for plan members.

premenstrual syndrome (PMS) (prē-me′n-strə-wal sin′-drōm)(†) A syndrome that is a collection of symptoms that occur just before the menstrual period.

premium (prē′mē-əm) The basic annual cost of health-care insurance.

prenatal period (prē-nā′tăl pîr′ē-əd)(†) The period that includes the embryonic and fetal periods until the delivery of the offspring.

preoperative (prē-ŏp′ər-ə-tĭv) Taking place prior to surgery.

prepuce (prē′pūs)(†) A piece of skin in the uncircumcized male that covers the glans penis.

presbyopia (prez-bē-ō′pē-ă) A common eye disorder that results in the loss of lens elasticity. Presbyopia develops with age and causes a person to have difficulty seeing objects close up.

prescribe (prĭ-skrīb′) To give a patient a prescription to be filled by a pharmacy.

prescription (prĭ-skrĭp′shən) A physician's written order for medication.

prescription drug (prĭ-skrĭp′shən drŭg) A drug that can be legally used only by order of a physician and must be administered or dispensed by a licensed health-care professional.

primary care physician (prī′měr′ē kâr fĭ-zĭsh′ən) A physician who provides routine medical care and referrals to specialists.

primary germ layer (prī′měr′ē jûrm lā′ər) An inner cell mass that organizes into layers: the ectoderm, mesoderm, and endoderm.

prime mover (prīm mōō′vər) The muscle responsible for most of the movement when a body movement is produced by a group of muscles.

primordial follicle (prī-mōr′dĕl-ăl fŏl′ĭ-kəl)(†) A structure that develops in the ovarian cortex of a female infant before she is born.

Privacy Rule (prī′və-sē rōōl) Common name for the **HIPAA** Standard for Privacy of Individually Identifiable Health Information, which provides the first comprehensive federal protection for the privacy of health information. The Privacy Rule creates national standards to protect individuals' medical records and other personal health information.

procedure code (prə-sē′jər kōd) Codes that represent medical procedures, such as surgery and diagnostic tests, and medical services, such as an examination to evaluate a patient's condition.

proctoscopy (prok-tos′kō-pē) An examination of the lower rectum and anal canal with a 3-inch instrument called a proctoscope to detect hemorrhoids, polyps, fissures, fistulas, and abscesses.

proficiency testing program (prə-fĭ′shən-cē tĕst′ĭng prō′grăm′) A required set of tests for clinical laboratories; the tests measure the accuracy of the laboratory's test results and adherence to standard operating procedures.

progesterone (prō-jĕs′tə-rōn′) A female steroid hormone primarily produced by the ovary.

prognosis (prŏg-nō′sĭs) A prediction of the probable course of a disease in an individual and the chances of recovery.

prolactin (PRL) (prō-lak′tin)(†) A hormone that stimulates milk production in the mammary glands.

proliferation phase (prə-lĭf′ər-ā′shən fāz) The second phase of wound healing, in which new tissue forms, closing off the wound.

pronation (prō-nā′shŭn)(†) Turning the palms of the hand downward.

pronunciation (prə-nun′cē-ā′shən) The sounding out of words.

proofreading (prōōf′rēd′ĭng) Checking a document for formatting, data, and mechanical errors.

prophase (prō′faz) Movement of the replicated centrioles to the opposite ends of the cell, creating spindle-like fibers during mitosis.

prostaglandin (pros-tă-glan′din)(†) A local hormone derived from lipid molecules. Prostaglandins typically do not travel in the bloodstream to find their target cells because their targets are close by. This hormone has numerous effects, including uterine stimulation during childbirth.

prostate gland (prŏs′tāt′ glănd) A chestnut-shaped gland that surrounds the beginning of the urethra in the male.

prostatitis (pros-tă-tī′tis) Inflammation of the prostate gland, which can be acute or chronic.

protected health information (PHI) (prə-tĕkt-əd hĕlth ĭn′fər-mă′shən) Individually identifiable health information that is transmitted or maintained by electronic or other media, such as computer storage devices. The core of the **HIPAA Privacy Rule** is the protection, use, and disclosure of protected health information.

proteinuria (prō-tē-nū′rē-ă) An excess of protein in the urine.

protozoan (prō′-tə-zō′ən) A single-celled eukaryotic organism much larger than a bacterium; some protozoans can cause disease in humans.

protraction (prō-trăk′shən) Moving a body part anteriorly.

proximal (prok′si-măl)(†) Anatomic term meaning closer to a point of attachment or closer to the trunk of the body.

proximal convoluted tubule (prok´simăl kon´vō-lū-ted tū´byūl)(†) The portion of the renal tubule that is directly attached to the glomerular capsule and becomes the loop of Henle.

psoriasis (sə-rī´ə-sĭs) A common skin condition characterized by reddish-silver scaly lesions most often found on the elbows, knees, scalp, and trunk.

puberty (pyōō´bər-tē) The period of adolescence when a person begins to develop secondary sexual traits and reproductive functions.

pulmonary circuit (pōol´mə-nĕr´ē sûr´kĭt) The route that blood takes from the heart to the lungs and back to the heart again.

pulmonary semilunar valve (pŭl´mənerē sem´ē loonər valv) A heart valve that is a semilunar valve. It is situated between the right ventricle and the pulmonary trunk.

pulmonary trunk (pōol´mə-nĕr´ētrŭngk) A large artery that branches into the pulmonary arteries and carries blood to the lungs.

pubis (pyü´-bəs) The area that forms the front of a hip bone.

pulmonary function test (pōol´mə-nĕr´ēfŭngk´shən tĕst) A test that evaluates a patient's lung volume and capacity; used to detect and diagnose pulmonary problems or to monitor certain respiratory disorders and evaluate the effectiveness of treatment.

puncture wound (pŭngk´chər wound) A deep wound caused by a sharp, pointed object.

punitive damages (pyōō´nĭ-tĭv dăm´ĭjz) Money paid as punishment for intentionally breaking the law.

pupil (pyōō´pəl) The opening at the center of the iris, which grows smaller or larger as the iris contracts or relaxes, respectively;

it regulates the amount of light that enters the eye.

purchase order (pûr´chĭs ôr´dər) A form that authorizes a purchase for the practice.

purchasing groups (pur´chĭs-ĭng grōops) Groups of medical offices associated with a nearby hospital that order supplies through the hospital to obtain a quantity discount.

Purkinje Fibers (per´kin-jē fī´bərz) Cardiac fibers that are located in the lateral walls of the ventricles.

pyelonephritis (pī´ĕ-lō-ne-frī-tis)(†) A urinary tract infection that involves one or both of the kidneys.

pyloric sphincter (pī-lôrĭk sfingk´ tər) The valve-like structure composed of a circular band of muscle at the juncture of the stomach and small intestine.

pyothorax (pī ōt hôr' aks) Pus or infected fluid in the pleural cavity causing collapse of the lung.

pyrogens (pī´ō-jenz)(†) Fever-producing substances released by neutrophils.

qi (chē) According to traditional Chinese medicine, a vital energy that flows throughout the body.

quadrants (kwŏd´rəntz) Four equal sections, such as those into which the abdomen is figuratively divided during an examination.

qualitative analysis (kwŏl´ĭ-tā-tĭv-ənăl´ĭ-sĭs) In microbiology, identification of bacteria present in a specimen by the appearance of colonies grown on a culture plate.

qualitative test response (kwŏl´ĭ-tā´tĭvtĕst rĭ-spŏns´) A test result that indicates the substance tested for is either present or absent.

quality assurance program (kwŏl´ĭ-tēə-shōor´əns prō´gram´) A required program for clinical laboratories designed to monitor the quality of patient care, including quality control, instrument and equipment

maintenance, proficiency testing, training and continuing education, and standard operating procedures documentation.

quality control (QC) (kwŏl´ĭ-tē kən-trōl´) An ongoing system, required in every physican's office, to evaluate the quality of medical care provided.

quality control program (kwŏl´ĭ-tē kəntrōl´ prō´grăm´) A component of a quality assurance program that focuses on ensuring accuracy in laboratory test results through careful monitoring of test procedures.

quantitative analysis (kwŏn´tĭ-tā´tĭvə-năl´ĭ-sĭs) In microbiology, a determination of the number of bacteria present in a specimen by direct count of colonies grown on a culture plate.

quantitative test results (kwŏn´tĭ-tā´tĭvtĕst rĭ-zŭlt´) The concentration of a test substance in a specimen.

quarterly return (kwŏr´tar-lē rĭ-tûrn´) The Employer's Quarterly Federal Tax Return, a form submitted to the IRS every 3 months that summarizes the federal income and employment taxes withheld from employees' paychecks.

qui tam **(kē -´təm)** Latin, meaning "to bring action for the king and for one's self."

radial artery (rā´dē-əl är´tə-rē) An artery located in the groove on the thumb side of the inner wrist, where the pulse is taken on adults.

radiation therapy (rā´dē-ā´shən thĕr´ə-pē) The use of x-rays and radioactive substances to treat cancer.

radiologist (rā´dē-ŏl´ ə-jĭst) A physician who specializes in taking and reading x-rays.

radius (rā-dā-əs) The lateral bone of the forearm.

rales (ralz) Noisy respirations usually due to blockage of the bronchial tubes.

random access memory (RAM) (răn′dəmăk′sĕs mĕm′ə-rē) The temporary, or programmable, memory in a computer.

random urine specimen (răn′dəm yoŏr′ĭn spĕs′ə-mən) A single urine specimen taken at any time of the day; the most common type of sample collected.

range of motion (ROM) (rānj mō′shən) The degree to which a joint is able to move.

rapport (ră-pôr′) A harmonious, positive relationship.

read only memory (ROM) (rĕd ōn′lēmĕm′ə-rē) A computer's permanent memory, which can be read by the computer but not changed. It provides the computer with the basic operating instructions it needs to function.

reagent (rē-ā′jənt) A chemical or chemically treated substance used in test procedures and formulated to react in specific ways when exposed under specific conditions.

reconciliation (rĕk′ən-sīl′ē-ā′shən) A comparison of the office's financial records with bank records to ensure that they are consistent and accurate; usually done when the monthly checking account statement is received from the bank.

records management system (rĭ-kôrdz măn′ĭj-mənt sĭs′təm) How patient records are created, filed, and maintained.

recovery position (rĭ-kŭv′ər-ē pə-zĭsh′ən) The position a person is placed in after receiving first aid for choking or cardiopulmonary resuscitation.

rectum (rĕk′təm) The last section of the sigmoid colon that straightens out and becomes the anal canal.

reference (rĕf′ər-əns) A recommendation for employment from a facility or a preceptor.

reference laboratory (rĕf′ər-əns lăb′rə-tôr′ē) A laboratory owned and operated by an organization outside the physician's practice.

referral (rĭ-fûr′əl) An authorization from a medical practice for a patient to have specialized services performed by another practice; often required for insurance purposes.

reflex (rē′flĕks′) A predictable automatic response to stimuli.

reflexology (rē-flĕk-sŏl′-ə-jē) Manual therapy to the foot and/or hand in which pressure is applied to "reflex" points mapped out on the feet or hands.

refraction (rĭ-frāk′shən) The bending of light by the cornea, lens, and eye fluids to focus light onto the retina.

refraction examination (rĭ-frāk′shən ĭg-zăm′ə-nā′shən) An eye examination in which the patient looks through a succession of different lenses to find out which ones create the clearest image.

refractometer (rē-frak-tom′ĕ-ter)(†) An optical instrument that measures the refraction, or bending, of light as it passes through a liquid.

Registered Medical Assistant (RMA) (rĕj′ĭ-stərd mĕd′ĭ-kəl ə-sĭs′tənt) A medical assistant who has met the educational requirements and taken and passed the certification examination for medical assisting given by the American Medical Technologists (AMT).

Reiki (ray-key) The use of visualization and touch to balance energy flow and bring healthy energy to affected body parts.

relaxin (rē-lak′sin)(†) A hormone that comes from the corpus luteum. It inhibits uterine contractions and relaxes the ligaments of the pelvis in preparation for childbirth.

remedy (rĕm′-ī-dē) A treatment prescribed by a homeopath in small amounts that in large doses would produce the same symptoms seen in the patient.

remittance advice (RA) (rĭ-mĭt′ns˘ ad-vīz′) A form that the patient and the practice receive for each encounter that outlines the amount billed by the practice, the amount allowed, the amount of subscriber liability, the amount paid, and notations of any service not covered, including an explanation of why that service is not covered; also called an explanation of benefits.

renal calculi (rē′nəl kăl′kyə-lī′) Kidney stones.

renal column (rē′nəl kŏl′əm) The portion of the **renal cortex** between the **renal pyramids.**

renal corpuscle (rē′nəl kôr′pə-səl) Corpuscle that is composed of the glomerulus and the glomerular capsule. The filtration of blood occurs here.

renal cortex (rē′nəl kôr′tĕks′) The outermost layer of the kidney.

renal medulla (rē′nəl mĭ-dŭl′ə) The middle portion of the kidney.

renal pelvis (rē′nəl pĕl′vĭs) The internal structure of the kidney. Urine flows from the renal pelvis down the ureter.

renal pyramids (rē′nəl pĭr′ə-mĭdz) Triangular-shaped areas in the medulla of the kidney.

renal sinus (rē′nəl sī′nəs) The medial depression of a kidney.

renal tubule (rē′nəl tū′byūl) Structure that extends from the glomerular capsule of a nephron and is composed of the proximal convoluted tubule, the loop of Henle, and the distal convoluted tubule.

renin (ren′in)(†) A hormone secreted by the kidney that helps to regulate blood pressure.

repolarization (rē′pō-lăr-i-zā′shŭn)(†) The process of returning to the original polar (resting) state.

reputable (rĕpyə-tə-bəl) Having a good reputation.

requisition (rĕk′wĭ-zĭsh′ən) A formal request from a staff member or doctor for the purchase of equipment or supplies.

res ipsa loquitur (reez ip-suh loh-kwi-ter) Latin, meaning "the thing speaks for itself," which is also known as the doctrine of common knowledge.

reservoir host (rĕz´ər-vwär´ hōst) An animal, insect, or human whose body is susceptible to growth of a pathogen.

resident normal flora (´re-zə-dənt, ´nŏr-məl, ´flōr-ə) Bacteria, fungi, and protozoa that have taken up residence either in or on the human body. Some of these organisms neither help nor harm the host and some are beneficial, creating a barrier against pathogens.

resource-based relative value scale (RBRVS) (rē´sôrs´ bāst rĕl´ə-tĭvvăl´yōō skāl) The payment system used by Medicare. It establishes the relative value units for services, replacing the providers' consensus on usual fees.

respiratory distress syndrome (res´pərətôr´ə distres sin'drəm) Condition found usually in premature babies, who lack the substance surfactant in their lungs, causing the lungs to collapse on expiration.

respiratory volume (rĕs´pər-ə-tôr´ē vŏl´yōōm) The different volumes of air that move in and out of the lungs during different intensities of breathing. These volumes can be measured to assess the healthiness of the respiratory system.

respondeat superior (rehs-pond-dee-at soo-peer-e-or) Latin, meaning "let the master answer," a doctrine under which an employer is legally liable for the acts of his or her employees, if such acts were performed within the scope of the employee's duties.

résumé (rĕz´ōō-mā´) A typewritten document summarizing one's employment and educational history.

retention schedule (rĭ-tĕn´shən skĕj´ōōl) A schedule that details how long to keep different types of patient records in the office after they have become inactive or closed and how long the records should be stored.

retina (rĕt´n-ə) The inner layer of the eye; contains light-sensing nerve cells.

retraction (rĭ-trăk´shən) Moving a body part posteriorly.

retrograde pyelography (rĕt´rə-grād´pī´ē-log´rə-fē)(†) A radiologic procedure in which the doctor injects a contrast medium through a urethral catheter and takes a series of x-rays to evaluate function of the ureters, bladder, and urethra.

retroperitoneal (re-trō-per-ə-ə-nē´əl) An anatomic term that means behind the peritoneal cavity. It is where the kidneys lie.

return demonstation (rĭ-tûrn´ dĕm´ən-strā´shən) Participatory teaching method in which the technique is first described to the patient and then demonstrated to the patient; the patient is then asked to repeat the demonstration.

rhabdomyolysis (rab´dō-mī-ol´i-sis)(†) A condition in which the kidneys have been damaged due to toxins released from muscle cells.

Rh antigen (är´ach an´tī-jən) A protein first discovered on the red blood cells of rhesus monkeys, hence the name Rh.

RhoGAM (rō´găm) A medication that prevents an Rh-negative mother from making antibodies against the Rh antigen.

ribosomes ((rībəsomz) The organelle within the cytoplasm responsible for protein synthesis.

RNA (är´ĕn-ā´) A nucleic acid used to make protein.

rods (rŏdz) Light-sensing nerve cells in the eye, at the posterior of the retina, that function in dim

light but do not provide sharp images or detect color.

rosacea (rō-zā´shē-ă)(†) A condition characterized by chronic redness and acne over the nose and cheeks.

rotation (rō-tā´shən) Twisting a body part.

route (rōōt) The way a drug is introduced into the body.

rugae (rōō´gā) The expandable folds of an organ. The folds of the stomach lining.

sacrum (sa´-krəm) A triangular-shaped bone that consists of five fused vertebra.

sagittal (saj´i-tăl)(†) An anatomic term that refers to the plane that divides the body into left and right portions.

salutation (săl´yə-tā´shən) A written greeting, such as "Dear," used at the beginning of a letter.

sanitization (săn´ĭ-tĭ-zā´shən)(†) A reduction of the number of microorganisms on an object or a surface to a fairly safe level.

sarcolemma (sar´kō-lem´ă) The cell membrane of a muscle fiber.

sarcoplasm The cytoplasm of a muscle fiber.

sarcoplasmic reticulum (sar-kō-plaz´mik re-tik´yū-lŭm) The endoplasmic reticulum of a muscle fiber.

SARS (severe acute respiratory syndrome) (särz; sivēr əkyōōt res´pərətôr´ē sin´drəm) A severe and acute respiratory illness characterized by fever and a nonproductive cough that progresses to the point at which insufficient oxygen is present in the blood.

saturated fat (săch´ə-rā´tĭd făt) Fats, derived primarily from animal sources, that are usually solid at room temperature and that tend to raise blood cholesterol levels.

scabies (skā´bēz) Skin lesions that are very itchy and caused by a burrowing mite. Scabies is most commonly found between the fingers and on the genitalia.

scanner (skăn´ər) An optical device that converts printed matter into a format that can be read by the computer and inputs the converted information.

scapula (skă´-pyə-la) Thin, triangular-shaped, flat bones located on the dorsal surface of the rib cage; also called shoulder blades.

Schwann cell (shwahn sĕl)(†) A neuroglial cell whose cell membrane coats the axons.

sciatica (sī-ăt´ĭ-kə) Pain in the low back and hip radiating down the back of the leg along the sciatic nerve.

sclera (sklîr´ə) The tough, outermost layer, or "white," of the eye, through which light cannot pass; covers all except the front of the eye.

scoliosis (skō´lē-ō´sĭs) A lateral curvature of the spine, which is normally straight when viewed from behind.

scratch test (skrăch tĕst) An allergy test in which extracts of suspected allergens are applied to the patient's skin and the skin is then scratched to allow the extracts to penetrate.

screening (skrēn´ĭng) Performing a diagnostic test on a person who is typically free of symptoms.

screen saver (skrēn sāv´ər) A program that automatically changes the monitor display at short intervals or constantly shows moving images to prevent burn-in of images on the computer screen.

scrotum (skrō´təm) In a male, the sac of skin below the pelvic cavity that contains the testes.

sebaceous (sĭ-bā´shəs) A type of oil gland found in the dermis.

sebum (sē´bŭm)(†) An oily substance produced by sebaceous glands.

Security Rule (sĭ-kyoŏr´ĭ-tē roŏl) The technical safeguards that protect the confidentiality, integrity, and availability of health information covered by **HIPAA.** The Security Rule specifies how patient information is protected on computer networks, the Internet, disks, and other storage media.

seizure (sē´zhər) A series of violent and involuntary contractions of the muscles; also called a convulsion.

sella turcica (sel´ă tŭr´sē-kă)(†) A deep depression in the sphenoid bone where the pituitary gland sits.

semen (sē´mən) Sperm and the various substances that nourish and transport them.

semicircular canals (sĕm´ē-sûr´kyə-lər kə-nălz´) Structures in the inner ear that help a person maintain balance; each of the three canals is positioned at right angles to the other two.

seminal vesicles (sem´-năl ves´i-klz)(†) A pair of convoluted tubes that lie behind the bladder. These tubes secrete a fluid that provides nutrition for the sperm.

seminiferous tubules (sem´i-nif´er-ŭs tū´byūlz)(†) These tubes contain spermatogenic cells and are located in the lobules of the testes.

sensorineural hearing loss (sen´sōr-i-nūr´ăl hîr´ĭng lôs) This type of hearing loss occurs when neural structures associated with the ear are damaged. Neural structures include hearing receptors and the auditory nerve.

sensory (sĕn´sə-rē) Afferent neurons that carry sensory information from the periphery to the central nervous system.

sensory adaptation (sĕn´sə-rē ăd´ăp-tā´shən) A process in which the same chemical can stimulate receptors only for a limited amount of time until the receptors eventually no longer respond to the chemical.

septic shock (sĕp´tĭk shŏk) A state of shock resulting from massive, widespread infection that affects the blood vessels' ability to circulate blood.

sequential order (sĭ´kwĕn´shəl ôr´dər) One after another in a predictable pattern or sequence.

serosa (se-rō´să)(†) The outermost layer of the alimentary canal; also known as the visceral peritoneum.

serous cells (sēr´ŭs sĕlz)(†) One of two types of cells that make up the salivary glands. These cells secrete a watery fluid that contains amylase.

serum (sēr´ŭm)(†) The liquid portion of blood (plasma) when all of the clotting factors have been removed.

service contract (sûr´vĭs kŏn´trăkt´) A contract that covers services for equipment that are not included in a standard maintenance contract.

sex chromosome (sĕks krō´mə-sōm´) Chromosome of the 23rd pair.

sex-linked trait (sĕks lĭngk trāt) Traits that are carried on the sex chromosomes, or X and Y chromosomes.

sigmoid colon (sig-mŏid ko-lən) An S-shaped tube that lies between the **descending colon** and the **rectum.**

sigmoidoscopy (sig´moy-dos´kŏ-pē) A procedure in which the interior of the sigmoid area of the large intestine, between the descending colon and the rectum, is examined with a sigmoidoscope, a lighted instrument with a magnifying lens.

sign (sīn) An objective or external factor, such as blood pressure, rash, or swelling, that can be seen or felt by the physician or measured by an instrument.

signature block (sig´-nuh-cher blok´) The writer's name and business title found four lines below the complimentary closing in a business letter.

silicosis (sil´ i kō´ sis) Chronic lung disease caused by the inhalation of silica dust.

simplified letter style (sĭm´plə-fīd´ lĕt´ər stīl) A modification of the full-block style in which the salutation and complimentary closing are omitted and a subject line typed in all capital letters is placed between the address and the body of the letter.

single-entry account (sĭng´gəl-ĕn´trē-ə-kount´) An account that has only one charge, usually for a small amount, for a patient who does not come in regularly.

sinoatrial node (sī´nō-ā´trē-ăl nōd)(†) A small bundle of heart muscle tissue in the superior wall of the right atrium that sets the rhythm (or pattern) of the heart's contractions; also called sinus node or pacemaker.

sinusitis (sī´nə-sī´tĭs) Inflammation of the lining of a sinus.

skinfold test (skĭn´ fōld tĕst) A method of measuring fat as a percentage of body weight by measuring the thickness of a fold of skin with a caliper.

slander (slăn´ dər) The speaking of defamatory words intended to prejudice others against an individual in a manner that jeopardizes his or her reputation or means of livelihood.

sleep apnea (slēp ap-ne´ah) A condition characterized by pauses in breathing during sleep.

slit lamp (slĭt lămp) An instrument composed of a magnifying lens combined with a light source; used to provide a minute examination of the eye's anatomy.

smear (smîr) A specimen spread thinly and unevenly across a slide.

SOAP (sōp) An approach to medical records documentation that documents information in the following order: S (**subjective** data), O (**objective** data),

A (assessment), P (plan of action).

software (sôft´wâr´) A program, or set of instructions, that tells a computer what to do.

sole proprietorship (sōl prə -prī´-tər shĭp) A form of medical practice management in which a physician practices alone, assuming all benefits, and liabilities for the business.

solution (sə-lōō´shən) A homogeneous mixture of a solid, liquid, or gaseous substance in a liquid, such as a dissolved drug in liquid form.

somatic (sō-măt´ĭk) A division of the peripheral nervous system that connects the central nervous system to skin and skeletal muscle.

somatic nervous system (SNS) (sō-măt´ĭk nûr´vəs sĭs´təm) A system that governs the body's skeletal or voluntary muscles.

SPECT (spĕkt) Single photon emission computed tomography; a radiologic procedure in which a gamma camera detects signals induced by gamma radiation and a computer converts these signals into two- or three-dimensional images that are displayed on a screen.

speculum (spĕk´yə-ləm) An instrument that expands the vaginal opening to permit viewing of the vagina and cervix.

spermatids (sper´mă-tidz)(†) Immature sperm before they develop their flagella (tails).

spermatocytes (sper´mă-tō-sīts)(†) The cells that result when spermatogonia undergo mitosis.

spermatogenesis (sper´mă-tō-jen´ĕ-sis)(†) The process of sperm cell formation.

spermatogenic cells (sper´mă-tō-jen´ik sĕlz)(†) The cells that give rise to sperm cells.

spermatogonia (sper´mă-tō-gō´nē-ă)(†) The earliest cell in the process of **spermatogenesis.**

sphenoid A bone that forms part of the floor of the cranium.

sphincter (sfĭngk´tər) A valve-like structure formed from circular bands of muscle. Sphincters are located around various body openings and passages.

sphygmomanometer (sfig´mō-mănom´ĕter)(†) An instrument for measuring blood pressure; consists of an inflatable cuff, a pressure bulb used to inflate the cuff, and a device to read the pressure.

spinal nerves (spī´năl nûrvs)(†) Peripheral nerves that originate from the spinal cord.

spirillum (spī-ril´ŭm)(†) A spiral-shaped bacterium.

spirometer (spī-rom´ĕ-ter)(†) An instrument that measures the air taken in and expelled from the lungs.

spirometry (spī-rom´ĕ-trē)(†) A test used to measure breathing capacity.

splenectomy (splən ek´ tō me) Surgical removal of the spleen.

splint (splĭnt) A device used to immobilize and protect a body part.

splinting catheter (splĭnt´ing kăth´ĭ-tər) A type of catheter inserted after plastic repair of the ureter; it must remain in place for at least a week after surgery.

sprain (sprān) An injury characterized by partial tearing of a ligament that supports a joint, such as the ankle. A sprain may also involve injuries to tendons, muscles, and local blood vessels and contusions of the surrounding soft tissue.

stain (stān) In microbiology, a solution of a dye or group of dyes that impart a color to microorganisms.

standard (stăn´dərd) A specimen for which test values are already known; used to calibrate test equipment.

standardization (stăn-dər-dĭ-zā´-shən) The consistency of the active ingredient(s) in a supplement from batch to batch and from manufacturer to manufacturer.

Standard Precautions (stăn´dərd prĭ-kô´shənz) A combination of Universal Precautions and Body Substance Isolation guidelines; used in hospitals for the care of all patients.

stapes (stā´pēz) A small bone in the middle ear that is attached to the inner ear; also called the stirrup.

statement (stāt´mənt) A form similar to an invoice; contains a courteous reminder to the patient that payment is due.

State Unemployment Tax Act (SUTA) Some states are also governed by this act; these taxes are filed along with FUTA taxes.

statute of limitations (stăch´ōot lĭm´ĭ-tā´shənz) A state law that sets a time limit on when a collection suit on a past-due account can legally be filed.

stent (stĕnt-) A metal mesh tube used to hold a vessel open.

stereoscopy (ster-ē-os´kŏ-pē) (†) An x-ray procedure that uses a specially designed microscope (stereoscopic, or Greenough, microscope) with double eye-pieces and objectives to take films at different angles and produce three-dimensional images; used primarily to study the skull.

sterile field (stĕr´əl fēld) An area free of microorganisms used as a work area during a surgical procedure.

sterile scrub assistant (stĕr´əl skrŭb ə-sĭs´tənt) An assistant who handles sterile equipment during a surgical procedure.

sterilization (stĕr´ə-lĭ-zā´shən) The destruction of all microorganisms, including bacterial spores, by specific means.

sterilization indicator (stĕr´ə-lĭ-zā´shən ĭn´dĭ-kā´shən) A tag, insert, tape, tube, or strip that confirms that the items in an autoclave have been exposed to

the correct volume of steam at the correct temperature for the correct amount of time.

sternum (st´ər-nəm) A bone that forms the front and middle portion of the rib cage; also called the breastbone or breast plate.

steroid al hormone (stîr´oid´ə hôr´mōn´) A hormone derived from steroids that are soluble in lipids and can cross cell membranes very easily.

stethoscope (stĕth´ə-skōp´) An instrument that amplifies body sounds.

strabismus (strə-bĭz´məs) A condition that results in a lack of parallel visual axes of the eyes; commonly called crossed eyes.

strain (strān) A muscle injury that results from overexertion or overstretching.

stratum basale (strat´ŭm bā-sā´le) (†) The deepest layer of the epidermis of the skin.

stratum corneum (strat´ŭm kōr´nē ŭm) (†) The most superficial layer of the epidermis of the skin.

stratum germinativum (strat´ūm jur´minə tē´vūm) The deepest layer of the epidermis; also known as staratum basale.

stressor (stres´or) (†) Any stimulus that produces stress.

stress test (strĕs tĕst) A procedure that involves recording an electrocardiogram while the patient is exercising on a stationary bicycle, treadmill, or stair-stepping ergometer, which measures work performed.

striations (strī-ā´shŭns) (†) Bands produced from the arrangement of filaments in myofibrils in skeletal and cardiac muscle cells.

stroke (strōk) A condition that occurs when the blood supply to the brain is impaired. It may cause temporary or permanent damage.

stylus (stī´ləs) A pen-like instrument that records electrical impulses on ECG paper.

subarachnoid space (sŭb-ă-rak´noydspās) (†) An area between the arachnoid mater and the pia mater.

subclinical case (sŭb-klĭn´i-kăl kās) (†) An infection in which the host experiences only some of the symptoms of the infection or milder symptoms than in a full case.

subcutaneous (SC) (sŭb´kyōo-tā´nē -əs) Under the skin.

subject line (sŭb´jĭkt līn) Optional line of two to three words that appear three lines below the inside address of a business letter.

subjective (səb-jĕk´tĭv) Pertaining to data that is obtained from conversation with a person or patient.

sublingual (sŭb-ling´gwăl) (†) Under the tongue.

sublingual gland (sŭb-ling´gwăl glănd) (†) The smallest of the salivary glands.

submandibular gland (sŭb-man-dib´yu-lăr glănd) (†) The gland that is located in the floor of the mouth.

submucosa (sŭb-mū-kō´s ă) (†) The layer of the alimentary canal located between the mucosa and the muscular layer.

subpoena (sə-pē´nə) A written court order that is addressed to a specific person and requires that person's presence in court on a specific date at a specific time.

***subpoena duces tecum* (suh-pee-nuh doo-seez tee-kuh)** Latin; a legal document that requires the recipient to bring certain written records to court to be used as evidence in a lawsuit.

substance abuse (sŭb´stəns ə-byōoz´) The use of a substance in a way that is not medically approved, such as using diet pills to stay awake or consuming large quantities of cough syrup that contains codeine. Substance abusers are not necessarily addicts.

sucrase (sū′krās)(†) An enzyme that digests sugars.

sudoriferous (soo′dərif′ərəs) The sweat glands.

sulci (sŭl′si)(†) The grooves on the surface of the cerebrum.

superbill (soo′pər-bĭl′) A form that combines the charges for services rendered, an invoice for payment or insurance copayment, and all the information for submitting an insurance claim; also known as an encounter form.

superficial (soo′pər-fĭsh′əl) Anatomic term meaning closer to the surface of the body.

superior (soo′-pîr′-ē-ər) Anatomic term meaning above or closer to the head; also called cranial.

supernatant (sū-per-nā′tănt)(†) The liquid portion of a substance from which solids have settled to the bottom, as with a urine specimen after centrifugation.

supination (sū′pi-nā′shŭn)(†) Turning the palm of the hand upward.

surfactant (sər fak′ tənt) Fatty substance secreted by some alveolar cells that helps maintain the inflation of the alveoli so that they do not collapse in on themselves between inspirations.

surgeon (sûr′jən) A physician who uses hands and medical instruments to diagnose and correct deformities and treat external and internal injuries or disease.

surgical asepsis (sûr′jə-kəl ă-sep′sis)(†) The elimination of all microorganisms from objects or working areas; also called sterile technique.

susceptible host (sə-sĕp′təbal hōst) An individual who has little or no immunity to infection by a particular organism.

suture (soo′chər) Fibrous joints in the skull. (25) A surgical stitch made to close a wound.

symmetry (sĭm′ĭ-trē) The degree to which one side of the body is the same as the other.

sympathetic (sĭm′pə-thĕt′ĭk) A division of the autonomic nervous system that prepares organs for fight-or-flight (stressful) situations.

symptom (sĭm′təm) A subjective, or internal, condition felt by a patient, such as pain, headache, or nausea, or another indication that generally cannot be seen or felt by the doctor or measured by instruments.

synaptic knob (si-nap′tik nŏb)(†) The end of the axon branch.

synergist (sĭn′ər-jist′) Muscles that help the **prime mover** by stabilizing joints.

synovial (sin-ō-vā-əl) A type of joint, such as the elbow or knee, that is freely moveable.

systemic circuit (sĭ-stĕm′ĭk sûr′kĭt) The route that blood takes from the heart through the body and back to the heart.

systemic lupus erythematosus (SLE) (si-stĕm′ĭk loo′p s er the′to′s s) An autoimmune disorder in which a person produces antibodies that target the person's own cells and tissues.

systolic pressure (sĭ-stŏl′ĭk prĕsh′ər) The blood pressure measured when the left ventricle of the heart contracts.

tab (tăb) A tapered rectangular or rounded extension at the top of a file folder.

Tabular List (tăb′yə-lər lĭst) One of two ways that diagnoses are listed in the **ICD-9.** In the Tabular List, the diagnosis codes are listed in numerical order with additional instructions.

tachycardia (tak′i-kar′dē-ă)(†) Rapid heart rate, generally in excess of 100 beats per minute.

tachypnea Abnormally rapid breathing.

targeted résumé (tär′gĭt-əd rĕz′oo-mā′) A résumé that is focused on a specific job target.

tarsals (tär′-səlz) Bones of the ankle.

taste bud (tāst bŭd) A structure that is made of taste cells (a type of chemoreceptor) and supporting cells.

tax liability (tăk lī′ə-bĭl′ĭ-tē) Money withheld from employees' paychecks and held in a separate account that must be used to pay taxes to appropriate government agencies.

telephone triage (tĕl′ə-fōn′ trē-äzh′) A process of determining the level of urgency of each incoming telephone call and how it should be handled.

teletherapy (tel-ĕ-thār′ăpē)(†) A radiation therapy technique that allows deeper penetration than brachytherapy; used primarily for deep tumors.

teletype (TTY) device (tĕl′ə-tīp) A specially designed telephone that looks very much like a laptop computer with a cradle for the receiver of a traditional telephone. It is used by the hearing impaired to type communications onto a keyboard.

telophase (tel′əfāz) The final stage of mitosis; chromosomes reach the centrioles and the division creating two cells, each with a complete set of chromosomes is completed.

template (tĕm′plĭt) A guide that ensures consistency and accuracy.

temporal (tem′-p(a)-rəl) Bones that form the lower sides of the skull.

temporal scanner (temp′-or-al skăn-ĕr) An instrument used to measure the body temperature by scanning the temporal artery in the forehead.

tendon (tĕn′dən) A cord-like fibrous tissue that connects muscle to bone.

tendonitis (ten dŭn ĭ tis) Inflammation of a tendon.

terminal (tûr′mə-nəl) Fatal.

terminal digit (tûrmə-nəl dĭjĭt) A small group of two to three numbers at the end of a patient number that is used as an identifying unit in a filing system.

testes (tĕs´tēz) The primary organs of the male reproductive system. Testes produce the hormone **testosterone.**

testosterone (tĕs-tŏs´tə-rōn´) A hormone produced by the testes that maintains the male reproductive structures and male characteristics such as deep voice, body hair, and muscle mass.

tetanus (tĕt´n-əs) A disease caused by *clostridium tetani* living in the soil and water; more commonly called lockjaw.

thalamus (thăl´ə-məs) Structure that acts as a relay station for sensory information heading to the cerebral cortex for interpretation; a subdivision of the **diencephalon.**

thalassemia (thal´əē´mēaə) An inherited form of anemia with a defective hemoglobin chain causing micocytic (small), hypochromic (pale), and short-lived red blood cells.

therapeutic team (thĕr´ə-pyōō´tĭk tēm) A group of physicians, nurses, medical assistants, and other specialists who work with patients dealing with chronic illness or recovery from major injuries.

therapeutic touch (thĕr´ -ə-pyōō-tĭk tŭch) The use of touch to detect and correct an person's energy fields, thus promoting healing and health.

thermography (ther-mog´ră-fē)(†) A radiologic procedure in which an infrared camera is used to take photographs that record variations in skin temperature as dark (cool areas), light (warm areas), or shades of gray (areas with temperatures between cool and warm); used to diagnose breast tumors, breast abscesses, and fibrocystic breast disease.

thermometer (ther-mom´ə-ter) An instrument, either electronic or disposable, that is used to measure body temperature.

thermotherapy (ther´mō-thār´ă-pē) (†) The application of heat to the body to treat a disorder or injury.

third-party check (thûrd pär´tē chĕk) A check made out to one recipient and given in payment to another, as with one made out to a patient rather than the medical practice.

third-party payer (thûrd pär´tē pā´ər) A health plan that agrees to carry the risk of paying for patient services.

thoracocentesis (thôr´ə kō´sen tē´ sis) Medical procedure where a sterile needle is introduced into the chest to remove fluid and pus.

thoracostomy (thor´ ə kos´ tə mē) The surgical insertion of a chest tube to provide continuous drainage of the thoracic (chest) cavity.

thorax (thôr´aks) The chest cavity.

thrombocytes (throm´bō-sīts) See **platelets.**

thrombophlebitis (thrŏm´bō-flĕ-bī´tis) (†) A medical condition that most commonly occurs in leg veins when a blood clot and inflammation develop.

thrombus (thrŏm´bəs) A blood clot that forms on the inside of an injured blood vessel wall.

thymosin (thī´mō-sin)(†) A hormone that promotes the production of certain lymphocytes.

thymus gland (thī´məs glănd) A gland that lies between the lungs. It secretes a hormone called **thymosin.**

thyroid cartilage (thī´roid´ kär´tl-ĭj) The largest cartilage in the larynx. It forms the anterior wall of the larynx.

thyroid hormone (thī´roid´ hôr´mōn´) A hormone produced by the thyroid gland that increases energy production, stimulates protein synthesis, and speeds up the repair of damaged tissue.

thyroid-stimulating hormone (TSH) (thī´roid´stim´yū-lā-ting hôr´mōn´) A hormone that stimulates the thyroid gland to release its hormone.

tibia (ti-bē-ə) The medial bone of the lower leg; commonly called the shin bone.

tickler file (tĭk´lər fīl) A reminder file for keeping track of time-sensitive obligations.

timed urine specimen (tīmd yōōr´ĭn spĕs´ə-mən) A specimen of a patient's urine collected over a specific time period.

time-specified scheduling (tīm spĕs´ə-fīd skĕj´ōol-ĭng) A system of scheduling where patients arrive at regular, specified intervals, assuring the practice a steady stream of patients throughout the day.

tinea (tin ē´ə) A fungal infection.

tinnitus (ti-nī´tus)(†) An abnormal ringing in the ear.

tissue (tĭsh´ōo) A structure that is formed when cells of the same type organize together.

T lymphocyte (tē lĭm´fə-sīt) A type of nongranular leukocyte that regulates immunologic response; includes helper T cells and suppressor T cells.

topical (tŏp´ĭ-kəl) Applied to the skin.

tort (tôrt) In civil law, a breach of some obligation that causes harm or injury to someone.

torticollis (tôr´tikol´is) A muscular disease causing a cervical deformity in which the head bends toward the affected side while the chin rotates to the opposite side.

touchpad (tūch păd) A type of pointing device common to laptop and notebook computers that directs activity on the computer screen by positioning a pointer or cursor on the screen. It is a small, flat device or surface that is highly sensitive to touch.

touch screen (tŭch skrēn) A type of computer monitor that acts as an intake device, receiving information thought the touch of a pen, wand, or hand directly to the screen.

tower case (tou´ər kās) A vertical housing for the system unit of a personal computer.

toxicology (tŏk´sĭ-kŏl´ə-jē) The study of poisons or poisonous effects of drugs.

trachea (trā´kē-ə) The part of the respiratory tract between the larynx and the bronchial tree that is tubular and made of rings of cartilage and smooth muscle; also called the windpipe.

trackball (trăk bôl) A pointing device with a ball that is rolled to position a pointer or cursor on a computer screen. It can be directly attached to the computer or can be wireless.

tracking (trăk´ĭng) (financial) Watching for changes in spending so as to help control expenses.

traction (trăk´shən) The pulling or stretching of the musculoskeletal system to treat dislocated joints, joints afflicted by arthritis or other diseases, and fractured bones.

trade name (trād nām) A drug's brand or proprietary name.

traditional Chinese medicine (TCM) (trə-dĭsh´-ə-nəl chĭ-nĕz mĕd´-ĭ-sĭn) An ancient system of medicine originating in China that involves herbal and animal source preparations to treat illness. TCM includes various treatments such as acupuncture and acupressure.

transcription (trăn-skrĭp´shən) The transforming of spoken notes into accurate written form.

transcutaneous absorption (trans-kyū-tā´nē-ŭs əb-sorp´shən)(†) Entry (as of a pathogen) through a cut or crack in the skin.

transdermal (trans-der´mel) A type of topical drug administration that slowly and evenly releases a systemic drug through the skin directly into the bloodstream; a transdermal unit is also called a patch.

transfer (trăns-fûr´) To give something, such as information, to another party outside the doctor's office.

transurethral resection of prostate (trans´yŏŏ rĕ thrəl rĕ-sak´ shən) Removal of the prostate through the urethra.

transverse (trăns-vŭrs´) Anatomic term that refers to the plane that divides the body into superior and inferior portions.

transverse colon (trăns-vûrs´ kō´lən) The segment of the large intestine that crosses the upper abdominal cavity between the ascending and descending colon.

traveler's check (trăv´əlz chĕk) A check purchased and signed at a bank and later signed over to a payee.

treatment, payments and operations (TPO) (trēt´mənt pā´mənts ŏp´ə-rā´shəns) The portion of **HIPAA** that allows the provider to use and share patient health-care information for treatment, payment, and operations (such as quality improvement).

triage (trē-äzh´) To assess the urgency and types of conditions patients present as well as their immediate medical needs.

TRICARE (trī´kâr) A program that provides health-care benefits for families of military personnel and military retirees.

trichinosis (trik-i-nō´sis)(†) A disease caused by a worm that is usually ingested from undercooked meat.

tricuspid valve (trī-kŭs´pid vălv)(†) A heart valve that has three cusps and is situated between the right atrium and the right ventricle.

triglycerides (trī-glĭs´ə-rīd´z) Simple lipids consisting of glycerol (an alcohol) and three fatty acids.

trigone (trī´gōn)(†) The triangle formed by the openings of the two ureters and the urethra in the internal floor of the bladder.

troubleshooting (trŭb´əl-shōō´tĭng) Trying to determine and correct a problem without having to call a service supplier.

trypsin (trip´sin)(†) A pancreatic enzyme that digests proteins.

tubular reabsorption (tū´byū-lăr)(†) The second process of urine formation in which the glomerular filtrate flows into the proximal convoluted tubule.

tubular secretion (tū´byū-lăr sĭ-krē´shən)(†) The third process of urine formation in which substances move out of the blood in the peritubular capillaries into renal tubules.

tutorial (tōō-tôr´ē-əl) A small program included in a software package designed to give users an overall picture of the product and its functions.

tympanic membrane (tĭm-păn´ĭk mĕm´brān´) A fibrous partition located at the inner end of the ear canal and separating the outer ear from the middle ear; also called the eardrum.

tympanic thermometer (tim-pan´ik ther-mom´ĕ-ter) A type of electronic thermometer that measures infrared energy emitted from the tympanic membrane.

ulna (əl´-nə) The medial bone of the lower arm.

ultrasonic cleaning (ŭl´trə-sŏn´ĭk klēn´ĭng) A method of sanitization that involves placing instruments in a cleaning solution in a special receptacle that generates sound waves through the cleaning solution, loosening contaminants. Ultrasonic cleaning is safe for even very fragile instruments.

ultrasound The noninvasive theraputic or diagnostic use of ultrasound for examination of internal body structures.

umami (oo-mom´ē) Savory taste produced by glutamic acid (monosodium glutamate), recognized as the fifth taste sensation.

umbilical cord (ŭm-bĭl´ĭ-kəl kôrd) The rope-like connection between the fetus and the placenta. It contains the umbilical blood vessels.

underbooking (ŭn´dər-bŏŏk´ĭng) Leaving large, unused gaps in the doctor's schedule; this approach does not make the best use of the doctor's time.

uniform donor card (yōō´nə-fôrm´ dō´nər kärd) A legal document that states a person's wish to make a gift upon death of one or more organs for medical research, organ transplants, or placement in a tissue bank.

unit (yōō´nĭt) A part of an individual's name or title, described in indexing rules.

unit price (yōō´nĭt prīs) The total price of a package divided by the number of items that comprise the package.

Universal Precautions (yōō´nə-vur´səl prĭ-kô´shənz) Specific precautions required by the Department of Health and Human Services' Centers for Disease Control and Prevention (CDC) to prevent health-care workers from exposing themselves and others to infection by blood-borne pathogens.

unsaturated fats (ŭn-săch´ə-rā´tĭd făts) Fats, including most vegetable oils, that are usually liquid at room temperature and tend to lower blood cholesterol.

upper respiratory (tract) infection (upper res´pərətôr´ē tract infek´ shən) The common cold.

urea (yōō-rē´ə) Waste product formed by the breakdown of proteins and nucleic acids.

ureters (yōō-rē´tərz) Long, slender, muscular tubes that carry urine from the kidneys to the urinary bladder.

urethra (yōō-rē´thrə) The tube that conveys urine from the bladder during urination.

uric acid (yōōr´ĭk as´id) Waste product formed by the breakdown of proteins and nucleic acids.

urinalysis (yōōr´ə-năl´ĭ-sĭs) The physical, chemical, and microscopic evaluation of urine to obtain information about body health and disease.

urinary catheter (yōōr´ə-nĕr´ē kăth´ĭ-tər) A sterile plastic tube inserted to provide urinary drainage.

urinary pH (yōōr´ə-nĕr´ē pē´äch) A measure of the degree of acidity or alkalinity of urine.

urine specific gravity (yōōr´ĭn spĭ-sĭf´ĭk grăv´ĭ-tē) A measure of the concentration or amount (total weight) of substances dissolved in urine.

urobilinogen (yūr-ō-bī-lin´ō-jen)(†) A colorless compound formed by the breakdown of hemoglobin in the intestines. Elevated levels in urine may indicate increased red blood cell destruction or liver disease, whereas lack of urobilinogen in the urine may suggest total bile duct obstruction.

urologist (yōō-rŏl´ə-jĭst) A specialist who diagnoses and treats diseases of the kidney, bladder, and urinary system.

use (yōōz) The sharing, employing, applying, utilizing, examining, or analyzing of individually identifiable health information by employees or other members of an organization's workforce.

uterus (yōō´tər-əs) A hollow, muscular organ that functions to receive an embryo and sustain its development; also called the womb.

uvula (yōō´vyə-lə) The part of the soft palate that hangs down in the back of the throat.

uvulotomy (yoo´vyəlot´əmē) Surgical procedure removing all or part of the uvula of the soft palate.

vaccine (văk-sēn´) A special preparation made from microorganisms and administered to a person to produce reduced

sensitivity to, or increased immunity to, an infectious disease.

vagina (və-jī´nə) A tubular organ that extends from the uterus to the labia.

vaginal introitus (vaj´ i-nəl in trō´ təs) The vaginal os or orifice. The opening of the vagina to the outside of the body.

vaginitis (vaj-i-nī´tis)(†) Inflammation of the vagina characterized by an abnormal vaginal discharge.

varicose veins (văr´i-kōs vānz)(†) Distended veins that result when vein valves are destroyed and blood pools in the veins, causing these veins to dilate.

vas deferens (văs´ dĕf´ər-ənz) A tube that connects the epididymis with the urethra and that carries sperm.

vasectomy (və-sĕk´tə-mē) A male sterilization procedure in which a section of each vas deferens is removed.

vasoconstriction (vā´sō-kon-strik´shŭn)(†) The constriction of the muscular wall of an artery to increase blood pressure.

vasodilation (vā-sō-dī-lā´shŭn)(†) The widening of the muscular wall of an artery to decrease blood pressure.

V code (vē kōd) A code used to identify encounters for reasons other than illness or injury, such as annual checkups, immunizations, and normal childbirth.

vector (vĕk´tər) A living organism, such as an insect, that carries microorganisms from an infected person to another person.

venipuncture (ven´i-pŭnk-chŭr)(†) The puncture of a vein, usually with a needle, for the purpose of drawing blood.

ventilation (vĕn´tə-lā´shən) Moving air in and out of the lungs; also called breathing.

ventral (vĕn´trəl) See **anterior**.

ventral root (vĕn´trəl rōōt) A portion of the spinal nerve that contains axons of motor neurons only.

ventricle (věn′trĭ-kəl) Interconnected cavities in the brain filled with cerebrospinal fluid.

ventricular fibrillation (VF) (ven-trik′yū-lăr fĭ-bri-lā′shŭn) An abnormal heart rhythm that is the most common cause of cardiac arrest.

verbalizing (vûr′bə-līz′-ĭng) Stating what you believe the patient is suggesting or implying.

vermiform appendix (ver′mi-fōrm ə-pěn′dĭks)(†) A structure made mostly of lymphoid tissue and projecting off the cecum. It is commonly referred to as simply the appendix.

vertical file (vûr′tĭ-kəl fĭl) A filing cabinet featuring pull-out drawers that usually contain a metal frame or bar equipped to handle letter- or legal-sized documents in hanging file folders.

vertigo (vûr′tĭ g ō) Dizziness.

vesicles (věs′ĭ-kəlz) Small sacs within the synaptic knobs that contain chemicals called neurotransmitters.

vestibule (ves ti b′yule) The space enclosed by the labia minora.

vestibule (věs′tə-byōōl′) The area in the inner ear between the semicircular canals and the cochlea.

vial (vī′əl) A small glass bottle with a self-sealing rubber stopper.

vibrio (vib′rē-ō) (†) A comma-shaped bacterium.

Virtual Private Network (VPN) (vur - choo-ul prahy-vit net-wurk) These are used to connect two or more computer systems.

virulence (vîr′yə-ləns) A microorganism's disease-producing power.

virus (vī′rəs) One of the smallest known infectious agents, consisting only of nucleic acid surrounded by a protein coat; can live and grow only within the living cells of other organisms.

visceral pericardium (vis′er-ăl per-i-kar′dē-ŭm)(†) The innermost layer of the pericardium that lies directly on top of the heart; also known as the epicardium.

visceral peritoneum (vīs′er-ăl per-ə-tōnē′əl) Also known as the serosa, the outermost layer of the abdominal organs that secretes serous fluid to keep the organs from sticking to each other.

visceral smooth muscle (vĭs′ər-əl smōōth mŭs′əl) A type of smooth muscle containing sheets of muscle that closely contact each other. It is found in the walls of hollow organs such as the stomach, intestines, bladder, and uterus.

vitamins (vī′tə-mĭnz) Organic substances that are essential for normal body growth and maintenance and resistance to infection.

vitreous humor (vĭt′rē-əs hyōō′mər) A jelly-like substance that fills the part of the eye behind the lens and helps the eye keep its shape.

voice mail (vois māl) An advanced form of answering machine that allows a caller to leave a message when the phone line is busy.

void (void) (legal) A term used to describe something that is not legally enforceable.

volume (vŏl′yōōm) The amount of space an object, such as a drug, occupies.

vomer (vō′-mər) A thin bone that divides the nasal cavity.

voucher check (vou′chər chĕk) A business check with an attached stub, which is kept as a receipt.

vulva (vul′ vah) External female genitalia.

vulvovaginitis (vul vō vaj′i-nī′tis) Inflammation of the external female genitalia and vagina.

walk-in (wôk′ĭn) A patient who arrives without an appointment.

WAN (wŏn) Abbreviation for Wide Area Network.

warranty (wôr′ən-tē) A contract that specifies free service and replacement of parts for a piece of equipment during a certain period, usually a year.

warts (wôrts) Flesh-colored skin lesions with distinct round borders that are raised and often have small finger-like projections; also called verruca.

wave scheduling (wāv skĕj′ōōl-ĭng) A system of scheduling in which the number of patients seen each hour is determined by dividing the hour by the length of the average visit and then giving that number of patients appointments with the doctor at the beginning of each hour.

Western blot test (wěs′tərn blŏt tĕst) A blood test used to confirm enzyme-linked immunosorbent assay (ELISA) test results for HIV infection.

wet mount (wět mount) A preparation of a specimen in a liquid that allows the organisms to remain alive and mobile while they are being identified.

white matter (hwīt măt′ər) The outer tissue of the spinal cord that is lighter in color than **gray matter.** It contains myelinated axons.

whole blood (hōl blŭd) The total volume of plasma and formed elements, or blood in which the elements have not been separated by coagulation or centrifugation.

whole-body skin examination (hōl bŏd′ē skĭn ĭg-zăm′ə-nā′shən) An examination of the visible top layer of the entire surface of the skin, including the scalp, genital area, and areas between the toes, to look for lesions, especially suspicious moles or precancerous growths.

Wood's light examination (wŏŏdz līt ĭg-zăm′ə-nā′shən) A type of dermatologic examination in which a physician inspects the patient's skin under an ultraviolet lamp in a darkened room.

written-contract account (rĭt´n kŏn´trăkt´ ə-kount´) An agreement between the physician and patient stating that the patient will pay a bill in more than four installments.

X12 837 Health Care Claim (hĕlth kâr klām) An electronic claim transaction that is the **HIPAA** Health Care Claim or Equivalent Encounter Information ("HIPAA claim").

xeroradiography (zē´rō-rā´dē-og´ră-fē)(†) A radiologic procedure in which x-rays are developed with a powder toner, similar to the toner in photocopiers, and the x-ray image is processed on specially treated xerographic paper; used to diagnose breast cancer, abscesses, lesions, or calcifications.

xiphoid process (zif´oyd prŏs´ĕs)(†) The lower extension of the breast-bone; the cartilaginous tip of the sternum.

yeast (yēst) A fungus that grows mainly as a single-celled organism and reproduces by budding.

yoga (yō´-gə) A series of poses and breathing exercises that provide awareness of the unity of the whole being. The practice of yoga also increases flexibility and strength.

yolk sac (yōk săk) The sac that holds the materials for the nutrition of the embryo.

zip drive (zĭp drīv) A Zip drive is a high-capacity floppy disk drive developed by Iomega®. Zip drives are slightly larger and about twice as thick as a conventional floppy disk. Zip drives can hold 100 to 750 MB of data. They are durable and relatively inexpensive. They may be used for backing up hard disks and transporting large files.

zona pellucida (zō´nă pe-lū´sid-ă)(†) A layer that surrounds the cell membrane of an egg.

Z-track method (zē´trăk mĕth´əd) A technique used when injecting an intramuscular (IM) drug that can irritate subcutaneous tissue; involves pulling the skin and subcutaneous tissue to the side before inserting the needle at the site, creating a zigzag path in the tissue layers that prevents the drug from leaking into the subcutaneous tissue and causing irritation.

zygomatic (zī-gə-m´a-tik) The bones that form the prominence of the cheeks.

zygote (zī´gōt) The cell that is formed from the union of the egg and sperm.

PHOTO CREDITS

CHAPTER 1
Fig. 1.11b, Fig. 1.12b, Fig. 1.13b, Fig. 1.14b:
© Ed Reschke.

CHAPTER 2
Fig. 2.3: © Victor B. Eichler, Ph. D.; Fig. 2.6a: © SPL/
Custom Medical Stock Photos, Fig. 2.6b, Fig. 2.6c:
© John Radcliff/Photo Researchers, Inc.; Fig. 2.7a-b:
© Biophoto Associates/Photo Researchers, Inc.;
Fig. 2.7c: © SPL/Photo Researchers, Inc.

CHAPTER 3
Fig. 3.2: © Ed Reschke; Fig. 3.11b: © Martin M. Rotker.

CHAPTER 5
Fig. 5.7: © Carolina Biological/Visuals Unlimited;
Fig. 5.9: © Don W. Fawcett, from Bloom, W. and
Fawcett, D.W., *Textbook of Histology*, 10th edition.
W.B. Saunders Co., 1975. Photo by T. Kuwabara;

Fig. 5.14b: © Bill Longcore/Photo Researchers, Inc.;
Fig. 5.15, Fig. 5.16, Fig. 5.17, Fig. 5.18, Fig. 5.19:
© Ed Reschke; Fig. 5.22: © SPL/Photo Researchers,
Inc.; Fig. 5.23c: © G.W. Willis/Visuals Unlimited;
Fig. 5.23d: © George Wilder/Visuals Unlimited.

CHAPTER 6
Fig. 6.2: © CNR/Phototake.

CHAPTER 7
Fig. 7.1: © Ed Reschke; Fig. 7.7b: The McGraw-Hill
Companies, Inc./Rebecca Gray, photographer.

CHAPTER 12
Fig. 12.4a: © Trapper Frank/Corbis/Sygma;
Fig. 12.4b: © Robert Eric/Corbis Sygma, Fig. 12.4c-f:
Reprinted by permission of publisher from: Albert
Mendeloff, "Acromegaly, diabetes, hypermetabolism,
proteinura and heart failure" *American Journal of*

Medicine, 20:1, 01-56, p. 135. © by Excerpta Medica,
Inc.; Fig. 12.5-I: Addison's Disease: a: © Associated
Press/AP; Addison's disease b: © Corbis; Fig. 12.5-2:
Cushing's syndrome: a-b: © Kathy Carbone, 4107
Hemingway Drive, Venice, FL 34293; Cretinism:
© Mediscan; Hyperthyroidism: © Dr. M. A. Ansary/
Photo Researchers, Inc.; Goiter: © L.V. Bergman
Collection.

CHAPTER 13
Page 200: © Ken Lax; Fig. 13.7a: © James P. Gilman,
C.R.A./Phototake; Fig. 13.7b: © Dr. P. Marazzi/
Photo Researchers, Inc.; Fig. 13.7c-d:
© Photo Disc/Getty Images; Fig. 13.8a-b: © Photo
Disc/Getty Images; Fig. 13.11: © Bonnie Kamin/
Photo Edit.

TEXT AND LINE ART CREDITS

CHAPTER 1
Fig. 1-10: From Shier, Butler, Lewis, *Hole's Anatomy,*
8th edition, pp. 89, Fig. 3.36. Copyright © 2003
by the McGraw-Hill Companies.

CHAPTER 2
Fig. 2-2: From Thierer and Breitbard, *Medical
Terminology,* 2nd edition, pp. 81, Fig 4.5. Copyright
© 2006 by the McGraw-Hill Companies.

CHAPTER 3
Fig. 3-3: From McKinley and O'Loughlin, *Human
Anatomy,* pp.151, Fig. 6.3. Copyright © 2006 by the
McGraw-Hill Companies; Fig. 3-4: From Shier,
Butler, Lewis; *Hole's Anatomy,* 8th edition, pp. 153,
Figs. 7.29 & 7.30. Copyright © 2003 by the
McGraw-Hill Companies; Fig. 3-7: From Shier,
Butler, Lewis, *Hole's Anatomy,* 8th edition, pp. 89,
Fig. 3.36. Copyright © 2003 by the McGraw-Hill
Companies; Fig. 3-9: From Stephen, Seeley, and Tate,
Anatomy and Physiology, 8th edition, pp. 228, Fig.
7.21. Copyright © 2004 by the McGraw-Hill
Companies; Fig. 3-10: From Shier, Butler, Lewis,
Hole's Anatomy, 8th edition, pp. 136, Fig. 4.9.
Copyright © 2003 by the McGraw-Hill Companies;
Fig. 3-12 From Shier, Butler, Lewis; *Hole's Anatomy,*
8th edition, pp. 232, Fig. 7.52. Copyright
© 2003 by the McGraw-Hill Companies.

CHAPTER 7
Fig. 7-7: From McKinley and O'Loughlin, *Human
Anatomy,* pp. 475, Fig. 15.24. Copyright © 2006 by
the McGraw-Hill Companies; Fig. 7-9: From McKinley
and O'Loughlin, *Human Anatomy,* pp. 498, Fig. 16-6.
Copyright © 2006 by the McGraw-Hill Companies;
Fig. 7-11: From McKinley and O'Loughlin, *Human
Anatomy,* pp. 549, Fig. 18.3. Copyright © 2006 by the
McGraw-Hill Companies.

CHAPTER 9
Fig. 9-2: From Stephen, Seeley, and Tate, Anatomy
and Physiology, 8th edition, pp. 1041, process fig.
A. Copyright © 2004 by the McGraw-Hill Companies;
Fig. 9-3: From Shier, Butler, Lewis, *Hole's Anatomy,*
8th edition. Copyright © 2003 by the McGraw-Hill
Companies.

CHAPTER 11
Fig. 11-11: From McKinley and O'Loughlin Human
Anatomy pp. 815 Fig. 26.8. Copyright © 2006 by the
McGraw-Hill Companies.

CHAPTER 12
Fig. 12-1: From McKinley and O'Loughlin,
Human Anatomy, pp. 615, Fig. 20.1. Copyright
© 2006 by the McGraw-Hill Companies; Fig. 12-2:
From McKinley and O'Loughlin, *Human Anatomy,*

pp. 616, Fig. 20.2. Copyright © 2006 by the
McGraw-Hill Companies.

CHAPTER 13
Fig. 13-3: From McKinley and O'Loughlin,
Human Anatomy, pp. 582, Fig. 19.12. Copyright ©
2006 by the McGraw-Hill Companies; Fig. 13-4:
From McKinley and O'Loughlin, *Human Anatomy,*
pp. 588 & 592, Fig. 19.17 and Clinical View Figure.
Copyright © 2006 by the McGraw-Hill Companies;
Fig. 13-6: From McKinley and O'Loughlin, *Human
Anatomy,* pp.593, Clinical View and Clinical View
Figure. Copyright © 2006 by the McGraw-Hill
Companies; Fig. 13-8: From McKinley and
O'Loughlin, *Human Anatomy,* pp. 587,
Clinical View Figure. Copyright © 2006 by the
McGraw-Hill Companies; Fig. 13-9: From
McKinley and O'Loughlin, *Human Anatomy,*
pp. 595, Fig. 19.21. Copyright © 2006 by the
McGraw-Hill Companies; Fig. 13-10: From McKinley
and O'Loughlin, *Human Anatomy,* pp. 597,
Fig. 19.23. Copyright © 2006 by the McGraw-Hill
Companies.

INDEX

Page numbers in **boldface** indicate figures. Page numbers followed by (b) indicate box features, (p) procedures, and (t) tables, respectively.

Tissue
  connective, 16, **17**
  defined, 4
  epithelial, 15–16, **16**
  muscle, 16–17, **17**
  nervous, 17, **18**
  tissue fluid and lymph, 153
Tissue hormones, 179
Toes
  bones of, 46, **46**
  muscles of, **58**, 61
Tongue, 164–165, **165**
  sense of taste, 193, **193**
Tonsils, 165, **165**
Torticollis, 63(b)
Trachea, 93–94, **94**
Transient ischemic attacks (TIAs), 118(b)
Transverse colon, 169, **170**
Transverse plane, 8, **8**
Trichimonas, 148(b)
Trichinosis, 63(b)
Tricuspid valve, 69, **69**
Triglycerides, 10, 172
Trigone, 124, **125**
Triiodothyronine, 184, 185(t)
Trisomy 21, 18(b)
Trochanter, 41(t)
True ribs, 43, **44**
Trypsin, 171
Tubal ligation, 146, **146**
Tubercle, 41(t)
Tuberculosis (TB), 102(b)
Tuberosity, 41(t)
Tubular reabsorption, 123, **124**
Tubular secretion, 124, **124**
Tumor, **24**, 25(t)
Turner's syndrome, 19(b)
Tympanic membrane, 205, **206**

U

Ulcer, **24**, 25(t), 176(b)
Ulna, 44, **45**
Umami, 193
Umbilical cord, 142
Universal donors, 83
Universal recipients, 83
Upper respiratory (tract) infection
    (URI), 102(b)
Urea, 124
Ureter, 121, **121**, 124
Urethra, **121**, 125, **125**

Uric acid, 124
Urinary bladder, **121**, 124, **125**
Urinary system, 120–127
  diseases and disorders, 126(b)–127(b)
  organs and function of, **121**, 121–123,
      122, 124–125
  preventing urinary cystitis in
      women, 125(b)
  structure and function of, **6**
  urine formation, 123–124, **123–124**
Urinary tract infection, preventing, 125(b)
Urine, formation, 123–124, **123–124**
Uterine cancer, 141(b)
Uterus, **136**, 137, **137**
Uvula, 165, **165**

V

Vagina, **136**, 137, **137**
Vaginal introitus, 137
Vaginal os, 137
Vaginitis, 140(b)–141(b)
Varicose veins, 72, 88(b)–89(b)
Vas deferens, **131**, 134
Vasectomy, 134, 146, **146**
Vasoconstriction, 72, **72**
Vasodilation, 72, **72**
Veins, 72, **72**
  major, 74, **76**, 77(t)
Vena cava, 74, **77**
Ventilation, 94, **95**
Ventral, 6, **7**, 7(t)
Ventral root, 112
Ventricle
  brain, 109
  heart, 68, **69**
Venules, 72, **72**
Vermiform appendix, 169, **170**
Verrucae, 32(b)
Vertebrae, 42, **43**
Vertigo, 212(b)
Very low-density lipoproteins (VLDL), 81
Vesicle, **24**, 25(t), 107
Vestibular glands, 138
Vestibule, 138, 205, **206**
Visceral pericardium, 67, **68**
Visceral peritoneum, 163
Visceral smooth muscle, 53
Vision. *See also* Eyes
  testing, 198–199
Vitamin, common vitamins and
    function, 172(t)

Vitamin A, 172(t)
Vitamin B, 172(t)
Vitamin B$_2$, 172(t)
Vitamin B$_6$, 172(t)
Vitamin B$_{12}$, 84(b), 172(t)
  red blood cell production, 78
Vitamin C, 172(t)
Vitamin D, 172(t)
  bone health, 38–39
  skin and production of, 22
Vitamin E, 172(t)
Vitamin K, 172(t)
Vitreous humor, 196
Vocal cords, 93, **94**
Voice box, 92
Voluntary nervous system, 112
Vomer, 42
Vulvovaginitis, 140(b)

W

Warts, 32(b)
  genital, 147(b)
Water, as molecule, 8
Wheal, **24**, 25(t)
White blood cells, 16
White matter, 106
  spinal cord, 108, **108**
Windpipe, 93
Women. *See also* Female reproductive system
  preventing urinary cystitis in, 125(b)
Workplace settings, ophthalmic
    assistant, 200(b)
Wrists, muscles of, 58–59, **58–59**

X

Xiphoid process, 43, **44**
X-ray
  for chest pain, 79(b)
  neurologic testing, 115

Y

Yolk sac, 142, **142**

Z

Zona pellucida, **141**, 142
Zygomatic, **41**, 42, **42**
Zygote, **141**, 142